Nutrition
for Dental
Health

ENHANCED THIRD EDITION

Rebecca Sroda, RDH, MS

Dean Emerita, Health Sciences
South Florida Community College
Avon Park, Florida

Tonia Reinhard, MS, RD, FAND

Director, Coordinated Program in Dietetics
Department of Nutrition and Food Science
Course Director Clinical Nutrition
School of Medicine
Wayne State University
Detroit, Michigan

JONES & BARTLETT
LEARNING

World Headquarters
Jones & Bartlett Learning
5 Wall Street
Burlington, MA 01803
978-443-5000
info@jblearning.com
www.jblearning.com

Jones & Bartlett Learning books and products are available through most bookstores and online booksellers. To contact Jones & Bartlett Learning directly, call 800-832-0034, fax 978-443-8000, or visit our website, www.jblearning.com.

Substantial discounts on bulk quantities of Jones & Bartlett Learning publications are available to corporations, professional associations, and other qualified organizations. For details and specific discount information, contact the special sales department at Jones & Bartlett Learning via the above contact information or send an email to specialsales@jblearning.com.

20943-3

Production Credits

VP, Product Management: Amanda Martin
Product Manager: Sean Fabery
Product Specialist: Rachael Souza
Product Coordinator: Elena Sorrentino
Digital Project Specialist: Angela Dooley
Director of Marketing: Andrea DeFronzo
Marketing Manager: Dani Burford
Production Services Manager: Colleen Lamy

VP, Manufacturing and Inventory Control: Therese Connell
Composition: S4Carlisle Publishing Services
Project Management: S4Carlisle Publishing Services
Cover Design: Kristin E. Parker
Senior Media Development Editor: Troy Liston
Rights Specialist: Rebecca Damon
Printing and Binding: LSC Communications

Library of Congress Cataloging-in-Publication Data
Library of Congress Cataloging-in-Publication Data unavailable at time of printing.

LCCN: 2020933114

6048

Printed in the United States of America
24 23 22   10 9 8 7 6 5 4 3

Dedication

This edition is dedicated to all the hard-working individuals at our publisher's company who gave permission to write the third edition, provided ideas for improvement, and assisted in elevating the final product to a new level. Sincerest thanks given to the following individuals:

Jonathan Joyce
John Larkin
Leah Thomson
Holly McLaughlin
Jennifer Clements
Kim Cox

Preface

Nutrition for Dental Health, Enhanced Third Edition, is a textbook for dental hygiene and dental assisting students as well as reference for practicing clinicians.

- Dental hygiene students who take only one nutrition course can use the text as all-encompassing for both a general and dental-related study of nutrition.
- Dental hygiene students who take a general nutrition course before enrolling in the program will find this book useful for a quick review of biochemistry before embarking on an in-depth study of nutritional counseling suggestions and techniques.
- Dental assisting students whose curriculum allows for only a few short weeks of nutritional study may select appropriate topics to cover information required in their curriculum.
- Practicing clinicians will find the 24-hour Food Recall, 3-day and 7-day diet diaries helpful in assessing clinical patients for nutritional inadequacies and for increased risk of oral disease. If change is needed, refer to the end of chapter "Relate to Patient" section that includes suggestions to improve nutritional content of the diet.

The driving force behind the work of this new edition was a need to update old content to reflect current research. Nutrition is not a static science and constantly adjusts to cultural and societal trends.

The writing style remains accessible for all levels of dental auxiliary students with interesting Food for Thought sections for practical understanding of content.

Nutrition is a complex, constantly evolving science, and it is this author's hope the new edition will stimulate natural curiosity in each reader to embark on their own path of nutritional inquiry.

CHAPTER FEATURES

Something new to this textbook is that each chapter was vetted for scientific accuracy by Tonia Reinhard, Registered Dietitian, author and professor of Nutrition and Food Science. With her contribution the reader can have confidence that all content is current and research supported.

This third edition presents consistent chapter organization. Each chapter begins with a related quote, learning objectives, and key terms that set the stage for learning. Every chapter has an introduction that is written to serve as a segue into more detailed content. At the end of each chapter is a Relate to Patient section that compiles and lists information for the reader, so they can incorporate lessons learned during patient education and nutritional counseling. The next section, Practice for Patients, offers an opportunity to critically think through a patient case, while applying information from the chapter. Finally, the Relate to You section includes challenges to the reader to self-apply the information, drawing from personal eating practices.

Nutritional content has been researched and referenced and is current for the moment. Even as you read this statement, new ideas are being discussed in the world of nutrition. As stated earlier, nutrition is not a static science, so it is very possible new trends are emerging.

NEW RESOURCES

New to this edition and available online is *Chapter 18*, Nutritive Value of Complimentary Therapies for Oral Care. This chapter complements information in Chapter 8, Dietary and Herbal Supplements. An introduction and history of holistic or complimentary therapies is explained. Content, including nutritional value, for progressive or nontraditional practices includes miswak, oil pulling, essential oils, aromatherapy, and teas. Step-by-step instructions for making a breathing inhaler, frozen oil bites, safety guidelines for using aromatherapy, and brewing tea for the best flavor and benefit are presented.

Five *Nutritional Counseling Videos* are posted for both students and instructors online. Chapter 16 teaches that Nutritional Counseling sessions are individualized according to patient need, allowing that each one is different. These videos are meant to serve as exercises for students to pick out good learning features and those that can be improved upon. A rubric is posted to assist instructors in guiding students to pick out important points.

Examples of personalized nutritional counseling *PowerPoint presentations* are provided that illustrate the variety of ways that information can be packaged for patients.

Faculty Calibration PowerPoint can be placed on the dental department's electronic learning platform, so instructors can access and view prior to grading students in clinic. This ensures consistent grading practices in clinic. Many instructors appreciate a refresher on nutrition as it relates to the oral cavity, especially if it has been many years since they completed their nutrition course.

Flash Cards serve as a learning aid to assist students with studying and learning. They prove to be very helpful when studying for National Boards as they include all the major key terms.

24-hour food recall and caries risk matrix is included in Chapter 16 and are also posted online for both students and instructors. These practical forms also relate to one of the new videos as their use is demonstrated while waiting for the doctor to check the patient.

New questions added to the test bank are in a format most likely to be seen on the National Board Exam. Questions from the previous edition remain allowing for different levels of assessing.

You will notice that *color photos* now adorn the chapters for enhanced learning. Tissue changes are discernable providing better examples than the previous black and white.

New and additional *full-color graphics* have been created for many chapters. New and previous illustrations assist students with understanding of more complex concepts.

Many chapters have suggestions for *further content exploration* through videos, Web sites, and books. Suggestions can be used to flip the classroom or used as part of online drop-box assignments and discussion threads.

Chapter Critical Thinking Challenges encourage students to process content and apply knowledge to a higher thinking order. These assignments can also be used to flip the classroom or be used for online assignments.

Basic new *PowerPoint slides* have been created to include new content. They are easy to customize to include or delete information or enhance with illustrations of your choosing. Special effects like progression/transition can be added to conform to instructor style.

Rebecca Sroda

Contributors and Reviewers

CONTRIBUTORS

Jill Gehrig, RDH, MA
Dean Emeritus
Division of Allied Health & Public
Service Education
Asheville-Buncombe Technical
Community College
Asheville, North Carolina

Deb Milliken, DMD
Professor and Faculty Chair
Department of Dental Education
South Florida State College
Avon Park, Florida

Dawn Pisarski, RN, MS, ANP-BC
Professor
Department of Nursing
South Florida State College
Avon Park, Florida

REVIEWERS

Judy Danielson, MDH
Clinical Assistant Professor
University of Minnesota School of
Dentistry
Golden Valley, Minnesota

Heather Doucette, MEd
Assistant Professor
Dalhousie University
Halifax, Nova Scotia, Canada

Pam Kawasaki, RDH, MBA
Associate Professor
Pacific University
Hillsboro, Oregon

Connie Kracher, PhD
Associate Professor of Dental Education
Indiana University—Purdue University
Fort Wayne, Indiana

Shawna Rohner, MS
Professor
Pacific University
Hillsboro, Oregon

Claire Tucker, MEd
Assistant Professor
University of Arkansas for Medical
Sciences
Little Rock, Arkansas

Cynthia P. Wampler, MS
Professor of Dental Hygiene
Florida State College at Jacksonville
Jacksonville, Florida

Contents

Introduction

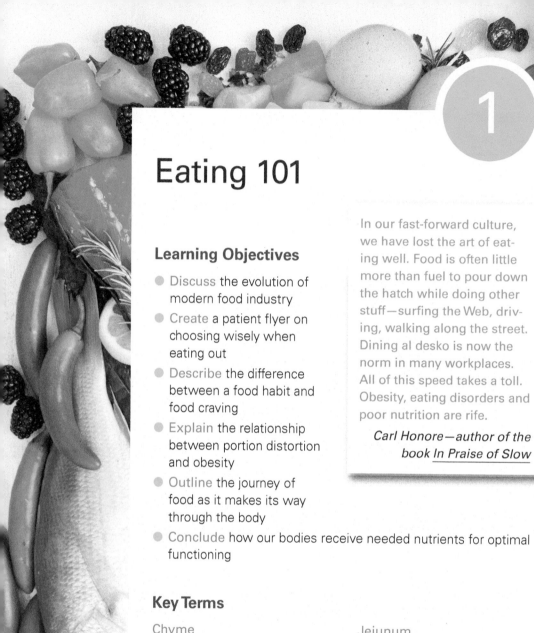

1

Eating 101

Learning Objectives

- Discuss the evolution of modern food industry
- Create a patient flyer on choosing wisely when eating out
- Describe the difference between a food habit and food craving
- Explain the relationship between portion distortion and obesity
- Outline the journey of food as it makes its way through the body
- Conclude how our bodies receive needed nutrients for optimal functioning

In our fast-forward culture, we have lost the art of eating well. Food is often little more than fuel to pour down the hatch while doing other stuff—surfing the Web, driving, walking along the street. Dining al desko is now the norm in many workplaces. All of this speed takes a toll. Obesity, eating disorders and poor nutrition are rife.

Carl Honore—author of the book In Praise of Slow

Key Terms

Chyme
Comfort Food
Consumption Norm
Enzyme
Food Craving
Food Habit
Gastrointestinal Tract

Jejunum
Nutrients
Nutrition
Peristalsis
Portion Distortion
Villi

INTRODUCTION

You are among the majority if you don't cook like your mother—you subscribe to a new generation's feeding patterns. How you nourish yourself and family is not the same experience as it was for your parents. Meal planning, preparation, and eating are very different in the 21st century, which makes your eating routines unique compared with that of previous generations. The 20th century mutated the concept of *family mealtime* with the help of food processing plants, a prolific fast-food industry, and targeted mass-marketing concepts.[1,2] Prepackaged meals and aisles of frozen meals predominate shopping carts and home pantries and freezers. Mom no longer spends hours in the kitchen preparing meals, and dinner is not always on the table when the *bread winner* returns home after a long, hard day at work.

(For better understanding of the major corporations that produce our food, watch the videos: Food, Inc. and Fed Up)

EATING IN THE 21ST CENTURY

Families find themselves without a chief cook in the kitchen and consuming one of every five meals (20%) in their cars.[3] You probably swing through a *drive-thru* for breakfast on your way to school or work, grab a *quick bite* for lunch, and stop for *fast food* in the evening before going to the next engagement scheduled in your *weekly planner*. Thanks to the food industry's 20th century influence, you can drink breakfast from a bottle, eat lunch out of a box, and dinner from a carton. With fast-food restaurants on every corner, you have the convenience your busy schedule demands, but beware….this new way of eating contributes to disease, and especially obesity.[4-6] Figure 1-1: Do you have a street in your city/town that looks like this? FAST FOOD ROW

Here are some *not-so-fun* facts on current eating habits:

- Consumption of soft drinks in the United States has more than doubled in the last 40 years. They are now the single most consumed food in the American diet.[7]
- Average person in the United States consumes about 126 g of sugar/day, which is over two times the 50 g/day recommended by the World Health Organization. Compare that to India's 5 g/day; Russia's 20 g/day; Singapore's 32 g/day; Canada's 89 g/day; United Kingdom's 93 g/day (www.euromonitor.com).
- The average American eats fast food 159 times a year. The average meal contains 1,200 calories, which is 190,000 calories a year. To burn that many calories you would need to run 1,700 miles equivalent from New York City to Denver, CO. (www.FastFoodNutrition.org).

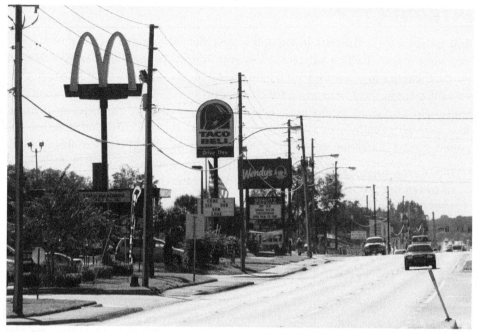

Figure 1-1   Fast Food Row. (Photo courtesy of Kevin Brown, Zolfo Springs, FL.)

FOOD FOR THOUGHT   **21ST CENTURY SNAPSHOT**

- Our days are lived according to planned schedules.
- Time scheduled for eating is minimal, and we prefer to eat on the run.
- Due to medical marvels, there is a vast geriatric population with their own unique set of health concerns.
- Population is increasing in numbers, and individuals are increasing in size.
- Portion norms are four times what they were 50 years ago.
- Although we are more aware of the benefits of daily exercise, we remain sedentary, spending more time in front of the TV or computer.
- More hours per day are spent at work, which puts more stress on the body.
- Most of us have other destinations than home after a busy day at work.
- According to the Centers for Disease Control and Prevention, Anthropometric Reference Data: Average American male is 5'9" tall and weighs 195.5 pounds and the average American woman is 5'3" and 166.2 pounds.

How does this compare to your height and weight? Read the following article for more information: www.npr.org, July 25, 2014. The Average American Man Is Too Big for His Britches by Serri Graslie.

YOU ARE WHAT YOU EAT

Nutrition is what you choose to eat and put into your body. The food you *select* contains nutrients, which are chemical substances that provide the body with energy and everything else it needs to function. Ninety-six percent of human body mass is composed of the elements:

Oxygen   Carbon   Hydrogen   Nitrogen

These elements also make up the six major nutrients found in food, making the saying "you are what you eat" really ring true. Food provides the body with a steady supply of fuel, which is created during digestion and absorption of six major nutrients: carbohydrates, proteins, lipids, water, vitamins, and minerals. Often, the body, in its own subtle way, will let you know which foods to eat in order to balance nutrients. When you are dehydrated, you feel thirsty and drink water (hydrogen and oxygen); when activity levels increase, you crave protein (carbon, hydrogen, oxygen, and nitrogen); and when you increase mental activity, your brain craves carbohydrates (carbon, hydrogen, and oxygen).

The first thing that usually comes to mind when thinking of a nutrient is one or two specific foods from the predominant food group. For example, something sweet for carbohydrates or meat and eggs for protein. In fact, most foods contain all six of the major nutrients. The proportion of the nutrients to each other in a specific food is what gives the food a label of either *carbohydrate rich*, *protein rich*, or *high (or low) fat*.

The food choices you make each day should be well thought out to keep your bodies healthy and functioning efficiently. Eating too much of any one food choice will usually *squeeze out* other food choices. For example, daily consumption of fast food decreases the chance of consuming more wholesomely prepared foods, and eating sweets throughout the day leaves less appetite for healthier snacks. This is not to say that you should never eat these foods; just don't eat them exclusively every day or for weeks on end.

Most of your daily food choices should be nutritious.

Occasionally indulge yourself in food that is delicious.

The relationship between food and the disease process happens when the body gets too much or too little of a particular nutrient over a period of time. Diabetes, cardiovascular disease, gross obesity, dental caries, and cancer (colon, esophageal, breast, and reproductive) are major diseases associated with unhealthy eating habits.[8–12] Consistently making unwise food choices can lead to major disease and a shorter life span.

PORTION DISTORTION

Studies show that portion sizes served in homes, fast food, and fine dining restaurants have increased over the last 20 years. This *increase in portion sizes*, coined **portion distortion**, has a direct cause-and-effect relationship with the obesity epidemic.

Consider the following examples at the U.S. Department of Health Web site: http://
www.nhlbi.nih.gov/health/educational/wecan/eat-right/portion-distortion.htm
    See Figure 1-2 PORTION DISTORTION for examples of changes in food
portions.

What you are served	What is one serving	Difference
630 calories 11 cups	− 275 calories 5 cups	= 35 calories = Vigorous calisthenics for 35 minutes

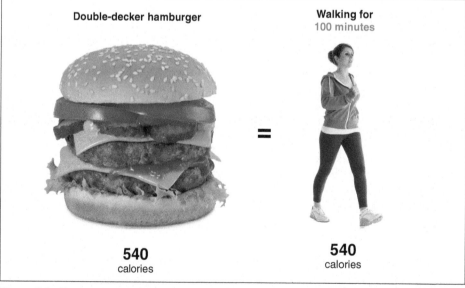

Double-decker hamburger	Walking for 100 minutes
540 calories	= **540** calories

Figure 1-2   Portion distortion.

If exercise efforts increased since the 1990s, the additional calories would burn off the increase in calories consumed. Instead, the population is much more sedentary.

We sit for hours in front of the television and computer screen.

We drive instead of walk and let modern appliances do our grunt work.

People have a tendency to eat what is put in front of them and typically do not consider that it might be too much. Consumers will equate bigger size with bigger value. **Consumption norm** is the *proper food unit to eat*. Mistakenly (and unfortunately), most consumers assume consumption norm is *what is placed before them*.

Consumption norm = what you should eat

Assumption norm = what is put before you to eat

FOOD FOR THOUGHT

One meal at a fast-food restaurant can add anywhere from 657 to more than 1,000 calories than a similar meal 20 years ago

- Today's fast-food cheese burger is 590 calories versus 333 calories 20 years ago. That means one would have to lift weights for 1.5 hours to burn off the additional 257 calories.
- Hardee's, Burger King, and Wendy's have 1,000+-calorie sandwiches. That is half or more of suggested caloric intake for a day.
- Twenty years ago, a 2.4 oz serving of French fries had 210 calories, and now an average serving of French fries is 6.9 oz for 610 calories.

NO *WASTE* or NO *WAIST*

Parents who condition children to eat everything on their plate need to think about what and how much to serve on the dish. With the gradual increase in portion distortion, we mindlessly consume the contents of a meal not until full, but rather until gone. Most diners are not conscious of calories consumed and get more satisfaction from a feeling of getting their money's worth.

Opt for NO WAIST! Do not be a victim of portion distortion. When eating out:
- Opt for the small—forget jumbo, king size, or even medium or large.
- Forget the sweet sodas and make water or unsweetened tea your beverage of choice.
- Ask for a to-go box when ordering your meal. Remove half of what is served on the plate and put it in the box for a later meal.

- At home, serve food on smaller plates and beverages in smaller glasses.
- Repackage foods bought at the big box store. The bigger package you pour from, the more you will eat.

Eat slower, savor every bite, and occasionally put the fork down, look around, and see what could happen if you do not become a conscious consumer.
For more reading on this topic—Mindless Eating—Why We Eat More Than We Think by Brian Wansink, PhD.

CHOOSE MYPLATE

The U.S. Department of Agriculture's (USDA) MyPlate, shown in Figure 1-3, is designed to serve as a guide to healthy eating and assist you in making healthy food choices. Visit www.choosemyplate.gov to set up a personal account. (See Chapter 11 for more information on MyPlate.) Serving suggestions for five food groups have been made to ensure a daily supply of important nutrients.

FRUITS   VEGETABLES   GRAINS   PRIOTEIN   DAIRY

MyPlate guidelines are suggestions and can be modified to accommodate specific diet requirements: vegetarians, lactose intolerant, specific cultural and religious practices.

Figure 1-3   MyPlate: a guide to daily food choices.

Following MyPlate guidelines configured specifically for you should include the following:

- Broad variety of foods from each category
- Three rich sources of calcium
- Three high-protein foods
- At least five servings of vegetables and fruits
- Whole grains for fiber
- Vegetable fats and omega-3 fatty acids
- *Also include plenty of water and daily moderate exercise*

FOOD HABITS/FOOD CRAVINGS

You may be choosing the food you eat out of **habit**, which is no more than mindless, routine eating. Habits are repetitive, and thought is not given to *what* you choose or *why* you choose a certain food. However, on a subconscious level, there is an association between eating the food and a comforting feeling or event. Some food habits are borne out of family traditions—like turkey for Thanksgiving, cake on birthdays, and cookies for Christmas. Other food habits are created out of social expectations like holding Starbucks coffee as you shop or beautifully displayed finger foods at a party to nibble on as you network and commiserate.

> *It has been said that:*
> *The human body has an*
> *innate wisdom. It lets us*
> *know when it needs a*
> *specific nutrient. When it*
> *talks to us like that, we*
> *experience craving.*

Food cravings can be either emotional or physiological. Not everybody gets them, but for those who do, they are very real. Unlike a food habit, food cravings are a conscious longing for something specific. If your craving is on an *emotional level*, it remains steady as long as the emotional need remains. Foods high in fat and carbohydrates tend to be chosen as comfort foods like chocolate candy, ice cream, or chocolate chip cookies. Once you fulfill the need, the craving disappears.[13,14]

If your craving is on a *physiological level*, it means hormones are in fluctuation.[15,16] You may go through phases, like eating peanut butter and crackers every day around 4:00 PM for 2 weeks and then smoked almonds at the same time for the next 2 weeks. This is neither accidental nor coincidental. If what you crave is based on a physiologic need, then your body will communicate when adequate levels are restored by eliminating the desire. If the craving is sustained, like having ice cream every night after dinner: it may start out as physiologic need and then turn in to habit. Table 1-1 gives examples of physiologic cravings.

Table 1-1	Manage Your Food Cravings	
Craving	**What Does It Mean?**	**Healthy Alternatives**
Chewing on ice	Low on iron	Meat, fish, poultry
Licorice	Adrenal function is low	A few pieces of licorice won't hurt
Chocolate	Deficient in magnesium	Raw nuts, seeds, fruit
Meat	Low on iron	Meat, prunes, figs
Cheese	Low in fatty acids	Salmon, flaxseed, walnuts
Salty foods	Stressed hormones	Meditation, stress management
Sweets	Low in chromium	Broccoli, cheese, grapes
Soda	Low in calcium	Kale, broccoli, dark greens

FOOD FOR THOUGHT   WHAT IS YOUR BODY TRYING TO TELL YOU WHEN YOU HAVE A CRAVING?

- Emotional balance is off, and comfort food is desired to help you cope.
- You need a mood adjustment—levels of neurotransmitters are fluctuating, and you need balance from a nutrient contained in the specific food you crave.
- Blood sugar level is low, and carbohydrates are needed to boost energy level.
- You lack a specific nutrient for optimal body functioning, and the food you crave will balance body chemistry.
- Chocolate is the single most craved food.[14] Some say it is not even food, but rather medicine because it contains *phenylethylamine*, a mood enhancer, and caffeine-like substances called *methylxanthine* and *theobromine*. Eating chocolate balances brain chemicals and boosts energy.

Ways to minimize a food craving:
- Move your body—exercise, stretch, or practice yoga to stave off depressive feelings.
- Choose complex carbohydrates for meals that will moderate blood sugar levels throughout the day.
- Eat frequent small nutritious meals throughout the day to minimize the sensation of hunger.
- Give in and eat a modest amount of what is craved.

DIGESTIVE PROCESS

The **gastrointestinal (GI) tract**, which supplies the body with nutrients and water, includes the following five *hollow* organs:

1. Esophagus
2. Stomach
3. Small intestine
4. Large intestine
5. Rectum

Three other *solid* organs along with the small intestine secrete enzymes that help reduce the food to micronutrients (Figure 1-4).

1. Pancreas
2. Liver
3. Gallbladder

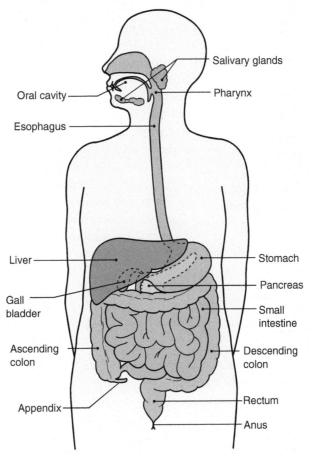

Figure 1-4 The digestive system.

The digestive process begins even before food or drink reaches the mouth. Low blood sugar level and sense of smell can stimulate the desire for food and drink. Just thinking about eating can wake up resting digestive organs and get the juices flowing.

The food and drink you put into your mouth is not in a form that the body can use for nourishment. It must go through a very complex process before nutrients can do their thing, like providing energy, repairing injured tissue, boosting immune system, and creating new cells and tissue. Digestion is an integrated process that requires teamwork from the body's voluntary and involuntary nervous systems that begins in the mouth, continues in the small intestines where most absorption of nutrients takes place, and ends in the large intestine where solid waste is excreted. You voluntarily put the food and drink in your mouth, rip and grind with your teeth, and swallow the soft mashed up food. Once it leaves the oral cavity, it is up to involuntary forces to guide the food on the rest of its journey.

The act of chewing reduces food to smaller particles, making it easier to swallow and pass through to the stomach. The human dentition crushes food with a force of almost 200 lb (90 kg), mashing the bolus of food, mixing it with enzymes excreted from salivary glands. The ability to chew well is vital to the digestive process because this is the first step in preparing food for enzyme action. Aside from breaking up food into smaller parts, the act of chewing causes involuntary secretion of enzymes from the pancreas, liver, gall bladder, and small intestine. An amylase called *ptyalin* is the first to be secreted in the digestive process, produced by salivary glands to break apart starch molecules into maltose.

Patients with limited chewing ability may complain of digestive problems, which is why they need to be encouraged to replace missing teeth and correct temporomandibular joint (TMJ) disorders.

Enzymes are of vital importance during the digestive process because they rearrange and divide food molecules, making them more bioavailable to the human body. If it were not for enzymes, nutrients in food could not be used by the body.

Digestive enzymes are specifically designed to do one particular job. Major enzyme groups are named to represent the job they do or the molecule they break down. (Notice enzyme names end with the *ase* suffix):

- Prote**ase** works on *protein*.
- Lip**ase** works on *lipids*.
- Amyl**ase** works on *carbohydrates*.
- Sucr**ase** works on *sucrose*.
- Lact**ase** works on *lactose*.

If a body <u>lacks</u> an enzyme, then that individual will be <u>intolerant</u> to the food it works on; lack of lactase would make someone unable to drink or eat dairy because of milk sugar called lactose. (You can read more about lactose intolerance in Chapter 2.)

Sometimes, it may take more than one type of enzyme to break apart food, as is the case when digesting protein. A protease called *pepsin*, secreted by the stomach, reduces protein into polypeptides, and then the process is continued by another protease called *trypsin*, manufactured by the pancreas, which continues to break down the protein while it is in the small intestine.

With advancing age, the body's ability to produce enzymes gradually diminishes, which limits nutrient absorption. Geriatric patients may report the use of food enzymes, to assist with digestion of all types of food.

Emotional and mental strain can influence the body's production of enzymes, stressing the importance for a positive, calm eating experience. (Read more about mindful eating in Chapter 11.)

After food has been chewed, swallowing pushes the mass into the esophagus, the *hallway* that funnels food into the stomach by way of peristalsis (alternating contractions and relaxation), until it hits the sphincter, the *door* that will open and admit the food to the stomach. The stomach stores the masticated food for about 1.5 hours and continues to reduce the mass to smaller particles with the aid of the enzyme pepsin and hydrochloric acid, which is secreted by the gastric gland. The contents being held in the stomach—food bolus, enzymes, and acids—have been turned into a mixture called chyme, which continues the journey into the small intestines. At this point, the liver produces bile to assist with breaking down fat and protein. The action of bile on fat and protein is similar to that of a degreaser. Proteins, carbohydrates, fats, vitamins, minerals, water, and alcohol have all been reduced to the smallest unit possible so that they can permeate the intestinal wall and find their way into the bloodstream.

FOOD FOR THOUGHT   WHY DOES HYDROCHLORIC ACID NOT DESTROY THE LINING OF THE STOMACH?

Hydrochloric acid is an aqueous solution of hydrogen chloride and gastric acid that protects us from harmful bacteria we may ingest with our food and harmful bacteria that may migrate from the colon into the small intestines. The stomach and intestines are lined with a healthy amount of bicarbonate-containing mucus, which protects organ linings from the effects of this caustic acid. Its industrial name is "muriatic acid" and can burn a hole if poured on wood.

Some uses are to etch concrete, clean lime residue, and process leather.

Stomach ulcers are painful sores that cause a dull ache in the stomach. Ulcers are created when the thick layer of protective stomach mucous becomes thin or absent. Reduction in stomach mucous can happen from an infection of the *Helicobacter pylori* bacteria, long-term use of aspirin or ibuprofen, excess acid from stress or spicy foods. Treatment includes prescribing antibiotics like metronidazole and taking Pepto-Bismol. Pepto-Bismol (bismuth) causes staining of the teeth and tongue. Patients may present with a black coating on their tongue and should be instructed to brush it every day.

The small intestine is divided into three sections: duodenum, jejunum, and ileum. Most digestion and absorption takes place in the small intestines, more specifically the **jejunum**. The lining of the intestines is variegated rather than smooth, with peaks called **villi**. The villi extensions increase the surface area of the small intestines, allowing for quicker passage of nutrients (3 to 10 hours). Once these small units of digested food pass into the bloodstream, they travel to all parts of the body, supplying it with fuel and nutrients needed for all metabolic processes.

Remnants of food that did not digest become waste and pass on to the large intestine, where water is absorbed from the waste, turning it to solid feces. Unlike the small intestine, the lining of the large intestine is smooth. Bacteria in the feces can manufacture vitamin K and biotin, which can be absorbed and used by the body. The rectum stores the feces until our brain gets the signal to eliminate it. Total *intestinal transit time* can be anywhere from 24 hours to 3 weeks.

We all know that energy can't be created, so we need to convert one form to another.

The digestive process breaks down large nutrient molecules (mainly carbohydrates and lipids) to create single molecules of glucose, then further breaks apart glucose to give us energy. This is done through an intricate function called the KREBS cycle, named for the British biochemist Hans Krebs, who discovered and wrote about the body's citric acid cycle. The citric acid cycle, synonymously called the Krebs cycle, is a very complex multistep chemical process that occurs in mitochondria of cells, and by using oxygen, changes the way molecules share electrons. For every glucose molecule that enters the cycle, our bodies give us two adenosine triphosphate (ATP) molecules.

ATP serves the body the same way gas serves an automobile; you don't move without it. You can only store enough ATP in muscle for a few seconds' worth of activity because it is a heavy molecule and would require extra body mass to carry around any excess. The daily food intake of 2,500 calories will produce about 180 kg of ATP.

Three body systems create energy by taking high-energy phosphates, (ATP), and converting them to low-energy phosphates, (ADP):

1. Phosphagen System—(anaerobic) for 1 to 30 seconds of high power needs for short-term intense activities like sprinting, throwing a pitch, throwing a discus—uses creatine phosphate to reconstitute ATP.
2. Glycolysis—(anaerobic) for 30 seconds to 3 minutes of high exertion like swimming laps—uses carbohydrates.
3. Aerobic System—(aerobic) must have oxygen because carbohydrates and fats are only burned in the presence of oxygen. A required supply of oxygen makes it the slowest system for sustained activities like marathon running.

The three systems do not work independently, but one can predominate at any one time depending on intensity and duration of activity.

NUTRITION CONCERNS

Since the 9/11 event, scientists are searching for ways to assure protection of our food crops from terrorist attacks. According to an article in the New York Daily News (AP Monday October 10, 2011), dozens of foreign insects and plant diseases slipped undetected into the United States since 9/11 due to officials being other-focused on preventing subsequent terrorist attacks. Agriculture experts usually assigned to preventing bug and disease invaders were reassigned to Homeland Security. One of the problems with the invasion of bugs and diseases is that chemicals will be used to eradicate them. More chemicals...do we need that?

There is much concern about the increase in atmospheric CO_2 levels from fossil fuels having an effect on nutritive value of our food crops. Carbon dioxide, methane, and nitrous oxide emissions into the atmosphere have increased in proportion to our industrialization and deforestation. This has created what is referred to as the greenhouse effect, which warms the earth. Wheat, rice, maize, and soybeans tested high for CO_2 levels, which reduced levels of iron, zinc, and level of protein. Reduced level of zinc and iron affect everyone but particularly babies and pregnant women, with resulting malnutrition, causing shorter life spans.[17]

RELATE TO PATIENTS

Preparing food and dining in the 21st century has its own unique challenges. You need to be mindful of current practices that are mainstream. Your patients are busy people, just like you, and need suggestions that are practical, quick, and convenient.

When counseling your patients, always consider the following:

- Delicious looking fruits and vegetables are probably not in the backyard ready to be picked off the vine or tree.
- Bread is not baking in the oven.
- Most patients do not eat *three square meals* a day.
- People heartily embrace convenience over prolonged meal preparation because sometimes busy schedules allow no choice.
- The Internet is full of fanciful trends that claim to prolong life. One Web site claims bone broth is one of three pillars of the LA Lakers official team diet and can even revive the dead! (www.shape.com Cooking Ideas, November 10, 2014).

CHAPTER
REVIEW

 PRACTICE FOR PATIENTS

Your patient has been historically good about making her 6-month recare appointments. She cancels her pending appointment twice but reschedules. When she arrives, her behavior indicates she is under stress and seems to be agitated. After initial conversation, she reveals she has taken on a part-time job as manager at a fast-food restaurant to save money for the fast approaching holiday. She reveals that food is free for workers so eating two hamburgers or pack of chicken nuggets usually serves as snacks to keep her going. Additionally, she sips on soda throughout her shift. Oral examination reveals heavy plaque at the gingival third throughout and incipient dental caries on the facial of tooth #s 6 and 11.

1. Explain how this new diet at work has impacted her oral health.
2. Write out a script of healthy advice that your patient should hear.

RELATE TO YOU

Assignment #1

The goal of this project is to jump-start your mind to begin thinking about nutrition and its relation to the body. Your assignment is to visit a grocery store of your choice with a relative or friend and passively observe their food choices and food selection process.

Answer the following questions about your observations:

1. List the food items in your selected person's shopping cart.
2. What body type do they have? Circle one:
   - Ectomorphic—light body build with slight muscular development
   - Mesomorphic—husky muscular body build
   - Endomorphic—heavy rounded body build with a tendency to become fat
3. Does body type match the food they have chosen to prepare/eat? Explain.
4. What would you add to their selection to balance out their diet?
5. What would you eliminate from their selection to make their diet more nutritious?
6. Did they read labels as they chose food for their carts?
7. Draw a conclusion about food choices and our bodies.

Assignment #2

Take a moment and think about your reasons for eating the foods you choose. Next time you grab something to eat, pay attention to how it changes your sense of being—physically and mentally. Determine if specific foods can elicit feelings of balance and well-being. When you feel like eating a snack, such as potato chips or candy, ask yourself if you are truly hungry, or if you are bored, upset, anxious, or tired. If you feel one of the first three states, then you desire comfort food because you are not balanced emotionally. If you choose the food because you are hungry or tired, then you have a physiologic need. Identifying the feeling before you eat can help you understand your eating habits. Make an inventory list of your favorite food selections and see if you can identify your comfort foods. Then complete Table 1-2 and see if foods you choose affect you in a certain way.

Table 1-2	Influence of Food

Keep a record of how your food selections make you feel. Check in with your body 30 minutes after consuming a particular food to determine what it does.

Food	Energetic	Happy	Clear Mind	Disoriented	Sleepy	Depressed

Assignment #3

Create a patient Nutrition Pamphlet that informs on nutritive value of fast-food selections and include information on choosing wisely when eating out at restaurants. Here are a few Web sites to get you started. Visit:

- www.webmd.com and search for the article on 10 Best Fast Food Meals
- www.calorieking.com to find number of calories in fast-food meals
- www.foodnetwork.com and read the article: How to Order Healthy at Any Restaurant by Kerri-Ann Jennings MS, RD
- www.fitnessmagazine.com and read the article Dine Out on a Diet: Your Restaurant Survival Guide by Brian Underwood

REFERENCES

1. Berkeley Media Studies Group. Target marketing soda and fast food: problems with business as usual. December 2010.
2. Schlosser E. *Fast Food Nation: The Dark Side of the All American Meal*. Boston, MA: Houghton Mifflin; 2000.
3. Delistraty C. The importance of eating together. *The Atlantic*. July 2014.

4. DeVogli R, Kouvonen A, Gimeno D. *Bull World Health Organ* 2014;92(2):99–107A.
5. Morris M, et al. Why is obesity such a problem in the 21st century? The intersection of palatable food, cues and reward pathways, stress, and cognition. *Neurosci Biobehav Rev* 2015;58:36–45.
6. Rigby N. Eating and obesity—the new world disorder. *Nutrients* 2013;5(10):4206–4210.
7. Jacobson M. *Liquid Candy—How Soft Drinks are Harming American's health.* Washington, DC: Center for Science in the Public Interest; 2005.
8. Donnenfeld M, et al. Prospective association between cancer risk and an individual dietary index based on the British Food Standards Agency Nutrient Profiling System. *Br J Nutr* 2015;114(10):1702–1710.
9. Johnson I. Understanding the association between diet and nutrition in upper gastrointestinal cancer. *Expert Rev Gastroenterol Hepatol* 2015;9(11):1347–1349.
10. Toledo E. Mediterranean diet and invasive breast cancer risk among women at high cardiovascular risk in the PREDIMED trial: a randomized clinical trial. *JAMA Intern Med* 2015;175(11):1752–1760.
11. Shivappa N, et al. Prospective study of dietary inflammatory index and risk of breast cancer in Swedish women. *Br J Cancer* 2015;113(7):1099–1103.
12. Kamran A, et al. Sodium intake, dietary knowledge, and illness perceptions of controlled and uncontrolled rural hypertensive patients. *Int J Hypertens* 2014;2014:245480.
13. VanDillen L, Andrade J. Derailing the streetcar named desire. Cognitive distractions reduce individual differences in cravings and unhealthy snacking in response to palatable food. *Appetite* 2016;96:102–110.
14. Hill A. The psychology of food craving. *Proc Nutr Soc* 2007;66(2):277–285.
15. Licino J, Negrano A, Wong M. Plasma leptin concentrations are highly correlated to emotional states throughout the day. *Transl Psychiatry* 2014;4:e475.
16. Holmes JL, Timko C. All cravings are not created equal. Correlates of menstrual versus non-cyclic chocolate craving. *Appetite* 2011;57(1):1–5.
17. Carrington D. Climate change making food crops less nutritious, research finds. *The Guardian.* May 2014.

WEB RESOURCES

Euromonitor International; Industry Reports www.euromonitor.com
Fast Food Nutrition; Restaurant Statistics www.FastFoodNutrition.org
Academy of Nutrition and Dietetics www.eatright.org
Centers for Disease Control and Prevention Division of Nutrition www.cdc.gov/nccdphp/dnpa
Government Information Food and Nutrition Information Center www.nal.usda.gov/fnic
Harvard School of Public Health www.hsph.harvard.edu

ADDITIONAL STUDY

Siegal A. *Promiscuous Eating: Understanding and Ending Our Self-Destructive Relationship with Food.* New York: Rogue Wave Press; 2011.
Video-Food, Inc. You'll Never Look at Dinner the Same Way Again. *Alliance Films Release;* 2008.
Wansink B. *Mindless Eating.* New York: Bantam Books; 2006.

Major Nutrients

Carbohydrates

2

Learning Objectives

- Name both chemical and nutritive classifications of carbohydrates
- Discuss the molecular difference between a monosaccharide, disaccharide, and polysaccharide
- Explain the digestion of carbohydrates in the body
- Describe maintenance of blood glucose level and outline the steps involved in reducing excess blood glucose and releasing glucose when the level is low
- Differentiate between an insoluble fiber and soluble fiber
- Explain what happens in the body when carbohydrates are restricted from the diet
- Give examples of foods that are rich in fiber and discuss their importance in the diet
- Counsel patients about the benefits of carbohydrates in the diet and guide them to choose those that are complex versus simple

> "I love being active and mentally present and aware. Therefore, I love carbs as they are what give me the energy I need to do all the things that I love to do. Choosing the right kind of carbohydrates allows me to get the most out of my day."
>
> *Cameron Diaz—Actress*

Key Terms

Amylose
Amylopectin
Complex Carbohydrate
Fiber
Glycemic Index
Glycogen

Homeostasis
Hyperglycemia
Hypoglycemia
Insoluble Fiber
Ketosis
Roughage

Satiety   Soluble Fiber
Simple Sugar   Spiking

INTRODUCTION

What is a carbohydrate?

If you answered "sugar," you would be half right. Carbohydrates are a *type* of sugar, but all carbohydrates are not *sweet* like that which you put in coffee or tea. Rice, pasta, bread, fruits, and vegetables are also carbohydrates. The size of the chemical arrangement is what determines the flavor and level of sweetness, but they all do pretty much the same thing for the body. And that is to provide fuel for your furnace.

Before the Industrial Revolution (1760–1840), foods most readily available for consumption were rich in carbohydrates and, therefore, the main source of nutrients for humans on the planet. Geographic regions each had their signature staple food that grew well on their land. These foods were consumed in the whole or natural form and were nutrient dense with vitamins, minerals, and fiber. Table 2-1 identifies the food staple by region.

The Industrial Revolution was a very creative time for man. Many machines were invented including those that refined wheat, sugarcane, and sugar beets into a fine powder. To get the fine white powder, the husks and pulp had to be removed. It was later learned that husks and pulp were the most nutritive part of the plant. Since the best part was removed (nutrients and fiber), the powdery flour and sugar lost nutritive value but retained calories. It was considered a luxury and a display of wealth to have a pantry full of bleached white flour and sugar. What once were *wealthy* sources of nutrients became *poor* sources, but their consumption remained the same. People began to prepare their food with

Almost one third of calories in the American diet are from refined sugar and corn syrup.

Table 2-1	Main Food Staples by Region
Region	**Food**
Asia	Rice
Middle East	Wheat
Great Britain	Barley and oats
Pacific Islands	Taro root
Africa	Cassava root and yams
America	Potatoes and corn
South America	Quinoa
Central America	Corn and rice

refined ingredients, and this led to the occurrence of obesity in people of wealth and position. Because of this refined flour and sugar/obesity connection, carbohydrates got a bad reputation of being fattening. This is erroneous thinking as all carbohydrates are not bad or unnecessary. The right kind of carbohydrates, when carefully selected, is an excellent low-fat source of fiber and nutrients.

| FOOD FOR THOUGHT | A SOUTHERN FOOD STAPLE: WHERE DO BELOVED SOUTHERN AMERICAN GRITS COME FROM? |

Grits are an indigenous carbohydrate-rich grain of the American southern states. The process for making hominy grits was learned from Native Americans. The same process is also used in the process of making Mexican tortillas.

Dried maize (corn) kernels are soaked in *lye*, which makes hominy. Ground-up hominy is used to make grits.

Lye = sodium hydroxide

Wait a minute... sodium hydroxide is in drain cleaner, good for dissolving hair and skin.

No worries... hominy is soaked in a weak solution of lye to soften and breakdown the husks and then thoroughly soaked and washed to remove the lye. Once dry, it is ground up into a course powder.

CARBOHYDRATES IN THE ECOSYSTEM

Lactose (milk sugar) is the only carbohydrate of animal origin.

With the exception of one sugar, plants are the source of all carbohydrates. Figure 2-1 illustrates where carbohydrates fit into the food chain.

1. Plant roots absorb water.
2. Foliage absorbs carbon dioxide (CO_2) from the air.
3. Plant absorbs rays from the sun.
4. Chloroplasts in the plant take all three—H_2O, sun, and CO_2—and through photosynthesis make monosaccharides.
5. Animals eat the plant and reduce the monosaccharides to glucose.

PRIMARY ROLE OF CARBOHYDRATES IN THE BODY

Carbohydrates are an important component of a balanced diet. Provided by most foods, especially grains, fruits, and vegetables, they are the most prolific source of energy for the body. The primary roles of carbohydrates are to:

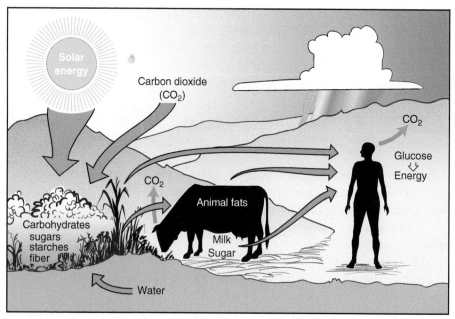

Figure 2-1 The carbon cycle.

- Supply the body with energy
- Maintain blood glucose levels
- Continue brain and nervous system function, even while sleeping
- Spare protein so the body does not burn dietary or body fat and protein for energy
- Help burn fat for fuel
- Provide bulk in the diet (fiber) and gives a sense of **satiety** (feeling full)

CLASSIFICATION OF CARBOHYDRATES

The word *carbohydrate* is Latin for hydrated water. Carbohydrates are often abbreviated CHO, which identifies three comprising elements:

<u>C</u>arbon   <u>H</u>ydrogen   <u>O</u>xygen

The chemical building blocks of CHOs are called *monosaccharides*, which are composed of:

$(C_6H_{12}O_6)$
6 carbon   12 hydrogen   6 oxygen atoms

Carbohydrates can be classified in two ways: either chemical or nutritive.

The *chemical classification* helps us understand how the molecules of carbohydrates link together, and the *nutritional classification* determines their value in our diet.

Table 2-2 outlines these two classification systems.

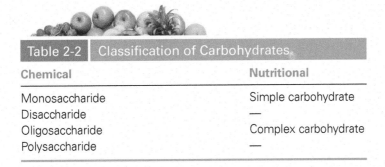

Table 2-2	Classification of Carbohydrates
Chemical	**Nutritional**
Monosaccharide	Simple carbohydrate
Disaccharide	—
Oligosaccharide	Complex carbohydrate
Polysaccharide	—

Chemical Classification of Carbohydrates

The main unit of carbohydrate is a monosaccharide (glucose molecule). One molecule of glucose consists of 6 carbon atoms, 12 hydrogen atoms, and 6 oxygen atoms: $C_6H_{12}O_6$. Figures 2-2 and 2-3 illustrate the chemical structures of monosaccharides and disaccharides, respectively.

1. Monosaccharide = 1 molecule of sugar
2. Disaccharide = 2 molecules of sugar
3. Oligosaccharide = 2 to 10 molecules of sugar
4. Polysaccharide = more than 10 molecules of sugar

Nutritional Classification

Simple Sugars

Monosaccharides and disaccharides are referred to as simple sugars and are usually those that are sweet to the taste. Candy, cookies, cake, soda, ripe fruits, and other baked goods fall in this category and are high in calories but lack the nutrients

Figure 2-2 Chemical structure of monosaccharides.

Figure 2-3   Chemical structure of disaccharides.

supplied by complex carbohydrates. Lactose (found in dairy products) and glucose (blood sugar) are also considered simple sugars but are not sweet to the taste.

Monosaccharides = One

Glucose is also called dextrose or **blood sugar**. It is the main agent for the body's fuel source that supplies energy to the body. Most other sugars are either converted or broken down to this single unit as it is small and soluble in water and can pass through cell membranes. Glucose can be stored as glycogen in muscle and the liver, or if consumed in excess, can be converted to fat for future energy supply.

Disaccharides = Two

Most sugars found in nature are disaccharides, which are two monosaccharides together. Unlike monosaccharides, they are too big to pass through cell membranes so are broken down to monosaccharides for use by the body. Some examples are as follows:

1. Sucrose, common table sugar, consists of one glucose and one fructose molecule, which gives our food the sweet taste.
2. Maltose consists of two glucose molecules and is created when larger carbohydrate molecules are broken down during digestion.
3. Lactose, the sugar found in milk, splits into the two monosaccharides glucose and galactose during digestion.

Complex Carbohydrates

Polysaccharides are referred to as **complex carbohydrates** and are the most nutrient dense of all carbohydrates providing vitamins, minerals, fiber, and water to the body. Grains with their husk intact like brown rice, whole grain bread, cereal, whole wheat pasta, legumes, fruits, and vegetables are foods rich in complex carbohydrates.

Table 2-3 lists common monosaccharides, disaccharides, and polysaccharides.

Figure 2-4A shows examples of simple and complex carbohydrates; Figure 2-4B shows examples of low nutrient simple carbohydrates (Table 2-4). Table 2-4 gives examples of complex carbohydrate substitutions for simple carbohydrates.

Table 2-3	Common names for chemical classification of carbohydrates

MONOSACCHARIDES

- Glucose—blood sugar
- Fructose—fruit sugar
- Galactose—milk

DISACCHARIDES

- Sucrose: glucose + fructose = table sugar
- Maltose: glucose + glucose = flavoring, breakdown product of starch
- Lactose: glucose + galactose = milk disaccharide

POLYSACCHARIDES

- Oligosaccharide
- Starch
- Glycogen

A   **B**

Figure 2-4   **A:** Examples of simple and complex carbohydrates. (Complex on left, simple on right: Photo courtesy of Kevin Brown, Zolfo Springs, FL.) **B:** Examples of low-nutrient simple carbohydrates—empty calories. (Photo courtesy of Kevin Brown, Zolfo Springs, FL.)

Oligosaccharides

Oligosaccharides are a unique type of carbohydrate because the body does not metabolize them in the usual way. They are larger than a disaccharide—at least two or more single sugar molecules—and are found in legumes (beans). Oligosaccharides pass

Table 2-4	Simple Carbohydrates versus Complex Carbohydrates	
Simple Carbohydrate	**Complex Carbohydrate**
White bread	Whole grain bread
White rice	Brown rice
Semolina pasta	Whole wheat pasta
Sugar-sweetened juices	100% fruit juice and vegetable juice
Flour tortillas	Wheat or spinach tortillas

through the stomach undigested into the intestines, where bacteria feed on the carbohydrate and create a gaseous end product, giving beans their unpleasant reputation.

Starch

Starch is the storage form of energy in plants, just as glycogen is the storage form of energy in animals (and man). The arrangement of glucose molecules determines whether the starch is amylose or amylopectin, the two most predominant starches.

Amylopectin is a series of highly branched chains of glucose molecules. It is sometimes referred to as a *waxy starch* that forms a stringy paste when heated, and this property makes it work well as a thickener in food. *Amylose* is composed of thousands of straight-chain glucose molecules. Foods that contain starch are grains, legumes, tubers (potatoes, yams, and turnips), and some fruits.

 FOOD FOR THOUGHT   EXPERIMENT WITH YOUR FOOD

One way to tell if a food contains starch is to add a drop of iodine. The unbranched helical shape of amylose reacts strongly to iodine and turns it blue-black. Amylopectin, cellulose, and glycogen will turn the iodine reddish-purple and brown.

Starch is used as a thickening agent in cooking and baking. A good example is cornstarch: when mixed with water over heat, it forms a sauce or gravy. When we consume starch, it gives us a sense of satiety or fullness, and the sense of being full stays with us for a longer period of time.

Glycogen

Glycogen is the most highly branched chain of glucose units and is the *storage form* of carbohydrates that is found in the liver and muscle.

In Liver—helps maintain blood glucose levels
In Muscle—provides quick supply of energy for working muscles

Fiber

Fiber is the ingredient in food that is usually referred to as **roughage** or *bulk* and is not used by the body for energy. Fiber is thousands of glucose units bonded together and is found exclusively in plants, which give them structure. A good example of fiber are stringy strips that run the length of celery and skin on a apple.

Fiber in plants is equal to bones in animals.

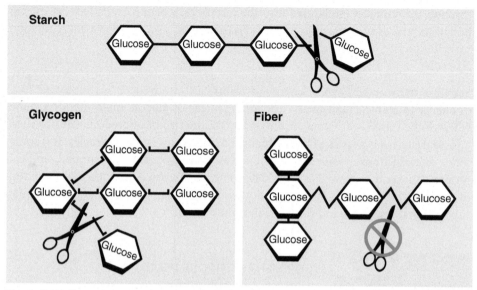

Figure 2-5   Enzymes cannot break apart fiber.

Humans do not have enzymes that can break down and digest fiber. The chemical links between fiber molecules are joined in such a way that they cannot be separated by human digestive enzymes. Vitamins and minerals in fiber-rich foods are not made available to the body and pass through unabsorbed. See Figure 2-5 for an illustration of enzyme activity. There are two general classes of fiber, and most foods contain both types—some have more soluble than insoluble. It is good to include both types in your diet as fiber feeds healthy bacteria that lives in the colon.

Soluble Fiber—dissolves in water.

Some examples of food high in soluble fiber are as follows:

- Black, kidney and navy beans
- Flaxseed
- Apricots, grapefruit, mangoes
- Turnips and sweet potatoes
- Oatmeal and oat bran

Function of Soluble Fiber

- Adds chewy or crunchy texture to foods
- Gives a sense of satiety—keeps the stomach full longer
- Stabilizes blood sugar—takes longer for the body to metabolize and slows release of glucose into bloodstream
- Helps lower cholesterol—binds fiber and carries it out of the body in waste

Insoluble Fiber—does *not* dissolve in water and passes through the body undigested.

Some examples of food high in insoluble fiber are as follows:

- Whole grains, brown rice, bran
- Corn, broccoli
- Dark leafy greens
- Skin on fruits and vegetables
- Seeds and nuts

Function of Insoluble Fiber

- Prevents disease by stimulating peristalsis and keeps colon muscles exercised and strong
- Decreases constipation
- Prevents hemorrhoids
- Prevents colon cancer—empties the colon so that the lining of the intestines and colon are not exposed to toxins for a long period of time. Think of undigested insoluble fiber scouring your intestines
- Decreases incidence of appendicitis

Table 2-5 lists the grams of the different types of fiber found in certain foods. When increasing the amount of fiber in your diet, do so gradually to allow your body time to adapt. Increasing the amount too fast will result in waste elimination problems. Drink plenty of fluids to keep stools hydrated, allowing for less constipation.

Table 2-5	Grams of Fiber in Food		
Food	Total Fiber	Soluble Fiber	Insoluble Fiber
Oat bran	28	14	14
Rolled oats	14	8	6
Wheat bran	43	3	40
Kidney beans	10	5	5
Pinto beans	11	5	6
Corn	3	2	1
Apple	2	1	1
Orange	2	1	1

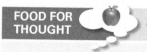

CAN LOW FIBER DIETS CAUSE GI DISEASE?

Dr. Denis Burkitt was an Irish physician who sought to discover why geographic areas had different incidence and distribution of cancer. He hypothesized and studied the causal relationship between gastrointestinal diseases and low-fiber diets. For more in-depth reading, access the biographical article in the *Journal of Nutrition* by Jon A. Story and David Kritchevsky.[1]

Modern man consumes on average 8 g of fiber per day. Our hunter–gatherer ancestors consumed close to 100 g/day because of diets rich in roots/tubers, grass/plants, and berries with seeds. Although it is hard to know for sure, researchers affirm that our ancestors were free of many of the diseases that affect modern man—cancer, heart disease, diabetes, and obesity. Paying attention to amount of fiber you consume on a daily basis and including more fiber-rich foods if deficient will improve your risk of common diseases.

When bacteria in the stomach are processing fiber, one of the by-products is short-chain fatty acids. Butyrate is a fat-chain fatty acid shown to have the ability to turn on an anticancer gene, which greatly reduces the risk of colon cancer—by about 30%.[2,3]

MAINTENANCE OF BLOOD GLUCOSE HOMEOSTASIS

A healthy blood glucose level is 80 to 100 mg/dL of blood. When blood glucose is higher, you have **hyperglycemia** (over). When blood glucose is lower, you have **hypoglycemia** (under).

Insulin and glucagon are the two hormones involved in keeping your blood glucose at an optimal level. When blood glucose level is too high or low, your sense of well-being is disturbed. If your body is circulating too much blood glucose, you feel an excess of energy and are nervous and excitable. When there is not enough blood glucose, you can feel lethargic, disoriented, and confused. Maintaining the right amount of glucose in the blood is called **homeostasis**. When the amount of glucose in your blood is in balance with what your body needs, there is an overall sense of well-being and you feel just the right amount of energy and alertness. Table sugar and foods rich in simple sugars will overdose your system with glucose, giving you the feeling of both extremes in a short period of time. This is called **spiking** (loading our bodies with sugar) and is a harmful pattern. You feel a rapid surge then subsequent decline in energy over a short time span. When you feel the drop in energy, the first inclination is to eat a candy bar or drink a soda to feel energetic again. This behavior greatly increases the amount of calories ingested (with no nutrients) and lends itself to detrimental long-term effects such as obesity and dental caries. Homeostasis works as follows and is illustrated in Figure 2-6:

Too much glucose in the blood stream: You are feeling jittery, anxious, hyperactive.

Receptor cells in the pancreas recognize that there is more glucose in the blood than the body currently needs for energy. The pancreas secretes the hormone *insulin*, which draws out the excess glucose, thus reducing the amount of blood glucose when the level gets too high. It attracts glucose from the bloodstream and stores it in the muscle and the liver where it is converted to **glycogen** (storage form of glucose). The glycogen stays in the muscle until the body needs it to move the muscle, or stores it in the liver for future energy use. There is a limit to the capacity of glycogen storing cells. Once the stores are filled, the overflow is routed to fat. Unused adipose (fat) cells begin to enlarge and fill with fat, and the storage capacity is *unlimited*.

Not enough glucose in the blood stream: You are feeling sleepy, lethargic, low energy.

Receptor cells in the pancreas recognize that the body is in need of energy so the pancreas secretes the hormone **glucagon**, which converts the *glycogen* in the liver to

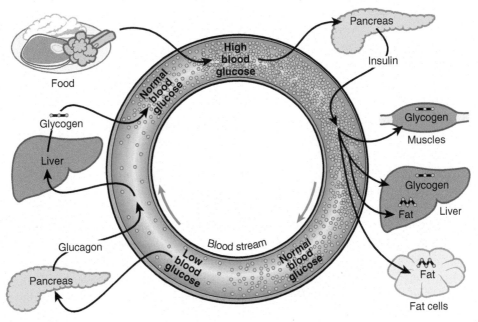

Figure 2-6 Blood sugar homeostasis.

glucose and releases it into the bloodstream, where it is carried through the body and used for fuel.

How the Body Regulates Blood Sugar

- Eating carbohydrates throughout the day will help maintain blood glucose levels. Eat a little with each meal.
- Whenever possible, choose the whole grain version of the food, because it is metabolized more slowly by the body.
- Avoid refined sugars—they are empty calories and cause spiking.

RECOMMENDED DIETARY INTAKE

There is no recommended dietary intake for carbohydrates, but it has been loosely recommended at 55% to 65% of total daily calorie intake, with 25 to 35 g being fiber. This amounts to about 300 g for a sedentary person and 500 g for a physically active person. It has also been suggested that we limit daily intake of refined sugar to less than 10% of total calorie intake, which includes the sugar present in processed foods like jams, jellies, baked goods, and beverages (2015 Guidelines for Health Americans). The average person consumes about 50 teaspoons of sugar each day including that which gets added to coffee, tea, and cereal, and that which is incorporated into recipes and processed foods. If you add that up, it is equivalent to a couple five-pound bags of sugar each month. According to the USDA Factbook Profiling Food Consumption in America, it is recommended you should have no more than 10 teaspoons a day, which is equivalent to slightly less than one can of soda.

FOOD FOR THOUGHT   **IS THERE REALLY SUCH A THING AS A SUGAR ADDICTION?**

Food manufacturers put sugar in just about all their products to stimulate appetite for more of the same. There are over 600,000 manufactured food products, and 80% of them contain sugar. The more you eat, the more you want.

Sugar addiction follows the same pattern as all other addictions—binge, withdrawal, craving. Studies conducted on lab mice showed that overtime, mice increased their sugar intake to twice the amount as at the beginning of the study. When sugar was withheld from them, they displayed signs of withdrawal like teeth chattering and body tremors. The mice needed to increase their intake to create the same initial feel-good effect.

In another study, scientists genetically altered lab mice without sugar receptors. They provided two bottles of water—one with and one without sugar. After a few hours, the mice began drinking exclusively from the sugar water bottles. Then they added a bottle with Splenda, and they still preferred the sugar water. Since mice are unable to communicate why they preferred the sugar water, scientists analyzed their brains and discovered that the mice released dopamine in response to sugar water. They could not taste it, but it made them feel good. Their brains, like ours, are slaves to feeling good.

Jonah Lehrer—McGriddles: http://scienceblogs.com/cortex/2009/07the_neuroscienceo_of_mc-griddles.php
de Araujo O-M, Sotnikova G, Caron N, et al. Food reward in the absence of taste receptor signaling. Neuron 2008;57(6):930–941.

DIGESTION OF CARBOHYDRATES

Monosaccharides do not require breakdown by enzymes, but disaccharides and polysaccharides must be reduced to monosaccharides by enzymes before they can be absorbed and used by the body. Polysaccharides are broken down to disaccharides, and disaccharides are broken down to monosaccharides. The s-p-l-i-t-t-i-n-g (or breaking apart) of molecules begins in the mouth when polysaccharides mix with salivary amylase and are reduced to disaccharides. Further degradation happens when the reduced molecules come in contact with stomach acids. Disaccharides are passed into the small intestine, where pancreatic amylase completes the breakdown to monosaccharides. These small monosaccharides then pass through the small intestinal villi into the bloodstream, where they travel to the liver for nutrient processing before being sent out to all parts of the body for use as energy.

- Sucrose is broken down by sucrase into glucose and fructose.
- Maltose is broken down by maltase into glucose units.
- Lactose is broken down by lactase into glucose and galactose.

GLYCEMIC INDEX

Glycemic Index is a numeric ranking system for carbohydrates based on their immediate effect on blood glucose levels. Foods high in fats and protein do not cause the rise in blood sugar levels as do carbohydrates. Carbohydrates that break down rapidly to supply the body with glucose are at the high end of the index, and those that take longer to break down and digest are at the low end. Some people make the mistake of thinking that only simple carbohydrates are at the high end when, in fact, some complex carbohydrates are also at the high end. The lower the glycemic index (GI), the less demand for insulin and slower the digestion and absorption rates. The less the demand for insulin, the better the blood glucose control. People who are diabetic need to learn the glycemic value of foods in order to prepare meals that will allow for slower release of glucose into the blood stream.[4,5] Some foods may surprise you where they fall on the spectrum. For example, a Coke has an index of 68, but Fanta Orange and Ocean Spray Cranberry juice cocktail also have 68. Athletes will appreciate knowing that Gatorade has 78 and banana has 62. Foods that are low on the spectrum that do a better job of maintaining blood glucose are grapefruit with 25, carrots 35, peanuts 7, and hummus 6. For more on how to calculate glycemic index, visit www.dummies.com/how-to/content/how-to-calculate-glycemic-load.html. Another Web site www.health.harvard.edu has a table of glycemic index for 100 + foods. Tables 2-6 through 2-9 gives a few examples of GI for foods.

Table 2-6	Glycemic Index (GI) of Foods (Glucose = 100)	
Low GI	**Medium GI**	**High GI**
Apples	Beets	Popcorn
Carrots	Cantaloupe	Watermelon
Grapes	Pineapple	Whole wheat bread
Kidney beans	Table sugar	While flour and bread
Peanuts	White and wild rice	Corn flakes
Lentils	Sweet potatoes	Cheerios
Corn	New potatoes	Baked potatoes

Table 2-7	Glycemic Index for Bread
Wonder bread	73
Kaiser Roll	73
Whole wheat bread	71
Whole wheat pita	57
Sour dough	52
Corn tortilla	52
Dark rye	51
Whole grain English muffin	45
Wheat tortilla	30

Table 2-8	Glycemic Index for Snacks
Fruit roll up	99
Pretzels (16)	83
Doritos	72
Microwave popcorn	72
Chewy Granola Bar	61
Snickers candy bar	55
Potato chips (11)	54
Peanut M&Ms (6)	33
Oreo cookies	64

Table 2-9	Glycemic Index for Beverages
12-oz can of beer	15
Red or white wine	15
8-oz glass whole milk	27
8-oz glass low-fat chocolate milk	49
12-oz can Coke	68
6-oz glass orange juice	71
6-oz glass unsweetened apple juice	57
6-oz glass tomato juice	54
6-oz glass carrot juice	61

CAUTIONARY ADVICE ABOUT CARBOHYDRATES

- **Lactose intolerance,** also referred to as *milk allergy,* occurs when there is an absence of the digestive enzyme lactase. Without lactase, the disaccharide lactose cannot be digested or absorbed. It passes undigested to the colon, where bacteria feed on the carbohydrate, resulting in cramping and diarrhea. People who are lactose intolerant must avoid dairy products or take lactase enzyme pills before consuming dairy products.
- Excessive fiber intake can decrease mineral absorption and cause cramping and gas. Be sure to increase fiber in the diet gradually and drink plenty of water.
- Carbohydrates are notorious for contributing to the development of dental caries with simple sugars being the most cariogenic. (See Chapter 9.)

- Excess consumption of simple carbohydrates can cause a temporary elevation in blood triglycerides, which can increase risk for heart disease.
- Loading up on simple sugars can cause blood glucose to spike and then drop below normal, causing a condition called rebound hypoglycemia.

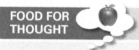

FOOD FOR THOUGHT   LACTOSE INTOLERANCE

Lactose-intolerant people can substitute fruit juices fortified with highly absorbable calcium citrate or take calcium supplements to supply the body with the daily requirement of calcium.

Certain ethnic groups are more prone to lactose intolerance: Asians, Native Americans, African Americans.

FOOD FOR THOUGHT   SUGAR AS PRESERVATIVE IN MANUFACTURED FOOD

Sugar is present in a wide array of processed foods, for example, cereal, canned food products, candy, and baked goods. Sometimes when you see it on a label, you wonder what it is doing in the recipe. The answer is: like salt, it can be used as a natural preservative because it pulls water from cells and disables bacteria. Most of the time, its taste is undetectable, as in canned goods, crackers, and processed foods.

CARBOHYDRATES ARE PROTEIN SPARING

Carbohydrates are called *protein sparing*. The function of protein in the body is varied but includes important tasks like creating antibodies, hormones, and building and repairing body tissue.(see Chapter 3). When the liver stores are depleted of glucose and carbohydrate consumption is restricted, the body will *create* needed glucose from amino acids found in protein through a process called **gluco*genesis***.

CARBOHYDRATE RESTRICTION

Carbohydrates are needed for many metabolic functions. If a diet restricts intake of carbohydrates (low carb), there is minimal glucose available for the body to use for vital processes. If there is not enough glucose to perform vital metabolic functions, the liver will convert fat into fatty acids using adipose cells (fat cells). The rapid release of all these fatty acids creates incomplete breakdown in the liver leading to formation of ketones. Glucose is the preferred energy source for all body cells, and ketones are the body's crisis reaction to lack of carbohydrates. With ketones circulating, the body enters a physiologic state of **ketosis**, which is a response to fuel shortage. Acetyl groups are also made during the production of ketones, which will give breath a distinctive *acetone smell* (fruity chemical odor).

Because our brain and heart need a steady supply of carbohydrates for proper functioning, a state of starvation will kick the body into *survival mode*, at which time it will use *ketones* for energy and brain and heart activity.

RELATE TO PATIENTS

When providing nutritional counseling for a patient and his or her diet diary reveals a deficiency in the food groups that supply the most carbohydrates (breads and cereals, dairy, and fruits and vegetables), encourage choosing and eating more complex versus simple carbohydrates. Some patients have difficulty making sudden switches or find that the more fibrous versions of bread, rice, etc., are less palatable. Suggest mixing simple and complex carbohydrates and gradually increasing the proportion of complex carbohydrates until they are able to make the change to healthier complex versions.

For example, you can suggest to your patient:

- Mix a few tablespoons of brown rice with white rice.
- Mix whole wheat pasta with semolina pasta.
- When preparing a sandwich, use one piece of white and one piece of whole grain bread, putting the white bread tongue side. Try the same with hamburger buns, rolls, and crackers.
- To increase the servings of fruits and vegetables, drink juice instead of soda.
- Add variety to meals with soft cooked and fresh vegetables.

CHAPTER
REVIEW

 PRACTICE FOR PATIENTS

Patient #1

Your patient has rampant facial caries on her six maxillary anterior teeth. She states that she has a problem staying awake for a 12-hour shift at the hospital and drinking a soda every other hour helps her stay alert. In addition to dental caries, you notice her blood pressure is higher than normal and she was recently diagnosed with asthma.

1. Would you consider the soda to be a simple sugar or a complex carbohydrate?
2. Give an explanation of what is happening in your patient's body to cause the cycle of low and high energy.
3. Suggest a drink substitution that would give her blood sugar homeostasis.
4. How does a diet high in simple sugars affect overall health?

Patient #2

Your patient is a night security guard at the local shopping mall. His food addiction is to fresh-baked doughnuts. Access to day-old doughnuts at the mall café is one of the job's benefits. He states that he has gained about 25 pounds since taking the job 3 years ago but that is OK because his girlfriend says there is "more to love."

1. Would you expect to find changes to his medical history? If so, what could be those changes?
2. Will his addiction to doughnuts affect the oral structures in any way?
3. What home care advice should you be sure to include during patient education?

RELATE TO YOU

Assignment #1

Evaluate your food and drink consumption over the last 2 days and determine if added sugar was less than 10% of the total calories in your diet. If your intake was higher, what changes can you make to better maintain your blood sugar level?

Assignment #2

Evaluate the amount of fiber in your diet. It has been suggested that our diets include 25 to 35 g of fiber per day. Locate a chart of fiber content of certain foods and add up the amount consumed on a typical day.

1. Did you meet your goal?
2. If not, how can you increase the amount of fiber in each meal?
3. Explain the necessity for adequate fiber in your diet—how does it improve your health?

Assignment #3

Spend a few days experimenting with different breakfast meals:

Using the chart from Chapter 1, complete the boxes an hour after your meal.
On one of the days, eat a meal that you enjoy that is high in simple sugars.
On another day, eat a meal that is rich with fresh fruit and complex cereal grains.
Both meals are carbohydrate—one simple and one complex. Does your body and
 mind know the difference?

REFERENCES

1. Story J, Kritchevsky D. Denis Parsons Burkitt (1911–1993). *J Nutr* 1994;124:1551–1554.
2. Borges-Canha M, et al. Role of colonic microbiota in colorectal carcinogenesis: a systematic review. *Rev Esp Enferm Dig* 2015;107(11).
3. Hu S, Liu L, Chang EB, et al. Butyrate inhibits pro-proliferative miR-92a by diminishing c-Myc-induced miR-17-92a cluster transcription in human colon cancer cells. *Mol Cancer* 2015;14(1):180.
4. Schulte EM, et al. Which foods may be addictive? The roles of processing, fat content, and glycemic load. *PLoS One* 2015;10(2):e0117959.

5. Augustin LS, et al. Glycemic index, glycemic load and glycemic response: an international scientific consensus summit from the international carbohydrate quality consortium (ICQC). *Nutr Metab Cardiovasc Dis* 2015;25(9):795–815.

WEB RESOURCES

Consumer Fact Sheet: Sugar in Your Diet www.sbreb.org/brochures/FactSheet/
Create your Plate for Diabetics http://www.diabetes.org/food-and-fitness/food/planning-meals/create-your-plate/?loc=ff-slabnav
Sugar Sweet by Nature www.sugar.org/consumers/sweet by nature.asp?id=279

Protein

Learning Objectives

- Discuss the benefits of protein in the diet
- Describe the difference between structural and functional protein and list examples of each
- Identify essential, nonessential, and semiessential amino acids from a list
- Explain the difference between dipeptide, tripeptide, and polypeptide bonds
- Outline the digestion of proteins
- Discuss disadvantages of both protein deficiency and excess and explain their effect on the body
- Define biologic value and give examples of foods with high value
- Discuss nitrogen balance and state situations when the body would be in positive or negative balance
- Differentiate between complete and incomplete protein, complementary and supplementary protein
- Compute your Recommended Dietary Intake of protein
- Counsel patients on consuming the recommended amount of protein for their weight

> Protein was the most valued ingredient 250 years ago: it was the rarest thing. Now the rarest thing we have is time: time to cook and time to eat.
>
> *Adam Gopnik—Author and staff writer for The New Yorker*

Key Terms

Amino Acid
Biologic Value
Complementary Protein

Complete Protein
Dipeptide
Essential Amino Acids (EAAs)

(continued)

Incomplete Protein

Kwashiorkor

Marasmus

Negative Nitrogen Balance

Nonessential Amino Acids

Peptide Bond

Polypeptide

Positive Nitrogen Balance

Sarcopenia

Supplementary Protein

Tripeptide

INTRODUCTION

If you are eating extra protein to help define your six-pack as you work out at the gym, proceed with caution! Consuming extra protein to build muscle mass and increase strength is a delicate science. The *quality* of protein you choose to add to your diet can impact your overall health: increasing fatty red meats can increase risk for heart disease, and eating more protein than your body needs circulates ketones that damage kidneys. Unless you are someone who runs marathons or are a professional body-builder, the recommended amount of daily protein is enough to support your energy needs.[1,2] Find your balance and don't overdo it.

Protein is *vital* for life and second only to water as the most important nutrient with which to nourish your body. Without protein you would not have muscle structure, and since muscle is what causes contractions that pump oxygen and nutrients throughout the body, you would not be able to breathe, much less stay alive.

Proteins, carbohydrates, and lipids are *similar* in composition as all three contain the elements carbon, hydrogen, and oxygen, but protein *differs* from them in that it has the added element of *nitrogen*. Unlike carbohydrates and lipids, protein is not identifiable as a single molecule but is made up of several amino acids. Nitrogen, the differing element, is part of the amino acid *building blocks* of protein. There are thousands of arrangements of amino acids that make protein, and each arrangement has a specific function in the body see Figure 3-1.

NITROGEN IN THE ECOSYSTEM

Figure 3-2 illustrates how nitrogen ends up in our food and is outlined below:

1. Nitrogen is constantly cycling through the earth's ecosystem and is absorbed from the air into the soil.
2. Plants absorb nitrogen from the soil and make amino acids by combining nitrogen absorbed from the ground with carbon fragments produced during photosynthesis.
3. Plants link amino acids together to form plant proteins.
4. Animals consume plant proteins, which convert to animal protein.
5. Animal waste returns nitrogen to the soil.
6. Humans consume plant proteins directly or indirectly while eating animal products.

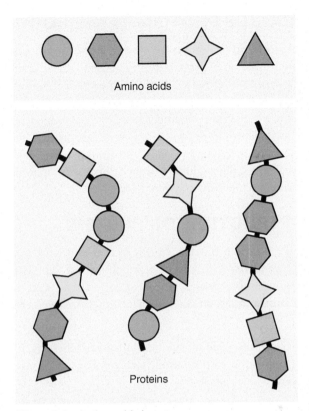

Figure 3-1 Amino acid shapes.

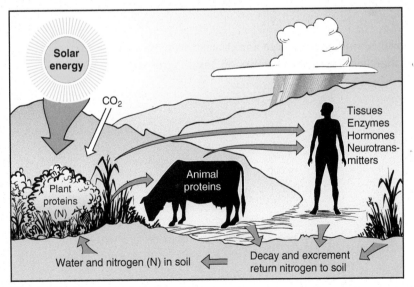

Figure 3-2 Proteins in the ecosystem.

PRIMARY ROLE OF PROTEIN IN THE BODY

The primary role of protein in the body is for *growth, maintenance, and repair*. Growth is the major metabolic function of protein during youth, with children requiring more than adults. During periods of growth, a body will need larger amounts of protein on a daily basis to build new body tissues and cells.

In maturity, protein's function is mainly for maintenance. As an adult, the amount required by an individual would depend on how much protein is lost each day in urine, feces, sweat, mucus, lost hair and nails, and sloughed skin cells. Persons under high levels of physical stress, illness, injury, or emotional stress may also require larger amounts of daily protein while the body repairs itself.

CHEMICAL STRUCTURE OF PROTEIN

Amino acids are the building blocks of protein that contain the elements of carbon, hydrogen, oxygen, *nitrogen*, and occasionally sulfur. The general configuration is as follows: one amino group, one acid group, and one functional group that attaches to a central atom of carbon. The functional group differs for each amino acid.

1. Amino radical group—one nitrogen atom and two hydrogen atoms: NH_2.
2. Carboxyl group—one carbon atom, two oxygen atoms, and one hydrogen atom: COOH.
3. Functional group that takes the place of one of the two hydrogens off the central carbon atom. The functional group is depicted as "R" in the pictorial graphic of amino acids and is what makes each amino acid unique and distinctive see Figure 3-3.

A protein molecule is large and usually made up of more than 100 amino acids linked together. There are 20 common amino acids that can join together to form a

Figure 3-3   Amino acid chemical structure.

protein molecule useful to the body. In order for amino acids to join together, two hydrogen and one oxygen are dropped (water molecule) forming a bond called a **peptide bond.**

When two amino acids link together, the resulting structure is called a **dipeptide,** and when three are linked, it is called a **tripeptide.** When there are several hundred amino acids linked together, they form a **polypeptide.** These structures can form long strands (structural protein) or a three-dimensional shape (functional protein). If you think of amino acids as jewelry beads that form bracelets, the arrangement for putting the beads together is endless.

Essential versus Nonessential

Amino acids can be either essential or nonessential. **Essential amino acids** are those that the body cannot synthesize from other compounds, so they must be obtained from food. However, the body can form **nonessential amino acids** from nitrogen and a carbon chain or from a similar essential acid. Four amino acids are considered semiessential during childhood because the metabolic pathways that synthesize these amino acids are not fully developed. The amounts required by the body depend on age and health, so it is difficult to make a general statement about dietary requirement. (See Table 3-1 for a list of essential, nonessential, and semiessential amino acids.)

Protein provides the body with many *structural* and *functional* processes, and it is the *shape* of the amino acid that determines how the body uses it.

Table 3-1	Essential, Nonessential, and Semiessential Amino Acids	
Essential	**Nonessential**	**Semiessential**
Isoleucine	Alanine	Cysteine[a]
Leucine	Aspartate	Tyrosine
Lysine	Asparagine	Histidine
Methionine[a]	Glutamate	Arginine
Phenylalanine	Glutamine	
Threonine	Glycine	
Tryptophan	Proline	
Valine	Serine	

[a]Contains sulfur.

Structural Proteins (Growth)

The structure of your body today is not the structure of your body tomorrow as we are constantly degrading and making new cells and tissue. For example, you lose cells when hair strands fall out, dry skin sloughs off, you sweat, and excrete body fluid. You gain cells with the growth of new hair and nail length. During periods of growth, the body will wake to a new morning with more bone and muscle tissue than it had upon retiring. Protein of good quality (containing all EAAs) is needed during periods of growth to assist our bodies in making complex structural parts.

- Skin
- Tendons
- Bone matrix
- Cartilage
- Connective tissue
- Teeth
- Eye lens

Functional Proteins (Maintenance and Repair)

Functional proteins do not follow the same molecular design as structural protein strands so they are more invisible and can dissolve in body fluids to be carried to all parts of the body to do their work. The amino acid chains twist and fold into a globular shape and do the following in the body:

- Regulate activity within the body's fluid compartments
- Synthesize hormones, enzymes, antibodies, transport proteins (lipoproteins), and chemical messengers (neurotransmitters)
- Regulate pH of the mouth

PROTEIN QUANTITY AND QUALITY

The body absorbs nitrogen from protein in the diet, which allows it to be measured to determine quantity present in your body at any given time. There are three states of nitrogen measurement, and all of us move from one state to another depending on our current situation; you can have a *balanced* amount of nitrogen or have *more* or *less* than your body needs. It is ideal for the body to be in nitrogen balance. Certain situations will cause your body to be in either positive nitrogen balance or negative nitrogen balance, both of which should be temporary conditions.

Quantity

The amount of nitrogen entering the body should be equal to the amount your cells need to replace parts.

- Nitrogen enters your body via food
- Nitrogen exits your body via urea, feces, sweat, mucus, sloughed skin, lost hair, lost nails

Positive nitrogen balance occurs when there is *more* nitrogen being absorbed and accumulated in the body than going out. This happens during periods of growth, pregnancy, muscle building, and repair of tissue after illness or injury. **Negative nitrogen balance** occurs when there is more nitrogen going *out* of the body than staying in, signifying loss of body protein. This state occurs during rapid weight loss, illness, fever, starvation, prolonged metabolic or emotional stress, and protein-deficient diets.

Positive Nitrogen Balance

Process occurs during periods of:

- Growth
- Pregnancy
- Muscle building
- Repair of tissue after injury

Negative Nitrogen Balance

Process occurs during periods of:

- Rapid weight loss
- Illness
- Fever
- Starvation
- Prolonged metabolic or emotional stress
- Protein-deficient diets

Quality

Protein quality is determined by the combination of essential amino acids (EAAs) in a single source of food. The more EAAs in its contents, the closer it is to a perfect protein and more useful to your body. Protein-rich foods have a **biologic value** based on a grading scale of 1 to 100 (see Table 3-2 for some examples). Its given number indicates how well nutrients from the food can be made into body protein. Foods that are closest to the value of 100 are mainly animal-derived proteins like eggs, meat, fish, poultry, and dairy. Although plant-derived proteins are lower in fat and digest more quickly than animal sources, most by themselves do not have all the amino acids needed to form a complete protein. Quinoa (keen-wa), is a plant protein with a biologic value close to 100 because it has high amounts of leucine and isoleucine. Just because a food does not have a high biologic value, does not mean that it should be avoided in the diet. Meal planners can be creative to combine foods that together will contain all the EAAs needed to form protein.

Complete proteins contain all the EAAs in the needed proportions. Animal protein provides complete proteins; most plant protein provides incomplete protein (see Table 3-3).

Table 3-2	Estimated Biologic Value in Foods of Animal and Plant Origin	
Source	**Estimated Biologic Value**
Animal Source	
Whole egg	100
Egg white	88
Cheese	84
Poultry	79
Fish	70
Lean red meat	69
Milk	60
Plant Source	
Quinoa	100
Brown rice	57
White rice	56
Peanuts	55
Peas	55
Corn	36
Potato	34

Table 3-3	Major Food Sources of Protein	
Animal Sources		**Plant Sources**
Meat		Legumes
Milk		Peas
Eggs		Beans
Fish		Grains
Crustaceans		Quinoa
Insects		

Incomplete proteins are low in one or more of the EAAs.

Complementary proteins form an amino acid pattern equal to that found in a complete protein by combining two foods in the same meal. An example would be combining grains and legumes; eaten together, they form a complete protein.

Supplementary protein is a small amount of a high-quality protein added to a meal that is otherwise marginal in terms of protein quantity. An example would be to add eggs, cheese, or milk to a high-carbohydrate meal, or incorporating quinoa in soup, casseroles, or baked goods.

It was once thought that for the body to utilize complementary or supplemental protein, both had to be consumed together in the same meal. Research has since revealed that the body can utilize foods that have been eaten within a few hours of each other to form complete proteins.

The quality of protein included in the diet makes a difference in overall health; fatty cuts of beef contributes saturated fat (see Chapter 4).

Processed meats (lunch meat) are a quick and easy source of protein, but be choosy with the brand and type you pick. Read the nutrition panels on labels to know which is healthiest for you. Some brands and types of lunch meat have more sodium and/or fat than others.[3] For example, three slices of a popular brand of turkey lunch meat is about 10 g of protein and, depending on the brand, up to 400 mg of sodium. A similar serving size of turkey roasted in your oven and then sliced can provide over 30 g of protein and about 50 mg of sodium. Although Salami, Bologna and hotdogs can provide grams of protein, they also provide higher amounts of fat. A 2010 research study at Harvard School of Public Health revealed a diet that included daily consumption of bacon, sausage, or processed deli meats was associated with a 42% risk of heart disease and 19% higher risk of diabetes.[4]

(**Vegetarian protein** is covered in Chapter 11).

The following is a list *lean* sources of animal protein:

- Beef—top round, flank, bottom round, round eye, sirloin
- Bison
- Eggs (especially whites)
- Seafood—rainbow trout, Alaskan salmon, scallops, shrimp, oysters
- Pork tenderloin
- Poultry—skinless chicken breast, turkey breast
- Venison
- Insects (couldn't resist)

See Figure 3-4 examples for lean sources of protein, Figure 3-5 for good sources of plant protein, and Figure 3-6 for poor sources of protein.

Figure 3-4   Lean sources of animal protein. (Photo courtesy of Kevin Brown, Zolfo Springs FL.)

Figure 3-5 Good sources of plant protein. (Photo courtesy of Kevin Brown, Zolfo Springs FL.)

Figure 3-6 Poor sources of protein—spam, salami, processed cheese food, lunch meat, hotdogs. Read product labels to assure highest grams of protein and lowest grams of sodium and fat. (Photo courtesy of Kevin Brown, Zolfo Springs FL.)

Is Quinoa the Vegetarian Replacement for Meat?

Quinoa, pronounced keen-wa, is a goose-foot, grain-like crop that is jam packed with nutrients. Goose-foot refers to plants that have split leaves resembling a goose's foot. Grown primarily in the Andes region of South America, quinoa is considered a perfect plant protein. It is rich in iron, magnesium, potassium, and fiber and is full of other anti-inflammatory phytonutrients. The leaves of the plant resemble spinach, and the seed grains can be bright red, purple, pink, tan, or black. Quinoa can be stored in an airtight container and will keep for up to 6 months in the refrigerator. Cooking the seed-grain is similar to cooking rice or oatmeal by boiling in water. Mixed in soup, cereal, or salad, it adds high amounts of lysine and isoleucine, two amino acid building blocks for protein, as well as some healthy fats including omega-3. Preliminary animal studies indicate that it has the ability to lower total cholesterol and maintain levels of good HDL cholesterol. Since it is not a true grain, there is decreased risk of allergies and is a good substitution for those following gluten-free diets. Visit www.simplyquinoa.com for a free Quinoa Starter Guide, containing recipes and information about this healthy, nutrient dense plant.

Buffalo—America's Original Meat Is Still a Healthy Choice

Buffalo is a lean, nutrient dense source of protein that is naturally low in saturated fat, cholesterol, and sodium. Compared to beef, buffalo offers only 2.4 g of fat per 100 g (the size of your palm—no fingers), whereas beef ranges from 10 to 18 g of fat/100 g, depending on the cut. If you are interested in saving calories, 100 g of cooked buffalo is 143 calories compared to beef's 283 for the same serving size. Although it is not stocked in every local food store, it is fairly easy to find at farmers markets and natural food stores. Since buffalo is so lean, it is cooked at lower temperatures for less time. To find out more about bison, visit www.bisoncentral.com, official Web site for the National Bison Association.

Entomophagy Is the Practice of Eating Insects

Humans have been eating insects all over the planet for thousands of years. Even today, over 2 million people worldwide eat insects as part of their daily diets.

Those who eat insects claim that they are a delicious source of protein and relished for their taste and texture, often considered a delicacy. However, in our part of the world, it gives us the eeww feeling, and we turn our noses up to it, and say things like "I'd rather starve." Perhaps we should be more open-minded and expand our food-selection horizons.

Insects pack a protein punch providing more nutrients per gram and contain fewer calories than beef or other mainstream source of protein. Grasshoppers, the most consumed insect of any type are equal in protein to ground beef. G-Hopper burger, anyone? According to National Geographic article published May 14, 2013, there are more than 1,900 edible insects. Report has it that ants are sweet and nutty, stinkbugs taste like apples, and red agave worms are spicy. For those of you who like pork rinds, try a tree worm for the same flavor. For more information on eating insects: visit www.insectsarefood.com.

RECOMMENDED DAILY ALLOWANCE

The RDA of protein is dependent on an individual's body size and physical activity and is estimated to be 40 to 65 g/day. The standard would be at the lower end for a slightly built, sedentary person and upper end for a person with a large frame with high activity level. Older adults should be encouraged to include high-quality protein in their daily diets to reduce effects of **sarcopenia**, which is loss of muscle mass due to aging.[5]

The amount is calculated as 0.8 g of protein/kg of body weight/day. Here are a few examples:

weight of 120 lb = 55 kg
0.8 × 55 = 44 g
200 lb = 90 kg
0.8 × 90 = 72 g

See the worksheet at the end of this chapter in the RELATE TO YOU section to determine your RDA for protein.

DIGESTION OF PROTEINS

Particles of protein-rich food are broken down to smaller pieces by chewing and grinding, but the enzymes secreted in the mouth do not affect the molecular structure. After the bolus of food is swallowed and deposited in the stomach, digestion of protein begins when hydrochloric acid and pepsin (a protease) react and break apart the molecules. When the mass of partially digested food passes into the small intestine (duodenum), trypsin and chymotrypsin continue to break down the protein into a single amino acid through a process called *hydrolysis*. Single amino acids can then pass through intestinal villi cells to be absorbed by the body and carried by blood to the liver. Liver cells use amino acids for protein synthesis or remove the amine group to use the carbon chain for fuel.

- Pepsin is the only protease that can digest collagen
- Hydrolysis is a process where a single water molecule is placed between two amino acids that are bonded together.

PROTEIN DEFICIENCY

Protein deficiency occurs when the diet is lacking in this nutrient and symptoms are seen in tissues that are replaced most often—red blood cells and cells lining the digestive tract, hair, and nails. Changes that occur in the body because of protein deficiency are as follows:

- Anemia
- Lowered resistance to infection
- Edema
- Brittle and slow-growing hair and nails
- Scaly appearance to the skin, with sores that will not heal

Our American diet supplies more than enough protein, so deficiencies are rare, but they are still documented in certain situations.

Examples of deficiency conditions are as follows:

1. Kwashiorkor—lack of dietary protein; edema accounts for the pot-bellied look on starving kids in undeveloped countries
2. Marasmus—near or total starvation due to low food supply
3. Anorexia Nervosa—refusal to eat due to psychological disorder (see Chapter 15)

PROTEIN EXCESS

How many times have you driven by a restaurant marquee advertising "all you can eat" or a "16-oz steak" on special? Unfortunately, the concept of protein excess is very common in most of our developed nations, sometimes to a gross extreme. MyPlate recommends no more than 6 oz of protein-rich food source twice each day.

Excess protein elevates levels of sulfates and phosphates in the body, which causes kidneys to excrete acid, and this can be harmful to the body. Studies have also shown excess protein causes calciuria, which is calcium in the urine. This happens when the body tries to buffer acid production with calcium generated during bone resorption.[6]

If your diet contains more protein than the daily requirement, your body has two options: *use it for energy or store it as fat.*

What happens when the body ingests more protein than it requires?

- Metabolic process dismantles protein into amino acids.
- Amino acids are metabolized, releasing energy and nitrogen.
- If the energy supply exceeds demand, the excess carbons are synthesized into fat and stored in adipose tissue.
- Excess nitrogen in the blood is processed through the liver and kidneys.
- Kidneys and liver work overtime to rid the body of excess nitrogen.

PROTEIN SUPPLEMENTATION

Body builders are the number one group supporting sales of protein supplements. Protein is needed for building and maintaining muscles or repairing them from heavy workouts. But your body also needs protein to make hormones, antibodies, and red blood cells to boost your immune system and to keep your hair, nails, and skin healthy. You cannot drink a protein supplement and *instruct* your body to make or enlarge muscle mass. Your body will take the amino acids and put them together to build the tissue needed most. Whatever is left gets excreted. Most individuals get enough protein through their diet and do not require protein supplements. However, athletes' protein needs will vary depending on whether they are growing, building muscle, dieting, or training for competition. A position paper published by the International Society of Sports Nutrition states that physically active individuals are able to obtain their daily need for protein as part of a balanced diet *but athletes should supplement with additional protein.*[7]

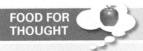

FOOD FOR THOUGHT   USE CAUTION WHEN BARBECUING MEATS!

When using a cooking method with muscle meat, poultry, or fish resulting in charring or blackening (e.g., barbecuing or grilling), fat drips onto the coals, forming a smoke that penetrates the meat. The effect of smoke penetrating the meat forms *heterocyclic amines* and *polycyclic aromatic hydrocarbons*—both of which are cancer-causing chemicals. It is recommended that you:

- Use lean cuts of meat when grilling
- Limit foods prepared this way
- Place foil between the meat and coals

RELATE TO PATIENTS

Most people report more than adequate servings for the meat group because of its abundance in our modern diets. If your patient reports *more* servings than suggested for this food group, advise as to what constitutes a serving size. Many people are unaware that restaurants are grossly over-serving so use a visual for reference. iPhone, deck of cards, a box of jello, or small digital camera. Other suggestions:

- Educate as to sources of alternative protein. For example, milk, beans, cheese, nuts, quinoa.
- Encourage meal preparation using chopped or shredded chicken, turkey, or beef with pasta or rice, versus large servings of each.
- Suggest two meatless dinners each week. (See Chapter 11 for information on vegetarianism.)
- If your patient is eating hot dogs or other processed meats, remind him or her to consume them with vitamin C to offset harmful effects of nitrosamines and inform that they are the poorest form of protein.

If your patient is *deficient* in the meat group, having prepared sources on hand makes it easy to incorporate more into meals. The following suggestions can be made:

- Boil eggs and store in the refrigerator to quickly add to salads and sandwiches.
- Include cheese, nuts, and beans with salads.
- Incorporate good sources of plant protein with meals-quinoa, beans, lentils.
- Prepare a pot of quinoa and use in prepared meals over a few days.
- Go ahead and order the 12-oz steak for dinner at a restaurant, but save half for a sandwich or casserole the next day.

CHAPTER
REVIEW

   PRACTICE FOR PATIENTS

Patient #1

A 36-year-old female presents to your office for an initial exam as part of treatment as a new patient. You strike up a conversation while taking a full mouth set of radiographs. She reveals that she has been following the Atkins Diet for about a year (see Chapter 11), and although she initially lost about 15 lb, she has gained it all back. When you question how much she is eating, she states she only eats protein-rich foods but is eating three eggs for breakfast, a stacked lunch meat sandwich on thin bread for lunch, and either large 12- to 16-oz steak, two chicken breasts, or link of kielbasa or three pork chop steaks for dinner. What advice would you give her about the quality and quantity of protein she is consuming and would this be detrimental to her teeth? (see Chapter 9—Cariostatic Foods)

Patient #2

Your patient is a young man who was in your high school graduation class and participated on the football and wrestling teams. He states he continues to work out at a gym on a daily basis—hardly misses a day—and is selling protein supplements as a side business. There are plenty of customers to purchase the product at the gym, and he asks if you would like to try a sample as well. He states the supplement seems to have helped his clients with their energy levels and to build well-defined muscles. How would you respond to his question?

 RELATE TO YOU

Assignment #1

Watch the video Vegucated—an experiment conducted on three meat-loving people who become vegans for 6 weeks. Answer the following questions:

1. How did the change in diet affect overall health?
2. Would you expect adopting the vegan diet to cause changes in oral health?
3. Think back to a time when your diet may have lacked enough protein and list symptoms of being in negative nitrogen balance.

Assignment #2

Compare your sense of well-being by eating a meal with quinoa as the main source of protein and a meal of your favorite meat or poultry.

1. Is there a different sense of satiety with plant protein versus animal protein?
2. Make a list of all the ways plant protein can be prepared as a main meal.

How much protein should you be eating each day? Calculate to see:

_____ lb/2.2 = _____ kg

_____ kg × 0.8 = _____ g of protein/day

Using the table below, calculate your protein intake for the day to see if you met your requirement.

Food	Grams of Protein
1 hard-boiled egg	6.3
1 chicken breast	36
4-oz turkey breast	34
2 slices turkey lunch meat	8
1 hamburger patty (70% lean/30% fat)	65
1 c. black beans	36
1 c. lentils	18
1 c. quinoa	24
3-oz prime rib	24
2 slices roast beef lunch meat	9
1 pork chop	24
1 slice cheddar cheese	7
1 slice Swiss cheese	8
3-oz tuna fish	25
5-oz cooked salmon	35
2 slice cotto salami	6
2 slices ham lunch meat	9
10 almonds	2.5
1 c. peanuts	38
2 T peanut butter	8
1 T hummus	2
8-oz skim milk	13
1 hot dog	5
2 slice bacon	6
2 slices bologna	6
1 c. cooked oatmeal	6
1-oz dark chocolate	1.5
5 oz wine	0.1
1 can beer	1.6

REFERENCES

1. Rankin J. Role of protein in exercise. *Clin Sports Med* 1999;18(3):499–511.
2. Helms E, Aragon A, Fitschen P. Evidence-based recommendations for natural bodybuilding contest preparation: nutrition and. supplementation. *J Int Soc Sports Nutr* 2014,11:20.
3. Agarwal S, Fulgoni VL, Berg EP. Association of lunch meat consumption with nutrient intake, diet quality and health risk factors in US children and adults: NHANES 2007–2010. *Nutr J* 2015:14:128.
4. Micha R, Wallace SK, Mozaffarian D. Red and processed meat consumption and risk of incident coronary heart disease, stroke, and diabetes: a systematic review and meta-analysis. *Circulation* 2010:121(21):2271–2283.
5. Paddon-Jones D, et al. Protein and healthy aging. *Am J Clin Nutr* 2015;101(6): 1339S–1345S.
6. Barzel U, Massey L. Excess dietary protein can adversely affect bone. *J Nutr* 1998;128(6):1051–1053.
7. Campbell B, et al. International society of sports nutrition position stand: protein and exercise. *J Int Soc Sports Nutr* 2007;4:8.

WEB RESOURCES

Protein Moving Closer to Center Stage www.hsph.harvard.edu/nutritionsource/protein.html
National Bison Association www.bisoncentral.com
Simplify Your Health and Energize Your Life www.simplyquinoa.com
Entomophagy Is the Future www.insectsarefood.com

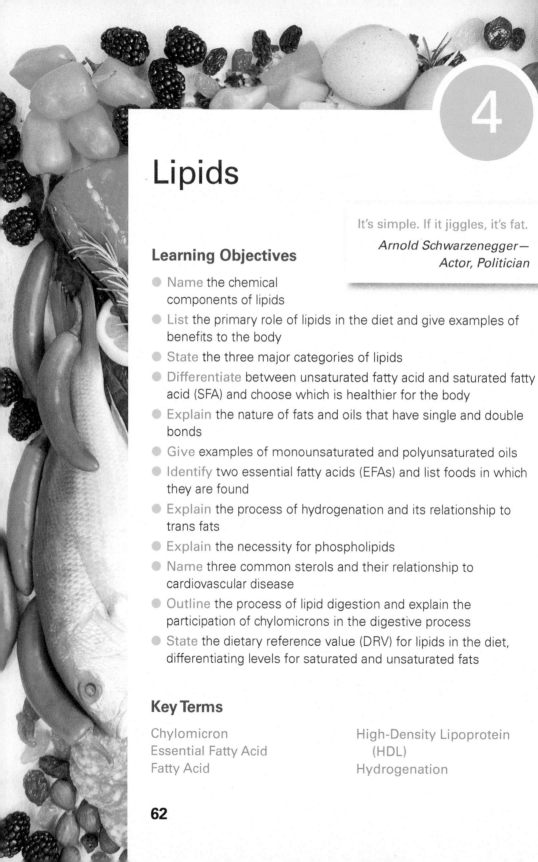

4

Lipids

> It's simple. If it jiggles, it's fat.
>
> *Arnold Schwarzenegger—*
> *Actor, Politician*

Learning Objectives

- Name the chemical components of lipids
- List the primary role of lipids in the diet and give examples of benefits to the body
- State the three major categories of lipids
- Differentiate between unsaturated fatty acid and saturated fatty acid (SFA) and choose which is healthier for the body
- Explain the nature of fats and oils that have single and double bonds
- Give examples of monounsaturated and polyunsaturated oils
- Identify two essential fatty acids (EFAs) and list foods in which they are found
- Explain the process of hydrogenation and its relationship to trans fats
- Explain the necessity for phospholipids
- Name three common sterols and their relationship to cardiovascular disease
- Outline the process of lipid digestion and explain the participation of chylomicrons in the digestive process
- State the dietary reference value (DRV) for lipids in the diet, differentiating levels for saturated and unsaturated fats

Key Terms

Chylomicron
Essential Fatty Acid
Fatty Acid

High-Density Lipoprotein (HDL)
Hydrogenation

Lipoprotein
Low-Density Lipoprotein (LDL)
Monounsaturated
Partially Hydrogenated
Phospholipid
Polyunsaturated

Saturated
Sterol
Trans Fat
Triglyceride
Very-Low-Density Lipoprotein
(VLDL)

INTRODUCTION

The broad category of lipids includes oils and fats, although the word *lipid* is often used interchangeably with the word *fat*. Typically, when we think or say the word fat, we are talking about anatomical appearance of a human body. In the 19th century, being obese signified that a person had enough money to afford the luxury of a steady diet so the size of a man or woman was directly proportional to his or her status in society. The bigger their frame, the wealthier and more esteemed they were by their contemporaries. Men would actually stuff their shirts before venturing out to an important meeting. Just look at President Taft, our largest president who weighed in at 340 lb. He got stuck in the White House bathtub more than once until an *extra-large* size tub was installed to accommodate his *extra-large* body. Americans were proud to have a president of such status. Somewhere along the last 100 years, perceptions have changed, and it is neither desirable nor considered healthy to be large.

So how does *fat* in the diet relate to the size of your body?

Increase in total calorie consumption, especially from food choices high in fat, contributes to our growing size. Although the book, Fat Chance, by Dr. Robert Lustig, makes a point that it is primarily *sugar*, not necessarily lipids, that causes the obesity epidemic, excess of both contributes. This is a problem because as we are growing larger as a population, we are getting sicker with metabolic diseases: obesity, hypertension, lipid disorders, heart disease, and diabetes type 2.

Proliferation of fast-food industry and its skewed marketing are the primary culprits for making us *large* (see Chapter 11). Changes they created make us maybe not the walking dead but certainly the *walking unhealthy*.

- *Food-processing industry* contributes to the obesity epidemic by using sugar, sodium, and hydrogenated fat to keep food from becoming spoiled and rancid. Shelf life is important for storing food in pantries.
- *Fast-food industry* contributes to the epidemic by ramping up portion sizes to steal patrons from competing chains.

● *Technological invention* minimizes daily movements and offers more sedentary forms of entertainment. Think of the convenience offered by dishwashers, washing machines and dryers, microwaves, and entertainment offered by television, iPads, video games, etc. Compare the energy expended on the same tasks of the 19th century.

If *calories consumed* far outweigh *calories expended*, it leads to *weight gain*.[1] The most recent World Health Organization Obesity Report states that as of 2014, more than 1.9 billion adults are overweight, with 600 million clinically obese. Forty-two million children younger than 5 years are already overweight. Statistics of this magnitude are frightening and explain why medical care facilities claim they are overburdened with patients seeking care for obesity-related diseases and disabilities. Learning to manage the content of our diet and being aware of how your food is marketed to you play a huge role in reversing the mess. But let's get back to lipids (fat) in the diet.

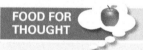

FOOD FOR THOUGHT — CAN YOU JUST SUCK THE FAT OUT?

Liposuction, the process of sucking out excess fat deposits in the body, is not a treatment for obesity or substitution for healthy diet and exercise. And it is not a quick fix for cellulite that causes dimpled-looking skin on the thighs and buttocks. Removing certain pockets of fat can reshape/recontour the body giving more desirable contours. According to www.plasticsurgery.org, more than 210,552 liposuction procedures were performed in 2014.

PRIMARY ROLE OF LIPIDS IN THE BODY

Lipids are an important major nutrient supplied by our diets and utilized for many purposes. Chemically, lipids contain carbon, hydrogen, oxygen, and sometimes phosphorus. They have the unique general characteristic of being insoluble in water and while in solution will either float or roll around in globules. Imagine mixing cooking oil or a pat of butter in a glass of water.

Intake of dietary fat has received a lot of public attention and is of special concern to those wishing to maintain a healthy body image. It is common knowledge that the fat you consume can be stored in the body and the more fat stored, the larger your pant size. But *dietary fat* may not necessarily deserve its universal bad reputation. The right kind of fat, when eaten in moderation, has value in both the diet and the body.

Completely eliminating fat from your diet is not a good idea as you need lipids for the following important functions:

- Insulate against the cold
- Cushion organs against injury
- Are components of every body cell
- Are a good source of energy
- Give a sense of satiety and slow digestion
- Carry fat-soluble vitamins A, D, E, and K
- Required to absorb beneficial fat-soluble phytonutrients like beta-carotene and lycopene
- Provides *essential* nutrients linoleic and linolenic acids (must provide in the diet)
- Make food taste good and give it a preferred smooth and creamy texture

TRIGLYCERIDES

Triglycerides are the largest category of lipids, constituting 95% of all fats found in food and body adipose tissue (fat depot). When stored in adipose tissue, they become the body's largest fuel reserve and provide vital insulation. Having fat stored in adipose cells is like having your own utility company to draw from during an energy crisis. And when it accumulates subcutaneously, it can act as a blanket that insulates against the cold or a shock absorber to cushion delicate organs such as the kidneys.

Triglyceride molecules contain carbon, oxygen, and hydrogen atoms arranged in two parts: the foundation molecule is *glycerol* and there are three *fatty acid* chains off the side. The fatty acid chains consist of carbon atoms with attached hydrogen and oxygen (COOH) (Figure 4-1).

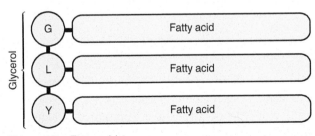

Figure 4-1 Fatty acid.

Fatty Acids

Triglycerides differ in their fatty acid composition, the difference being the number of carbon atoms in their chains and the number of double bonds. Fatty acid carbon chains can be short, medium, or long:

- Short—four or less carbons (short chains mix better in water—like milk)
- Medium—5 to 10 carbons
- Long—more than 12 carbons

Saturation of Fatty Acids

Fatty acids can be categorized as saturated, monounsaturated, or polyunsaturated, depending on how the carbon atoms are bonded together and whether they have a single or double bond. When a triglyceride is saturated, it means all carbon atoms have bonded to hydrogen (single bond) and there are no carbon atoms joining with the carbon next to it (double bond). When one carbon in the chain joins with another, it has a double bond and is called monounsaturated fat. If there is more than one place along the chain where a carbon bonds with another, it will have many double bonds and is called a polyunsaturated fat.

Single bonds between carbon and hydrogen result in a straight flexible chain that will pack into a hard fat such as lard, butter, and stick margarine. Think of toy blocks stacking neatly. Double bonds between carbons result in a bend at the site of the double bond. This bend does not allow the lipid to pack neatly, so it stays liquid at room temperature, like cooking oil. Think of several random toys thrown into a bag, unable to stack together. The more double bonds a fatty acid has, the softer the fat is at room temperature.

The saturation of fatty acids is as follows and is illustrated in Figure 4-2:

- **Saturated** fatty acids (SFAs)—no double bonds
- **Monounsaturated fatty acids** (MUFAs)—one double bond
- **Polyunsaturated fatty acids** (PUFAs)—more than one double bond

Saturated Fatty Acid

If the source of the lipid is from animals, it is considered a saturated fat and will be solid at room temperature, such as the marbling of fat in a piece of beef or pork. Examples of the different types of fatty acids are presented in Figure 4-3. This type of fatty acid is associated with increased cardiovascular disease (through inflammation) and breast and colon cancer.[2–5]

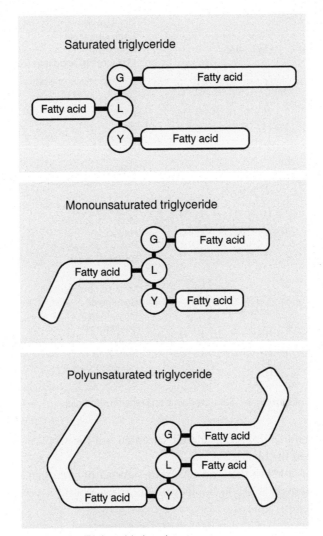

Figure 4-2 Triglyceride bond.

Carbon chains that hold the full number of hydrogen atoms are said to be saturated. Research continues into the relationship between saturated fats and cardiovascular disease and the benefits of it in the diet.[6-9]

Unsaturated Fatty Acid

If the source of fatty acid is from plants, it is considered monounsaturated or polyunsaturated and will be liquid at room temperature, such as olive, corn, and canola oils.

Figure 4-3   Saturated and unsaturated fats/oils.

The only plant source lipids considered saturated are the tropical oils coconut and palm, and are used mainly for baking.

Carbons that hold less than the maximum number of hydrogen atoms will double bond with themselves. (Carbon bonds with another carbon.) Two common unsaturated fatty acids are as follows:

1. Monounsaturated (oleic acid)
2. Polyunsaturated (linoleic acid)

An MUFA has one set of double carbon bonds. MUFAs have not been associated with any health problems. It is even thought that they may reduce the risk of cardiovascular disease by lowering low-density lipoprotein (LDL) cholesterol, the harmful cholesterol.[10]

PUFAs have two or more double carbon bonds. Although PUFAs have not been directly correlated with health problems, studies are ongoing as to their relationship with certain reproductive organ cancers.

OXIDATION OF FATTY ACIDS

Oxygen atoms can attach at the point where carbon would attach to hydrogen. When this happens, it causes the oil to smell and taste rancid. SFAs do not have open carbon bonds where oxygen can attach and are less likely to become spoiled. But an *unsaturated* fatty acid has *open* carbon bonds and is more likely to become rancid. The more unsaturated the fatty acid is, the more open bonds available and the more vulnerable it is to oxygen saturation. If the oxygenated fatty acid is ingested, it can promote oxidative damage in the body, which can lead to chronic diseases. Infusing *hydrogen* to the open bond in place of oxygen will make the unsaturated fatty acid more resistant to oxygenation and solid at room temperature. This process is called **hydrogenation**, which infuses hydrogen into the fatty acid chain so that any *vacant* double bonds become full. Hydrogenated lipid is referred to as a **trans fat** and affects the body in the same way a *saturated fat* does. Food manufacturers use this process to make their product more spreadable, for example, changing corn oil into margarine or making oily natural peanut butter creamy. Hydrogenation is what turns liquid oil into Crisco or stick margarines. Trans fats also make an oil more stable so that it can be reused (e.g., for deep frying).

Trans Fats

Most unsaturated fatty acids have the hydrogen atom (hydrogenation) on the same side of the double bond. This is called the *cis* form. In the *trans form*, the hydrogen atoms are on opposite sides of the double bond. This different configuration of the trans form causes the fatty acid to have a *kink*. Figure 4-4 shows the difference between cis and trans oleic acids. Fatty acids that are kinked do not stack as well as do those that are straight.

Trans fats are created when oils are *partially* hydrogenated. Once the food product has been infused with *hydrogen*, it is no longer considered saturated, monounsaturated, or polyunsaturated. All food labels must state whether a food product contains saturated fat as well as trans fat because they too alter blood cholesterol and there is strong evidence that they are even more detrimental to arteries than saturated fats.[11-17] Research also indicates that trans fats elicit inflammatory properties.[18,19]

Cut trans fats from your diet as follows:

- Avoiding foods listing *partially hydrogenated* oil as an ingredient
- Avoiding deep fried foods
- Use olive oil or canola oil when cooking
- Use margarine from a tub rather than from a stick

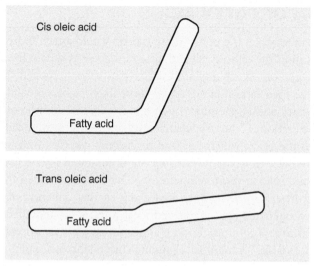

Figure 4-4   Cis and trans fats "kinks."

ESSENTIAL FATTY ACIDS

There are two **essential fatty acids (EFAs)** your body is unable to make, so you must get them from foods in your diet. They are commonly referred to as *omega oils*:

1. Omega-3: linolenic acid, found in flaxseed, canola, or soybean oil; walnuts; tuna; and salmon
2. Omega-6: linoleic acid, found in vegetable oils

The number after omega indicates on which carbon the double bond is located. Omega-3 has been referred to as the *anticardiovascular* disease nutrient.[14] Your body is always forming and destroying tiny blood clots, and omega-3 helps form substances that reduce blood clot formation, thereby keeping your blood thin.

PHOSPHOLIPIDS

Phospholipids are a second category of lipids in your food and body. Chemically, a phospholipid looks like a triglyceride except it contains a phosphorus-containing molecule attached in place of one of the fatty acids. Phospholipids function in our bodies as emulsifiers that keep molecules of fat and water in solution. They also make up the cell membrane and control movement of materials in and out of a cell. Phospholipids are great for cooking and baking because they can keep ingredients from separating.

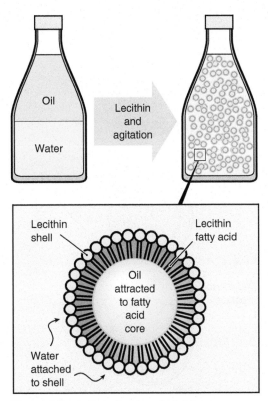

Figure 4-5   Action of a phospholipid.

A common phospholipid is lecithin (Figure 4-5), which is found naturally in soybeans and egg yolks.

STEROLS

Sterols are a third category of lipids with a distinction of carbon rings instead of chains and contain no fatty acids. Cholesterol is the most well-known sterol in food and the body and has the important function of serving as a precursor for manufacturing vitamin D and sex hormones like testosterone and progesterone. Eating foods rich in cholesterol is no longer a serious concern; for most people, *dietary* cholesterol does not significantly affect *blood* levels of cholesterol (Scientific Report of the 2015 Dietary Guidelines Advisory Committee). Many foods high in cholesterol like bacon, sausage, fast food, and red meat are also high in trans and saturated fats (Figure 4-6), which are associated with increased risk of cardiovascular disease.

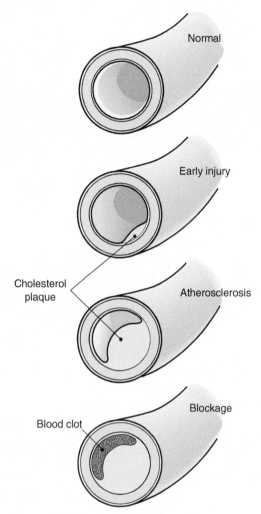

Figure 4-6   Stages of blocked arteries.

LIPOPROTEINS TRANSPORT LIPIDS

Because oil and water do not mix, the body has its own way of allowing fat to travel through the bloodstream to bring lipids to every body cell. **Lipoproteins** are soluble in both oil and water, so they can circulate freely through the blood. Packaged this way, fats can remain soluble and not separate from liquid blood. Lipoproteins are triglycerides coated with protein, cholesterol, and phospholipids.

1. Triglycerides
2. Protein
3. Phospholipids
4. Free cholesterol
5. Cholesterol bound to fatty acids

Chylomicron

Figure 4-7   Chylomicron.

Chylo means milky, and micron means small: after eating a high-fat meal, the blood is so full of chylomicrons it appears milky.

A chylomicron is a type of packaged lipoprotein that is formed during lipid absorption in the small intestines and transported by the lymph system into the bloodstream to be utilized by the body for energy (Figure 4-7).

Besides chylomicrons, there are three other types of important lipoproteins: HDLs, LDLs, very-low-density lipoproteins (VLDLs). HDLs are made in the liver and small intestine and consist of more protein than cholesterol. LDLs, on the other hand, are denser in cholesterol than protein. LDLs carry the cholesterol to the heart's arteries, where it can penetrate the vessel walls and narrows or "clogs" the arteries and restricts blood flow, giving LDL its bad reputation. HDLs are considered healthy because they actually have a protective factor against LDL. HDLs can remove cholesterol from vessel walls and take it back to the liver, where it is excreted with body waste. VLDL is mostly cholesterol and very little protein, and like LDL, contributes to cardiovascular disease. VLDL transports endogenous (made in the body) cholesterol, whereas the HDL and LDL transport dietary cholesterol.

Desirable blood cholesterol should be below 180 mg/dL. Much of its effect depends on genetics and other metabolic factors. Table 4-1 indicates the amount of cholesterol contained in certain foods.

Tips for keeping straight with the healthy and the bad

↑ LDL = ↑ risk of cardiovascular disease

↑ HDL = ↓ risk of cardiovascular disease

Think of the H in HDL as Heart Healthy

Table 4-1	Foods that Contain Cholesterol
Per Serving	**Milligrams Cholesterol**
1 cup	
Whole milk	33
Low-fat milk	10
Skim milk	4
Cheddar cheese	30
Cottage cheese	10
1 teaspoon	
Butter	11
Margarine	0
Vegetable oil	0
3–4 oz	
Lobster	71
Shrimp	194
Salmon	63
Crab	52
3–4 oz	
Beef sirloin	89
Beef short ribs	94
Beef liver	389
Veal	135
3–4 oz	
Skinless chicken	85
Chicken liver	631
Hot dog	100

FOOD FOR THOUGHT   RECOMMENDED CHOLESTEROL GUIDELINES FOR HEALTHY ADULTS

According to Cleveland Clinic's what do cholesterol numbers mean? Aim for:

Total cholesterol less than 180 mg/dL

LDL less than 130

HDL over 60

Triglycerides less than 150

In a 2013 report from American College of Cardiology, it suggests to keep HDL over 50 and total cholesterol lower than 170 mg/dL.[20] Although most guidelines recommend similar levels, if you are someone who is at high risk for heart disease, it is best to follow guidelines prescribed by your physician.

How do statins work?

We need cholesterol for important body functions. However, too much circulating in our bloodstream may lead to atherosclerosis of the arteries where cholesterol-laden plaques build tiny forts blocking good blood flow. A simple blood test can tell you if your numbers are in the healthy zone. If blood flow is severely restricted or completely blocked, it leads to heart attack or stroke, depending on where the clog develops. Taking a statin, known by common pharmaceutical names such as Lipitor, Zocor, and Crestor (there are more), inhibits an enzyme that controls the manufacture of cholesterol in the liver. When production slows down, other liver enzymes respond by building more LDL (bad cholesterol) receptors that kidnap and bind with passing LDL and VLDL and destroy it. The less cholesterol circulating in the blood, the fewer forts are built and less chance of clogging arteries.

Does eating foods high in cholesterol affect overall health?

According to Berkeley Wellness Letter, September 2011, many people believe the fallacy that cholesterol in their blood (their cholesterol level) comes from cholesterol in foods they eat. The truth is most of what circulates in your blood is made by your liver. Even a vegetarian who does not eat animal protein manufactures all the cholesterol his or her body needs to work efficiently. Cholesterol levels will not rise when you eat cholesterol-laden foods.

Typically, most diets provide 300 mg of cholesterol each day. This is equivalent to one egg for breakfast and one serving of meat for dinner. If that amount is more than your cells need, it is excreted. Rarely will a small amount be deposited in artery walls forming plaques that lead to atherosclerosis. You need cholesterol circulating as it is part of body cells, hormones, and other metabolic functions.

Dietary cholesterol has very little effect on the overall cholesterol levels, and it is much more important to pay attention to saturated fat content of food because that is what has a greater effect on your arteries. Avoid foods high in saturated fats to maintain good cholesterol levels (Table 4-2).

Table 4-2	Foods High in Saturated Fat

Bacon
Lard
Palm oil
Corned beef
Pastrami
Ground beef
Hot dogs
Bologna (processed meats)
Bacon
Sausage
Egg yolks
Baked goods
(Fast Food)
Hamburgers
French fries
Tacos

RECOMMENDED DIETARY ALLOWANCE

The American Heart Association recommends, based on a 2,000-calorie diet:

- Reducing saturated fat to less than 7% of daily calories
- Reducing trans fats to 1%
- Keeping fats between 25% and 35% of your daily diet (fish, nuts, and vegetable oils)
- Majority of fats should be monounsaturated and polyunsaturated

Another way to figure the amount of fat in a diet is to count grams. When counting grams, there should be no more than 65 total grams and limiting saturated fat to 20 g (2,000-calorie diet).[21]

DIGESTION OF FATS

Fats begin their digestion in the mouth with the help of lingual lipase secreted from oral salivary glands and then with gastric lipase that gets secreted when it enters the stomach. Fat remains in the stomach longer than carbohydrates and proteins, which gives the sense of fullness for a longer period of time. Digestion continues in the small intestine (duodenum), where chyme (a mixture of food, acids, and enzymes) is emulsified by bile and further broken down by pancreatic lipase. The liver produces bile and stores it in the gallbladder until it is needed for digestion of fat. Bile enters the small intestine via the bile duct. Emulsification by bile turns fat molecules into smaller particles, making it easier for lipase to break fat molecules into fatty acids and glycerol. Short-chain and medium-chain fatty acids make their way to the liver, and the long-chain fatty acids are converted into chylomicrons and dumped into the lymph system, which carries the chylomicrons through the bloodstream. Any fatty acids not used for fuel are repackaged and stored in adipose tissues. Unabsorbed cholesterol is bound by soluble fiber and eliminated from the body. (Eating soluble fiber keeps cholesterol levels low.) The mixture of reduced fat and bile is absorbed through the small intestinal villi.

Plants and animals absorb fat-soluble chemicals, such as pesticides, that are stored in fat and oil. People who consume these plants and animals will absorb some of the stored chemicals, such as dichlorodiphenyltrichloroethane (DDT).

RELATE TO PATIENTS

When analyzing a patient's diet diary, consider if your patient's food choices are high or low fat. Demonstrate to them how to configure 25% to 35% RDA for fat with only greater than 7% saturated fat. Sections of MyPlate that contain the most lipids are the dairy and meat group. Inquire if they consciously choose low-fat dairy products or choose lean cuts of meat.

The following are examples of how to encourage low-fat food selections:

- FiRST is an acronym to remember when choosing meat, which stands for flank, round, sirloin, and tenderloin. These four cuts are considered the leanest and have the least amount of marbled saturated fat.
- Vegetarians may choose cheese, nuts, or legumes as a protein substitution. If cheese predominates, inform that 85% to 90% of the calories in cheese come from fat, much of which is saturated.[22]
- If your patient is drinking whole milk, a sudden switch to skim or fat-free milk may be too big of a change and result in failure. Suggest gradually switching by drinking 2% for a few weeks, then switching to 1% for a few weeks, and then eventually working down to fat-free. Sometimes there is greater success by mixing the two—whole and skim. There is just as much calcium in skim milk as there is in whole milk.
- If your patient is using high-fat spreads, suggest trying some of the fat-free margarines and cream cheeses.

- When choosing a topping for baked potatoes and in pasta salads, fat-free salad dressings and salsa are good substitutions.
- Encourage using monounsaturated and polyunsaturated cooking oils.
- Identify food sources of EFAs—omega-3 and omega-6.
- Educate about trans fats, and teach your client how to spot them on food labels.
- Almost any food from the fruit and vegetable food group is fat free. Three exceptions are olives, avocados, and coconuts, but they still have beneficial nutrients.

FOOD FOR THOUGHT   Avocados are accused of being laden with fat. According to www.avocado.org, the fruit contributes 20 vitamins, minerals, and beneficial plant compounds. The fat content is monounsaturated and polyunsaturated, which means it is healthier than saturated fat.

CHAPTER REVIEW

PRACTICE FOR PATIENTS

Patient #1

Your patient has periodontal disease, and the dentist asked that you provide nutritional counseling to support and supplement her restorative treatment plan. When comparing her diet diary to what MyPlate recommended for her, it appears she is deficient in dairy and reports using unhealthy fats when cooking. She keeps a can of animal lard (from bacon grease) on the stove as it gives great flavor to most dishes.

1. What type of fatty acid is the animal fat?
2. Give examples of healthier substitutions
3. What health issues are related to using animal fats?

Patient #2

Your patient is the 20-year-old son of the office manager. His weight is not proportional to his height: at this young age, he weighs in at 247 lb and his cheeks are enlarged so that it makes brushing the maxillary posterior teeth difficult. He is unable to adequately reach the posterior most tooth due to facial musculature. His blood pressure records on borderline high, and his health history indicates his physician is monitoring him for diabetes.

1. Explain the process of adipose accumulation in the body.
2. How has excess adipose accumulation impacted your patient's oral health status?
3. Explain the responsibility of a dental health care professional in counseling obese patients.

 RELATE TO YOU

Assignment #1

1. Do a search to determine which is better for health—butter or margarine.
2. Visit www.mayoclinic.org and read which spread is better for my heart—butter or margarine.
3. Visit www.Health.clevelandclinic.org to see what they suggest.
4. Write a paragraph on why you choose to use butter or margarine.

Assignment #2

Gather together cans, boxes, and cartons of foods you routinely eat or use in recipes. Look at the label and see if it states partially hydrogenated oil or hydrogenation under ingredients.

1. What food has partially hydrogenated listed to describe an ingredient?
2. What effect does this have on your body when consumed?
3. Is there a healthier choice for you?

Assignment #3

Experiment with butter/substitute spreads.

1. Leave a teaspoon of your favorite spread on the counter. What is the consistency after 1 hour? If it remains solid, what does this mean? If it is soft and oily, what does this mean?
2. Is there a "best choice" for you?

REFERENCES

1. Bray GA, Popkin BM. Dietary fat intake does affect obesity! *Am J Clin Nutr* 1998;68(6):1157–1173.
2. Blekkenhorst LC, et al. Dietary saturated fat intake and atherosclerotic vascular disease mortality in elderly women. *Am J Clin Nutr* 2015;101(6):1263–1268.
3. Kris-Etherton PM, Fleming JA. Emerging nutrition science on fatty acids and cardiovascular disease: nutritionists' perspectives. *Adv Nutr* 2015;6(3): 326S–337S.
4. Hodge A, et al. Dietary and biomarker estimates of fatty acids and risk of colorectal cancer. *Int J Cancer* 2015;137(5):1224–1234.
5. Khodarahmi M, Azadbakht L. The association between different kinds of fat intake and breast cancer risk in women. *Int J Prev Med* 2014;5(1):6–16.
6. Siri-Tarino PW, Sun Q, Hu FB, et al. Meta-analysis of prospective cohort studies evaluating the association of saturated fat with cardiovascular disease. *Am J Clin Nutr* 2010;91(3):535–546.
7. De Souza RJ, et al. Intake of saturated and trans unsaturated fatty acids and risk of all cause mortality, cardiovascular disease, and type 2 diabetes: systematic review and meta-analysis of observational studies. *BMJ* 2015;351:h3978.
8. Malhotra A. Saturated fat is not the major issue. *BMJ* 2013;347:f6340.
9. Astrup A, et al. The role of reducing intakes of saturated fat in the prevention of cardiovascular disease: where does the evidence stand in 2010? *Am J Clin Nutr* 2011;93(4):684–688.
10. Schwingshackl L, Hoffmann G. Monounsaturated fatty acids, olive oil and health status: a systematic review and meta-analysis of cohort studies. *Lipids Health Dis* 2014;13:154.
11. Michas G, Micha R, Zampelas A. Dietary fats and cardiovascular disease: putting together the pieces of a complicated puzzle. *Atherosclerosis* 2014;234(2):320–328.
12. Rubinstein A, et al. Eliminating artificial trans fatty acids in Argentina: estimated effects on the burden of coronary heart disease and costs. *Bull World Health Organ* 2015;93(9):614–622.
13. Ganguly R, Pierce GN. The toxicity of dietary trans fats. *Food Chem Toxicol* 2015;78:170–176.
14. Endo J, Arita M. Cardioprotective mechanism of omega-3 polyunsaturated acids. *J Cardiol* 2016;67(1):22–27.
15. Estadella D, et al. Lipotoxicity: effects of dietary saturated and transfatty acids. *Mediators Inflamm* 2013.
16. Attia-Skhiri N, Fournier N, Pourci ML, et al. Trans fatty acids: effects son lipoprotein metabolism and cardiovascular risk. *Ann Biol Clin* 2009;67(5):517–523.
17. Mauger JF, et al. Effect of different forms of dietary hydrogenated fats on LDL particle size. *Am J Clin Nutr* 2003;78(3):370–375.
18. Esmaillzadeh A, Azadbakjt L. Home use of vegetable oils, markers of systemic inflammation, and endothelial dysfunction among women. *Am J Clin Nutr* 2008;88(4):913–921.
19. Mozaffarian D, et al. Trans fatty acids and systemic inflammation in heart failure. *Am J Clin Nutr* 2004;80(6):1521–1525.

20. Stone NJ, et al. 2013 ACC/AHA Guideline on the treatment of blood cholesterol to reduce atherosclerotic cardiovascular risk in adults; a report of the American college of cardiology/American heart association task force on practice guidelines. *J Am Coll Cardiol* 2014;63(25):2889–2934.
21. Hooper L, et al. Reduction in saturated fat intake for cardiovascular disease. *Cochrane Database Syst Rev* 2015;10:6.
22. National Dairy Council Cheese and Nutrition Bulletin. 2011.

ADDITIONAL STUDY

Fat Chance: The Bitter Truth about Sugar by Dr. Robert Lustig. Hudson Street Press; 2013.

Vitamins

> Faith and prayer are the vitamins of the soul; man cannot live in health without them.
>
> *Mahalia Jackson*

Learning Objectives

- Identify factors that distinguish between fat-soluble and water-soluble vitamins and list vitamins in each category
- Discuss the differences between absorption and storage of water-soluble and fat-soluble vitamins
- Explain how individuals can have a vitamin toxicity or imbalance
- Discuss the advantages and disadvantages of supplementation with vitamins
- State the major functions of vitamins in the body
- Discuss the impact that food preparation and processing have on nutrients available for use by the body
- Using tables and charts, identify source, recommended daily allowance (RDA), and excess and deficiency states of 13 vitamins
- Discuss the impact that medical conditions and medications can have on the absorption and effectiveness of vitamins

Key Terms

Antioxidants
Enriched
Essential
Fat Soluble
Fortification
Imbalance
Megadose

Precursor Molecules
Recommended Dietary
   Allowance
Toxicity
Water Soluble
Vitamins

INTRODUCTION: VITAMINS AND ORAL HEALTH

Most health care providers and scientists agree that vitamins play a crucial role in overall health. General health is often reflected in the health of the oral tissues as well. With the modern trend of associating inflammatory diseases with nutrient intake, the oral tissues are perfect starting places for the assessment of adequate nutrition. The inflammatory diseases of periodontitis and gingivitis and the biofilms that play a role are impacted by many factors, and vitamins are one such factor.

Vitamin Supplements: Needed or Not?

Supplementation is prolific in US culture. According to a recent search of the National Institutes of Health, Dietary Supplement Label Database, there are 135 products with folic acid as part of the product name and an additional 5,190 products that list folic acid somewhere on the label. Additionally, the database lists 738 products with vitamin D in the product name and 5,982 products that list vitamin D as an ingredient on the label.[1]

These are just two examples of the large numbers of products available for people who want to supplement their diet with additional vitamins. This example confirms that vitamin supplements are big business. But what role do vitamins play in human nutrition? Can sufficient vitamins be consumed in the foods we eat?

Popular opinion in the United States regards vitamin supplementation as important for optimal health. In fact, aside from a daily supplement of a multiple vitamin, some people will supplement with huge dosages of a particular vitamin to prevent disease. An example is vitamin C, or compound OTC drugs containing large amounts of vitamin C used to prevent or treat a cold.

Dental health care providers should be aware that vitamin supplementation may affect the tissues in the oral cavity positively or negatively:

- Supplementation may cause interactions with other medications the person is taking.
- Supplementation may cause systemic reactions that affect the entire body and health of the person taking them (Quintessence International Nutrition and Oral Health, and Access).

Dental health care providers must also keep in mind that tooth loss through caries or periodontal disease greatly impacts the person's ability to eat nutrient-rich foods. In that case, vitamin supplementation might be considered as a method of aiding in maintaining health.[2–5]

Vitamins are carbon-based, organic molecules needed by the body in very small quantities to help with metabolic processes and are found in biologic sources.

Ideally, vitamins will be supplied in the food you eat; in some cases, they may be a dietary supplement that is taken to supplement or increase the amount of a vitamin beyond what is obtained through the diet. Vitamins are necessary for cellular processes. Without vitamins in the correct amounts, at the correct time, being used by the correct cells, body processes will break down and the person will become ill.[2,6] The sources of vitamins have become a challenge in modern society. Most vitamins cannot be made within the body and must come from outside the body. These are **essential** vitamins. However, some are formed from precursor molecules in the skin or other organs. Many people believe that megadoses of vitamins will enhance body function. Usually, a **megadose** of a particular nutrient is consumed as a supplement in quantities greater than the recommended dietary allowance (RDA). For example, a common misconception is that "vitamins give you energy."[7] The truth is, some vitamins *help* with the metabolic reaction that releases energy from food molecules being processed inside cells. But if the body has an adequate supply of vitamins to help with the production of energy that cells can use, taking more vitamins will not make you more energetic or stronger or increase endurance. In fact, just the opposite might occur.

Discovery

For a 100 years, it was recognized that some disease conditions seemed to be alleviated by eating certain foods. Of course, the existence of these molecules, called vitamins, was not known until much later. Following the discovery of vitamins and their roles in debilitating and fatal diseases when people lacked sufficient amounts, the study of vitamins opened a new field of science and nutrition. Although it is true that vitamins will successfully treat specific diseases related to deficiency, more research is needed to ascertain their role in prevention of disease and maintenance of health.

The role of vitamins as protectors against cell deterioration was only recently discovered and occurs through a complex set of molecular interactions. Some vitamins shield cells from the effects of exposure to the environment that can cause cell death over time. Vitamins that protect cells in this way are called **antioxidants**.[8–10]

What are vitamins? They are

- Organic molecules
- Essential or from precursor molecules
- Noncaloric
- Prevent and treat vitamin deficiency–related diseases
- Needed in small amounts for cellular metabolism (energy production)
- Help prevent cellular breakdown in their role as antioxidants

CATEGORIES OF VITAMINS

Vitamins have alphabet/numeric and common names. Table 5-1 identifies both.

Vitamins are also divided into one of two solvent categories: **water soluble** or **fat soluble**. Water-soluble vitamins include vitamin C and all the B vitamins. Fat-soluble vitamins are A, D, E, and K. Figure 5-1 identifies water-soluble and fat-soluble vitamins.

Fat-soluble or water-soluble vitamins vary in each of the following aspects:

- Which foods supply the vitamin
- Vulnerability of the vitamin during cooking
- How the vitamin functions in the body
- How the body absorbs and distributes the vitamin in the body
- Whether the body can store the vitamin

RECOMMENDED NUTRIENT INTAKE

Only minute amounts of any one vitamin are required on a daily basis. Vitamins are found in all food groups, with fruits and vegetables being especially good sources for most vitamins. Vitamin B_{12} is the only vitamin found exclusively in animal food, whereas all other vitamins can be obtained from both plants and animals. (See individual vitamins for specific recommended intakes and food sources.)

Table 5-1	Alpha/Numeric and Common Names of Vitamins
Vitamin	**Name**
B_1	Thiamin
B_2	Riboflavin
B_3	Niacin, niacinamide
B_6	Pyroxidine
B_9	Folate, folic acid
B_{12}	Cobalamin
H	Biotin
C	Ascorbic acid
A	Retinols
D	Calciferol
E	Tocopherol
K	Coagulations

Figure 5-1   Water-soluble and fat-soluble vitamins.

Recommended dietary allowance (RDA) represents the amount of a vitamin thought needed for good health with variances for sex and age. The levels on vitamins recommended in this chapter are based upon the RDA.

DIGESTION AND ABSORPTION

Vitamins are *released* from food during the digestive process but are not *digested*. The way they are processed depends on their classification:

- *Water-soluble vitamins* used by the body for metabolic processes are absorbed through the small intestine into the blood stream and delivered to body cells. Any excess that is not used by cells right away is excreted by the kidneys in the urine.
- *Fat-soluble vitamins* (vitamins A, D, E, and K) and fatty acids pass into the cells of the small intestine with other fats and travel through the lymphatic system to eventually enter the blood stream and travel to body cells. They are circulated through the blood with the help of molecules called lipoproteins. Excessive amounts of fat-soluble vitamins are often stored in the body, and

small amounts are excreted in feces. The storage of fat-soluble vitamins can lead to toxicity.[11] Figure 5-2 identifies absorption and storage of fat-soluble vitamins.

In the case of both fat-soluble and water-soluble vitamins, conditions that alter absorption of foods from the digestive tract impact the absorption of the vitamins and can produce deficiency of the vitamins. Some of these conditions are the result of aging, medications, and disease processes.

TOXICITY/IMBALANCE

Vitamin **toxicity** can occur when excess amounts of a vitamin are absorbed into the body. Each vitamin has the potential for toxicity, but fat-soluble vitamins are the most likely to become toxic because they can be stored and accumulate in fat tissues. There is less danger of water-soluble vitamins exerting a toxic effect on the body because storage is limited, and usually the excess is excreted on a daily basis.

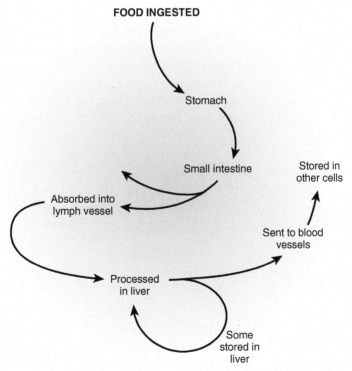

Figure 5-2 Absorption and storage of fat-soluble vitamins.

Some foods have vitamins added to them during processing. There is a potential for toxicity when a person eats too much of this type of food or takes *megadoses* of vitamin supplements—more than the RDA.

Vitamin D is the most toxic of all vitamins because of its addition to many highly processed foods that are readily consumed in the Western diet. Because vitamin D enhances the absorption of calcium, an excess of vitamin D causes an excess of calcium circulating in the blood, which can be detrimental to the heart and can cause calcifications in the kidneys and other parts of the body.[7]

Two water-soluble vitamins that can be somewhat toxic are vitamin B_6 and niacin (B_3). Both can have detrimental effects if the amount ingested is more than the kidney can handle and excrete. The following are facts about vitamin toxicity:

- Fat-soluble vitamins have the greatest potential for toxicity.
- Vitamin D, a fat-soluble vitamin, is the most toxic of all vitamins.
- Vitamin B_6 and niacin are the most toxic *water*-soluble vitamins.
- Consumption of excessive amounts of certain highly processed foods and megadoses of vitamin supplement can contribute to vitamin toxicity.

An **imbalance** of vitamins occurs when too much of one vitamin is added to an adequate diet, causing a deficiency of other vitamins or other components in the biochemical actions of the body. For example, the B-complex vitamins function as a group, with one no more important than the other. Excess of one of the B vitamins can throw off the biochemical balance, creating a deficiency in its partners.

B-complex vitamins act as coenzymes in many energy-producing reactions of the cell. Coenzymes participate with the cells in a reaction to produce energy molecules cells use to power cell processes. Figure 5-3 illustrates how vitamins function as coenzymes.

Figure 5-3 Vitamins as coenzymes assist cells make energy.

SYNTHESIZING VITAMINS

Most of the vitamins required by the body to function efficiently are essential, meaning that they cannot be manufactured by the body and must have external sources such as the food you eat. A few vitamins can be synthesized using existing chemicals in the body. The existing chemicals are called precursor molecules.[7] Examples of synthesizing vitamins from precursors are using tryptophan to make niacin (B_3), using a cholesterol compound in skin and UV sunlight to make vitamin D, and using carotene to make vitamin A. The body can also synthesize vitamin K, biotin (vitamin H), and pantothenic acid (B_5) with the help of resident bacteria in the colon. Once the diet remedies the vitamin deficiency, the body will stop producing the vitamin and use what is supplied in the food.

How the body uses precursors to make vitamins:

It uses	To make
Tryptophan	Niacin (B_3)
Cholesterol compound in skin + sun	Vitamin D
Carotene	Vitamin A
Normal bacteria in the colon	Vitamin K, Biotin (H), pantothenic acid (B_5)[12]

PRIMARY ROLE OF VITAMINS IN THE BODY

Vitamins perform the following functions in the body:

- Energy metabolism: B-complex vitamins participate in the chemical conversion of foods we eat into energy that can be used by our cells. Through a series of chemical reactions in each cell of the body, carbohydrates, lipids, and proteins are converted into glucose which in turn is converted into a form of chemical energy that cells can use to power their actions. The form of energy is called adenosine triphosphate (ATP). ATP is to the body what gas is to a car. Figure 5-3 further illustrates how cells make energy.
- Protein synthesis
  - Vitamins A, D, B_6 (pyroxidine), and C help form proteins used in epithelium, bone, and collagen.
  - Vitamins B_9 (folic acid), B_{12} (cobalamin), E, and K help form proteins used in bone marrow to form new red blood cells (RBCs). The life of an RBC is approximately 4 months, so maintenance of an adequate supply demands continual use of body resources. A lack of one or more vitamins at the time of development will manifest as anemia. The type of anemia depends on which vitamin the body is deficient in.
- Antioxidants

Vitamins A, C, and E serve as antioxidant protectors from damaging free radicals—made by reactions with oxygen atoms. As a rule, oxygen travels through the body in pairs in the form of an oxygen molecule (O_2). When oxygen molecule becomes a single atom (O), it is highly reactive and searches for other atoms with which to bond. Once an oxygen atom becomes a free radical with an unpaired electron looking for a partner, a chain reaction occurs, releasing other oxygen atoms to become free radicals, and body cells get damaged in the process.[8–10,13] Figure 5-4 illustrates antioxidants stabilizing free radicals.

Free radicals are readily formed when the body is

- Converting food to energy
- Exercising
- Exposed to pollutants such as tobacco smoke

The *oxidative stress* caused by the free radicals is responsible for cell damage related to cancer, some heart and blood vessel disease, eye diseases such as cataracts and macular degeneration, and even neurological conditions such as Parkinson's and Alzheimer's disease, as well as aging.[10] Antioxidant substances such as vitamins protect the body from oxidative stress intercepting the single oxygen atoms before the chain reaction is initiated, preventing the effect from occurring.

Co-Q 10 is an antioxidant that plays a role in energy production in cells. Recently, some high-quality research has been conducted, which indicates that co-Q 10 is found in several vital organs including the heart, liver, and kidneys. The coenzyme is found in small quantities in fish, meats, and whole grains. Research evidence suggests that the coenzyme supplement may benefit people who have heart failure, and improved recovery from heart

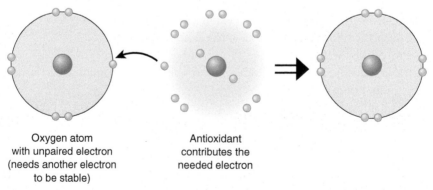

Oxygen atom
with unpaired electron
(needs another electron
to be stable)

Antioxidant
contributes the
needed electron

Figure 5-4   Radicals neutralized by antioxidants.

surgery. As with many nutritional supplements, more research is needed to determine the recommended levels, interactions, and possible benefits of the coenzyme.[14,15]

Numerous research studies and clinical trials have not provided sufficient evidence that high doses of dietary supplements of antioxidant vitamins really do prevent disease.[8] In fact, megadoses of some antioxidants such as vitamin A are linked to increased risks of cancer and other systemic diseases.[8] Additionally, consideration should be given to the interaction of large doses of antioxidants in combination with medications.[8]

Scientists speculate that health benefits from certain foods may be the result of other substances in the foods and not from the antioxidant vitamins. Scientists also speculate that smaller doses of antioxidant vitamins found naturally occurring in food may be more beneficial in preventing disease than the megadoses in supplementation. Undoubtedly, the relationship between antioxidants, free radicals, and good health is much more complicated than popping a pill to prevent disease.[8]

Research for antioxidants is ongoing, so it is important to review the literature frequently to give accurate advice to patients. Presently, there is more support *not* to recommend antioxidants because they may not have the desired effect and can be harmful for some people when taken in large doses. Figure 5-4 illustrates how antioxidants protect cells.

Other functions of vitamins include boosting the immune system, keeping the mind alert, helping with hormone production, and synthesizing genetic material.

Table 5-2 lists vitamins and their specific functions.

VITAMINS AND FOOD PROCESSING/PREPARATION

Processing fresh foods assists in preserving food and improves shelf life for the consumer as well as the industries that grow and sell food in large quantities. It is important for the consumer to understand how processing may affect the food. Processing natural foods often makes the food safer to eat and extends shelf life.[10,16] While some processing techniques cause degradation of the vitamin molecules and other nutrients so that they become fewer in number or less efficient at performing their functions in the body, processing may also eliminate harmful bacteria that can cause disease and help make food more affordable.[16]

To ensure that food remains vitamin rich after processing, manufacturers may enrich or fortify their products. **Fortification** occurs when vitamins and minerals are added to the food product, usually during or after processing has occurred. Fortification adds nutrients to the foods, which do not naturally occur in those particular foods. Examples of fortified foods include cereals and milk with added vitamins A and D. **Enriched** food products add nutrients that were lost during processing to the level present in the unprocessed product. As grains such as wheat and rice are

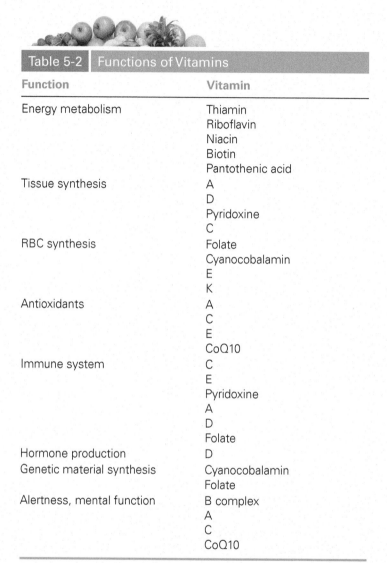

Table 5-2	Functions of Vitamins
Function	**Vitamin**
Energy metabolism	Thiamin
	Riboflavin
	Niacin
	Biotin
	Pantothenic acid
Tissue synthesis	A
	D
	Pyridoxine
	C
RBC synthesis	Folate
	Cyanocobalamin
	E
	K
Antioxidants	A
	C
	E
	CoQ10
Immune system	C
	E
	Pyridoxine
	A
	D
	Folate
Hormone production	D
Genetic material synthesis	Cyanocobalamin
	Folate
Alertness, mental function	B complex
	A
	C
	CoQ10

milled for bread and flour, much of the B vitamins, minerals, and fiber are removed when the grains are broken into smaller particles. Enriching the end product replaces some of the lost nutrients.

High temperatures, light, and oxygen—all detrimental to water-soluble vitamins—are common methods of processing foods. Even the fertilizers that are used in growing foods can make a difference in vitamin content![17] Boiling food on the stovetop causes nutrients to be released from the food into water; to retain these nutrients, this water can be used to cook something else—for example, rice, mashed potatoes, or soup. Prolonged exposure to heat, as in Crock-Pot cooking, roasting, and frying, can actually destroy water-soluble vitamins. Careful consideration of food preparation can preserve vitamins so that they will benefit the body when consumed in food. Stir frying at a high temperature seals in nutrients, and short cooking time reduces nutrient loss. Microwaving uses a small amount of water and high temperature for a short amount of time, also preserving most of the vitamins' properties.

The following are some healthful tips when choosing fruits and vegetables to ensure the maximum benefit from the vitamins provided:

- Select the freshest possible fruits and vegetables. As the food sits on the truck, shelf, or in the refrigerator, the more vitamin content is lost.
- Shop at farmer's markets for produce that is in season and has been recently harvested and inquire about the use of substances to alter ripening or shelf life.
- Purchasing fruits and vegetables from the frozen food section in a grocery store may be an excellent alternative to fresh foods that are not in season. For the best quality of nutrients, shake the bag to be sure it is not a frozen block of ice. One solid piece in the bag indicates that the product has thawed, which will cause nutrients to leach into the water and be less available in the food.
- Historically, canned produce has been considered the least desirable because of intense heat used to sterilize it. However, canned food may actually be a better choice than old fresh vegetables that have been stored for an extended time and lost much of the nutrient value. When selecting canned foods, be cautious about those with added salt and sugar, which are not truly needed to preserve the canned food.[18]
- Some food processors have begun using *high pressures* to preserve food. When done without *high temperatures*, this may be the best alternative to "fresh from the garden." Since heat is not used, vitamin content is stable, and the flavor and color of the food are retained.[18]
- Dehydrating requires that the food be dried out (desiccated). This concentrates some of the nutrients, but destroys others, such as vitamin C. Dehydrated foods that must be reconstituted prior to eating lose much of the nutrients to the cooking water, just as boiling the vegetables.[18]
- Wash fruits and vegetables instead of peeling them to preserve the availability of the nutrients just under the skin.
- Vitamins in fruits and vegetables are often reduced in any kind of processing.
- Water-soluble vitamins are the most vulnerable to loss during food processing/shelf time/cooking.

- Select the shortest cooking method with the lowest heat, which is essential to vitamin preservation in foods.
- Use herbs and spices in vegetables to enhance the flavor—you are more likely to eat them more often!

For more information on this topic, visit: www.betterhealth.vic.gov.au and www.foodinsight.org.

VITAMIN CHARTS AND LISTS

Most vitamins serve the body in more than one capacity and can be found in multiple foods. Reading charts and lists from textbooks and Web sites can cause the reader quite a bit of confusion. Sources vary in identifying what function a particular vitamin performs because the vitamin may be involved in MANY functions. One vitamin may be involved in blood cell synthesis and also involved in 100 different enzyme actions in protein synthesis. Another variation that frequently occurs is identification of foods that contain high levels of a vitamin. Often the variation results from the differences in environment in which the fruit or vegetable was grown (fertilizer, soil, climate, other conditions) that produce variations in nutrient content. It is almost impossible to make a complete and comprehensive vitamin document, so most references glean important facts and try to arrange them in an organized way. For the purpose of this textbook, an attempt has been made to provide the oral health care provider with basic information that may be helpful in counseling patients about oral conditions. The highlights of the *major* functions, sources, deficiency and excess states, and RDA are provided as a baseline for the reader's investigation into vitamin nutrition. The list is neither comprehensive nor all encompassing, but it can serve as a resource for initial vitamin inquiry.

Not mentioned among the sources for each of the vitamins is the supplementation with multivitamins and individual vitamins that are often taken in substitution for the food sources of vitamins. Although vitamins are molecules and can be taken into the body in the supplement form, some vitamins are not absorbed as readily by the body in that form and the available vitamin for use is not in the correct form or will not be absorbed to the same degree as the food source form. The person who chooses to use supplements should do further investigation to determine which form of the vitamin is best absorbed and used by the body.

Vitamin information has been organized into water-soluble and fat-soluble categories for study.

See Figures 5-5 and 5-6, vitamin-rich fruits and vegetables.

Substantial amount of the information about individual vitamins that follows is taken from the National Institutes of Health Office of Dietary Supplements at www.

Figure 5-5   Vitamin-rich fruits. (Courtesy of Kevin Brown, Avon Park, FL.)

Figure 5-6   Vitamin-rich vegetables. (Courtesy of Kevin Brown, Avon Park, FL.)

ods.od.nih.gov, MedlinePlus at http://www.nlm.nih.gov/medlineplus/druginfo/ natural, Harvard School of Public Health Nutrition Source at www.hsph.harvard. edu/nutritionsource, and the US Department of Health and Human Services Office on Women's Health at http://www.womenshealth.gov/fitness-nutrition/ nutrition-basics/vitamins.html.

WATER-SOLUBLE VITAMINS

Thiamin: B$_1$

Function

Thiamin functions as a coenzyme with the enzymes involved in the metabolism of glucose, amino acids, and fats to convert the major nutrients into calories. All can be used to produce energy. Thiamin also plays a role in the growth and development of cells and in their functions.

Absorption into the Body

Thiamin has a short lifespan in the body, so a constant daily supply is required. It is absorbed into the blood from the small intestine. Small amounts of the vitamin also can be produced by bacteria that live in the intestine.

Sources

In the United States, many breads and cereals are enriched or fortified with thiamin. Infant formula is also fortified. Best naturally occurring sources are pork, trout, and black beans.

Deficiency State

Thiamin is not a common vitamin deficiency in the United States because most people have sufficient amounts of the vitamin in their diet. The absolute vitamin deficiency is *beriberi*. However, certain conditions and medications predispose people to thiamine deficiency called Wernicke-Korsakoff syndrome.

   Wernicke-Korsakoff Syndrome—Associated with

- Chronic alcohol dependence or abuse
- Severe gastrointestinal disorders
- Blood-related malignancies
- HIV/AIDS
- Some medications

Wernicke-Korsakoff Syndrome—Signs and Symptoms

- Alterations of the brain structure
- Loss of sensation in the arms and legs
- Psychosis resulting in severe memory loss

Beriberi—Symptoms Include the Following

- Loss of muscle function and feeling in the extremities
- Mental confusion, memory loss, and disorientation
- Wasting
- Fatal if untreated

Groups at risk for thiamine deficiency include those with chronic diseases who require multiple medications. In many cases, this describes the elderly population in the United States. The diseases or conditions most associated with deficiency are those that alter absorption from the intestine. An example of an alteration of absorption is bariatric surgery in which parts of the digestive tract are removed to promote weight loss.

Excessive Thiamin Risks

Like most water-soluble vitamins, excess amounts of thiamine are excreted. Most scientists theorize that when excess thiamine is present, the excess is simply not absorbed from the intestine. That which is in excess in the blood is filtered and excreted in the urine. However, scientists do not recommend excessive intakes of thiamine just because the adverse effects are unknown at this time.[18]

Recommended Dietary Allowance

The amount of thiamine recommended is different for each age group and sex. For adults, the RDA is 1.2 to 1.1 mg.

Riboflavin: B$_2$

Function

Riboflavin is an essential part of major coenzymes that help with production of ATP and releasing energy from carbohydrates, lipids, and proteins. Riboflavin also plays a role in growth and development, the metabolism of drugs, and other cell functions.

Absorption into the Body

Riboflavin is absorbed into the blood from the small intestine. Only small amounts of the vitamin can be stored in the body. Some riboflavin is produced in the intestine by resident bacteria after eating vegetable-based foods.

Sources

Careful storage of foods rich in riboflavin is necessary to preserve the vitamin. The riboflavin molecule is easily destroyed by ultraviolet light. Since a common source of the vitamin is milk or milk products, most of these products are typically stored in opaque containers. It should also be noted that riboflavin is very sensitive to heat during cooking. Other sources of riboflavin are meat and fortified or enriched breads and cereals.

Deficiency State

Ariboflavinosis, the deficiency state of riboflavin, is rare in the United States. Most causes of deficiency are thyroid hormone deficiency or other endocrine disorders. People who have deficiency of riboflavin usually have deficiencies of other nutrients as well.

Ariboflavinosis—Symptoms Include the Following

- Skin lesions and hair loss
- Hyperemia (too much blood)
- Tissue inflammation resulting in edema around the mouth, throat, and eyes
- Angular cheilosis: cracks in corners of mouth and lips. (See Figure 5-7 for example of angular cheilosis.)
- Glossitis: atrophy of filiform papillae; swollen, dark red tongue
- Deterioration of the liver and nervous system

Groups at risk for riboflavin deficiency include physically active vegetarians, pregnant and lactating women and their infants, and people who do not eat milk products such as those who are lactose intolerant.

There is ongoing research about the role that riboflavin plays in other processes in the body such as its use in the prevention of migraine headaches or DNA damage from carcinogens. Do not jump to conclusions about research that is still being conducted![19]

Because riboflavin in excess of body needs is not absorbed but is excreted, toxicity is unknown.

Figure 5-7 Angular cheilosis. (Courtesy of Dr. Deb Milliken, Avon Park, FL.)

Recommended Dietary Allowance

Recommended intake for riboflavin depends on the person's age and sex. Requirements increase for pregnant and lactating women. For most healthy persons, the RDA is around 1.1 to 1.3 mg.

Niacin: B₃

Function

Niacin is needed for all cell functions and is a coenzyme and partner to riboflavin. It also participates in the conversion of glucose released from food into energy and assists with blood cell formation.

Absorption into the Body

Niacin is absorbed into the body in the digestive tract. It dissolves readily in the fluids of the digestive tract and is well absorbed. Niacin, especially in prescription dosages, has many drug interactions with OTC and prescription medications. Many of the combinations alter the level of absorption and availability of niacin (or the other drug). Examples include aspirin and the cholesterol-lowering drugs called "statins." More information is found in the drug interactions section for this vitamin.

There are several forms of vitamin B_3. The most common are niacinamide and niacin, which have very different roles in the body. In some cases, niacin is more effective, and in others, niacinamide is the form of choice. Niacin can be converted to niacinamide in the body when niacin is in excess.

Source

Both forms of B_3, niacin and niacinamide, can be found in food sources. Yeast, meat and fish, beans, nuts, coffee, and fortified grains are major sources. B_3 can also be found in vitamin supplements with other B vitamins.

Deficiency State

The deficiency state is rare in the United States, mostly due to the fortification of many popular food sources. The most likely candidates for niacin deficiency are abusers of alcohol.[19]

Pellagra—symptoms include the following:

- Dermatitis, skin irritation
- Diarrhea
- Dementia
- Death if left untreated

Excess State of Niacin or Niacinamide (B_3)

- Causes facial flushing at prescription dosages
- Liver dysfunction
- Gout
- Ulcers of the digestive tract
- Loss of vision
- High blood sugar
- Irregular heartbeat

Niacin is often used in excessive amounts by supplementation in order to treat or prevent specific conditions. Available well-founded evidence is limited for some indications; however, high doses of niacin are likely effective for lowering bad cholesterol and triglycerides and raising good cholesterol. Caution should be used in taking large doses of niacin because of drug interactions and side effects. Niacin also has many interactions with herbal supplements, and caution should be used in mixing them. Careful research is required.

Drug Interactions with B_3

The B_3 vitamins interact with alcohol and many drugs including those prescribed for gout, seizures, high cholesterol, and diabetes. When taken with large doses of aspirin, niacin can maintain toxic levels in the blood. Niacin also interacts with the nicotine patch by increasing the side effects of the niacin, particularly flushing and dizziness.

Recommended Dietary Allowance

Recommended intake varies with age and sex, as well as pregnancy and lactation. The RDA for most healthy adults is 14 to 16 mg/day.

Pyroxidine: B_6

Function

B_6 is a designation given to a group of six related molecules of the vitamin family. Pyroxidine is one of the molecules, which functions as an enzyme in over 100 reactions of protein metabolism. It also plays a role as a coenzyme in the breakdown of carbohydrates and fats for energy production. It also assists with nerve conduction and the immune system function. Pyroxidine promotes the formation of red and white blood cells and some of the chemical mediators of immune responses.

Absorption into the Body

B_6 is absorbed from the small intestine into the blood where it is altered into "free form" and becomes active in its roles in the body.

Source

Best food source of B_6 is chickpeas. However, very high sources include beef liver, tuna, salmon, chicken breast, fortified cereals, potatoes, bananas, and marinara sauce. B_6 can be found in a large variety of foods, and careful meal planning should result in adequate amounts in the diet.

Deficiency State

Deficiency states are microcytic anemia, depression, convulsions, depressed immune system, angular cheilosis, and glossitis.

Excess State

Vitamin B_6 is the most toxic water-soluble vitamin because it can be stored in the muscle and liver. Long-term megadosing may cause permanent neurologic damage that includes numbness in extremities and uncoordinated muscle movement.

Drug Interactions

The bioavailability of pyridoxine is affected by many different medications. Examples include

- Some drugs used to treat tuberculosis
- Some drug used to treat rheumatoid arthritis, asthma, depression
- Tetracycline, an antibiotic

The problem of bioavailability can be addressed with supplementation and taking the medication at a different time than the vitamin.

Other drug interactions with B_6 occur when the vitamin reduces the availability of the drug. Examples of reduced effectiveness for a drug in combination with B_6 are levodopa (L-dopa) used to treat Parkinson's disease and phenytoin used to treat seizures.

Recommended Dietary Allowance

Recommended intake for most healthy adults is 1.3 mg/day.

Folate: B_9 (Folacin, Folic Acid)

Function

Folate functions as a coenzyme in the synthesis of nucleic acids, DNA and RNA. It also is responsible in the metabolism of amino acids. Without vitamin B_9, cell division would be impaired.

Absorption into the Body

Vitamin B_9 is converted to an active form of the vitamin before it is absorbed into the blood stream from the intestine. It is unknown if the unchanged form of the vitamin that manages to make its way into the blood stream has any functional effect on body processes.

Source

The primary food source for folate and folic acid is beef liver. Barring that, other food sources include dark green leafy vegetables such as cooked spinach, black-eyed peas, asparagus, and Brussels sprouts. Fortified and enriched foods such as cereals, rice, and spaghetti noodles are also good choices.

Deficiency State

Although the deficiency of vitamin B_9 is uncommon in the United States, there are certain groups of people that are most at risk. People who have a poor diet, abuse alcohol, and suffer from diseases of the digestive tract are most susceptible. Pregnant women have greatest cause for concern because deficiency of B_9 is known to cause fetal neural tube defects, low birth weight, and fetal growth retardation. Other signs of deficiency in adults are ulcerated tongue and mucosal lesions, epidermal discolorations, headache, difficulty concentrating, and heart palpitations.

Severe forms of the deficiency can result in a condition called megaloblastic anemia.

Low levels of folate have been studied in people with cancer and depression and there are some indications that increasing folate intake may help with these condition. Research is ongoing, and results are not final.

Excessive State

Because of the relationship between B_9 and cell division, additional research must be conducted on the impact of excessive intake of the vitamin on precancerous lesions.

In combination with B_{12}, large doses of folic acid can correct megaloblastic anemia.

Drug Interactions

Folic acid supplements do not mix well with some drugs that persons may be taking for other conditions. For example, when folic acid supplement is taken with methotrexate, a drug commonly used to treat cancer and rheumatoid arthritis, the effects of both may be altered. The same kind of effect could occur when folic acid is taken with some antiseizure medications.

Recommended Dietary Allowance

Medications can interfere with bioavailability: aspirin, oral contraceptives, anticonvulsants, and some anticancer drugs. Recommended intake is approximately 400 µg daily, ideally from food sources.

Cobalamin: B_{12}

Function

Cobalamin participates in the production of many different essential components in the body. It is used to produce the hemoglobin found in RBCs, DNA and RNA, hormones, proteins, and lipids. Cobalamin also works in conjunction with other vitamins in synthesis and metabolism reactions.

Absorption into the Body

Food sources of B_{12} are processed in the body differently than supplement forms of the vitamin. Food source form of B_{12} requires action of stomach acid and enzymes to be converted to its free form. Supplements are already in the free form. Both are then absorbed into the blood stream in the large intestine. Absorption is regulated by the body's need. When excess is ingested, it is excreted readily.

Source

Sources are almost exclusively from animal foods such as clams, salmon, trout, and tuna. Beef is a reasonably good source as well. Fortified and enriched cereals and breads also contain good amounts of B_{12}.

Some people who have a malabsorption disorder must obtain B_{12} by regular injections because they cannot absorb the vitamin through the intestine in any of its oral forms.

Deficiency State

Pernicious anemia is a condition that causes deterioration of the intestinal lining and prevents absorption from the intestine. Deficiency in B_{12} may result from pernicious anemia, also known as megaloblastic anemia and nerve disorders, even if the person is taking adequate amounts of B_{12}. Signs of the vitamin deficiency include nerve damage that causes tingling of the hands and feet, constipation, depression, and memory loss. There are also oral signs with soreness of the tongue and mucosa.

People who are especially susceptible to the vitamin deficiency are those with gastrointestinal disorders such as celiac and Crohn's disease, who have had weight loss surgery, and vegans who do not consume animal protein or fortified foods.

Excess State

Cobalamin has a low potential for toxic side effects from excess ingestion either through food or supplement intake. Because of its pretty red color, it is used in research studies as a placebo.

Drug Interactions

Vitamin B_{12} does interact with some commonly used medications, many of which are OTC medications. Drugs used to treat gastric reflux or heartburn and peptic ulcers interfere with the absorption of the vitamin by altering the stomach acid and enzymes.

Recommended Dietary Allowance

The RDA for healthy adults is 2.4 mcg daily.

Biotin: H

Function

Biotin participates in cell growth in the synthesis of DNA and RNA. It also assists in releasing energy from carbohydrates, lipids, and proteins. Biotin is helpful in regulating a steady blood sugar level.

Absorption into the Body

Biotin is absorbed from the small intestine. Bacterial synthesis of the vitamin occurs in most people to a level that would prevent deficiency. Absorption may be inhibited by intestinal disorders such as removal of the stomach or part of the intestine and chronic inflammatory bowel disease.

Source

Along with bacteria making biotin in the intestine, biotin may also be obtained from food and supplement sources. Food sources are liver, cauliflower, salmon, carrots, bananas, soy flour, fortified cereals and yeast, molasses, and nuts. Biotin is heat sensitive and is easily lost during food preparation with heat.

Deficiency State

Deficiency is rare and is usually attributed to a genetic or digestive tract disorder. Inadequate levels of the vitamin cause several forms of skin conditions and rashes, fungal infections, depression, high blood sugar, and hair loss. An oral manifestation of the deficiency is inflammation of mucous membranes.

Excessive State

Though there is little evidence of any toxicity for biotin, many people believe that taking large supplemental doses can help with treatment of some conditions. Hair loss, brittle nails, and diabetic nerve pain are among them.

Drug and Supplement Interactions

A number of drugs interact with biotin in the body. Some of the interactions accelerate biotin breakdown and may result in a deficiency state of the vitamin. For example, some of the medications used to prevent seizures could reduce biotin levels.

Other drugs may cause increased levels of the drugs because of the supplementation of biotin. Examples are several antipsychotic and antidepressant drugs.

Recommended Dietary Allowance

For years, there was no RDA for biotin. However, today it is recognized as needed in tiny amounts, approximately 30 mcg daily.

Pantothenic Acid: B$_5$

Function

Pantothenic acid serves as a coenzyme that assists with the release of energy from carbohydrates, fats, and proteins. It also assists with synthesis of fatty acids, cholesterol, hormones, cell membranes, and the neurotransmitter acetylcholine. Pantothenic acid also helps to activate the enzymes needed for vitamin A and D synthesis.

Absorption into the Body

Pantothenic acid is absorbed from the small intestine. Interestingly, less absorption takes place when higher concentrations of the vitamin are present in the intestine. Excess of the vitamin is excreted in the urine and feces.

Source

Food sources for B$_5$ are numerous as the vitamin occurs naturally in many foods. They include yeast, chicken, beef, potatoes, oats, molasses, and whole grains. In general, vegetables are also good sources of the vitamin. The supplement, royal jelly, contains the highest amount of the vitamin of any naturally occurring source.

Deficiency State

Because this vitamin is commonly found in animal and plant tissue, deficiencies are rare. Pantothenic acid is known as the "antipellagra" vitamin because of its effects on skin. If a deficiency state exists, it might exhibit as loss of feeling in the arms and legs, muscle cramps, and loss of muscle coordination.

Drug Interactions

There are no documented drug interactions with vitamin B$_5$.

Recommended Dietary Allowance

RDA recommendation for dietary allowance is 5 mg for most healthy adults.

Vitamin C: Ascorbic Acid

Function

Vitamin C assists with formation of collagen fibers, strengthens immune system, aids with iron and calcium absorption, and helps with protein metabolism. Vitamin C is an antioxidant and helps to limit the effects of free radicals and oxidative stress on cells. Vitamin C seems to possess antihistamine qualities and can shrink swollen tissues. For this reason, increasing ingestion of vitamin C is thought to offer temporary relief from swollen tissues during a cold or flu, which gives it its curative reputation.

Absorption into the Body

Vitamin C undergoes intestinal absorption into the blood stream and then is converted into its active form within the cells. Remarkably, the absorption levels of vitamin C decrease when intake levels increase. Then, much of the vitamin C remains unchanged and excreted in urine and feces.

Sources

Food sources are largely fruits and vegetables. Among those with the highest concentrations are red and green peppers, citrus fruits and juices, kiwi, citrus fruits, cruciferous vegetables, tomatoes, cantaloupe, and strawberries. Vitamin C is also available in fortified cereals. It should be noted that vitamin C is easily destroyed with lengthy storage and heating during preparation.

Deficiency State

Scurvy—symptoms include the following:

- Initially seen as fatigue
- Gingival inflammation because of breakdown of collagen fibers, loose teeth
- Petechiae and bruising, poor healing
- Joint pain
- Secondary iron deficiency
- Fatal if untreated

Although the cause of scurvy is well known and uncommon in the United States, low levels of vitamin C are known to be common among smokers. Of course, smoking cessation is the best course of action, but otherwise, smokers should be advised to increase vitamin C intake above RDA by approximately 35 mg/day as noted in NIH, Office of Dietary Supplements.

Excess State

The eyes, adrenal glands, and brain have the ability to store high concentrations of vitamin C for about 3 months. Because it can be stored, excesses are possible. Symptoms include the following:

- Diarrhea and nausea with cramping
- Formation of kidney stones due to uric acid
- Iron toxicity

Some evidence indicates that at high levels, the antioxidant function of vitamin C may be reversed and the vitamin may contribute to cell damage instead of help to prevent it.

Drug Interactions

Vitamin C has the potential to interact with a number of medications, and caution should be used in combining the vitamin with any other substance. In particular, a group of drugs called "statins" that are used to increase good cholesterol in the body will interact with vitamin C to reduce the effect of the drug. Supplemental vitamin C has also been implicated in shielding cancer cells from anticancer therapies such as radiation and chemotherapy. While the research is ongoing and not fully supported by clinical evidence, caution should be used.[1]

Recommended Dietary Allowance

As mentioned, smokers need to consume more vitamin C than the RDA. It is possible that those exposed to secondhand smoke also need additional vitamin C, but the amount is unknown. RDA for the vitamin is 75 to 90 mg daily.

FAT-SOLUBLE VITAMINS

Vitamin A

Function

Vitamin A assists with formation of the tissues of the eye and the normal function of the membranes covering the eye and the cornea. Vitamin A is also involved in immune function, and formation of the heart, lungs, kidney, and other organs.

Absorption into the Body

The precursor molecule for vitamin A is commonly found in plants as a pigment called carotenoid. The precursor molecule is absorbed by the cells of the small intestine and sent to the body's cells where conversion the pigments into a group of several molecules known as vitamin A.

Sources

Vitamin A is available in supplement forms as well as food sources. There are several food sources with high levels of vitamin A. For example, sweet potatoes, beef liver, spinach, pumpkin, and carrots are exceptionally high in vitamin A. Additional sources include cantaloupe, red peppers, and mango. There are also a number of fortified cereals and dairy products with vitamin A added.

Deficiency State

Vitamin A deficiency is rare in the United States; however, it is common in many developing countries. Poverty often limits access to foods that naturally contain vitamin A. When deficiencies in vitamin A are present, poor health consequences during pregnancy and infancy may be present. Infants without sufficient levels of vitamin A have increased risk of eye disease and lung and digestive tract diseases in addition to slow growth and development.

Hypovitaminosis A—symptoms include the following:

- Dry, bumpy skin, poor immunity, slow growth
- Night blindness, exophthalmia (total blindness)
- Possible increases in periodontal diseases
- Macular degeneration
- Risk factor for severe measles
- Death, if untreated

Excess State

- Increased risk of lung cancer in smokers
- Symptoms are headache, vomiting, double vision, hair loss, pain in joints
- Reduced bone density and fractures
- Coma and death

Drug Interactions

Vitamin A in combination with medications that contain retinoids may result in excessive levels of both. Most of these drugs are used to treat skin conditions.

Recommended Dietary Allowance

Recommended intake is an RDA of 700 to 900 mcg/day for most healthy adults.

Vitamin D

Function

Vitamin D has been studied for its many effects on the human body in recent years. It has been studied for links to everything from tooth loss to depression and from its impact on brain function and to aging. Some things we know for certain, vitamin D:

- Promotes calcium absorption and aids with calcium levels in the blood
- Along with calcium and phosphate assists with bone formation, remodeling, and growth
- Aids in cell growth, nerve and muscle function, the immune system, and reduction of inflammation
- Plays a much greater role in fighting disease than was ever considered previously

Absorption into the Body

Vitamin D can be absorbed into the body from the intestine; however, most vitamin D is produced within the skin by a reaction between ultraviolet light and a precursor molecule. Then the molecule undergoes several reactions in the liver and kidney to become an active and functional molecule.

Sources

Aside from the body's own ability to make vitamin D, it has food sources as well. The flesh and oils of fatty fish such as swordfish, salmon, and tuna are the primary natural food sources. There are a number of fortified foods with vitamin D. They are mostly orange juice and milk products.

Deficiency State

Deficiency of vitamin D is one of the major reasons for the plethora of research on the topic. It is considered by some to be a worldwide problem connected to lifestyle, obesity, poverty, and autoimmune chronic diseases as noted in Harvard T.H. Chan of Public Health Nutrition Source.

Rickets (children) and osteomalacia (adult form of rickets); symptoms of rickets include the following:

- Pigeon breasted (prominent sternum) and bowlegged (poorly formed bones) and other bony deformities
- Bone pain and muscle weakness
- Delayed dentition and poorly calcified teeth

Fortified milk eliminated this problem in the United States, but it is still common worldwide. It is prevalent in countries where vitamin D-deficient mothers breast-feed infants. Vitamin D deficiency affects dark-skinned people more readily than it does light-skinned people. Lifestyles that preclude people from activities in the sun or require sunscreen are also contributors.

Excess State

The more vitamin D in the body, the more calcium is absorbed and circulating in the bloodstream. Excess calcium collects in soft tissues and can produce calcium stones in the kidneys. It also causes calcifications or hardening of blood vessels, which can be pathologic to the heart.[4,8]

Symptoms of excess are as follows:

- Anorexia, weight loss
- Frequent urination
- Cardiac dysfunction
- Calcification of vascular tissue

Drug Interactions

Vitamin D has the potential for several drug interactions. The most common occurs with steroids prescribed to reduce inflammation. The combination causes a reduction in calcium absorption and ultimately loss of bone or osteoporosis. In fact, any drug that causes a change in the absorption of vitamin D or calcium has the potential for creating a problem.

Recommended Dietary Allowance

Recommended intake is an RDA of 15 mcg daily for healthy adults.

Ongoing Research Related to Vitamin D Deficiency

- Worldwide deficiencies occurring with approximately 1 billion people affected
- In China alone, 69% to 75% of population among middle-aged and elderly[20]
- Lifestyle factors contributing to the deficiency: smoking behavior, alcohol consumption, daily time outdoors, physical activity[21]

Vitamin E

Function

Vitamin E acts as an antioxidant and is involved in the immune function and other metabolic processes. It works with enzymes that cause the dilation of blood vessels and inhibits blood clotting.

Sources

Supplemental vitamin E is available in many forms. However, studies indicate that only about half of the supplement form is absorbed compared to the same amount of the natural food source form (https://ods.od.nih.gov/factsheets/VitaminE-HealthProfessional). Food sources are mostly oils derived from wheat germ and various types of seeds. Specifically, sunflower seeds, almonds, and hazelnuts and their oils are excellent natural sources of vitamin E.

Absorption into the Body

Vitamin E is absorbed from the small intestine into the bloodstream where it travels to the liver. The liver processes the vitamin into one of several forms. Only the active form of the vitamin is retained to function in the body. The other forms are excreted.

Deficiency State

Deficiency is not common but can occur in infants and people who have digestive disorders affecting the absorption of the vitamin. Deficiency manifests as nerve pain, loss of muscle coordination, retina degeneration, and immune system disorders.

Excess State

Many claims about the vitamin's ability to prevent and treat disease have caused people to consider supplementation of the vitamin in large doses. In general, very little evidence exists that confirms that vitamin E can prevent any disease. A few studies suggest that it may be helpful in the treatment and prevention of age-related macular degeneration and cataracts of the eye.

Vitamin E excess is rare when consuming vitamin E from foods; however, supplementation of the vitamin in large amounts may cause an excess state.

Excess symptoms include the following:

- Nausea and diarrhea
- Increased risk of hemorrhagic stroke and bleeding

Drug Interactions

Vitamin E interacts with anticoagulant and antiplatelet medications to inhibit clotting. The vitamin also interacts with cholesterol reducing drugs such as the "statins" and niacin to reduce their overall effects.

Recommended Dietary Allowance

Recommended intake is an RDA of 11 to 15 mg daily for healthy adults.

Vitamin K

Function

Vitamin K functions as a cofactor for the synthesis of prothrombin required for blood clotting. It also has a function in bone metabolism.

Absorption into the Body

Vitamin K is naturally found in foods, but is mainly produced by bacteria that normally reside in the intestine. The pathway into the body is through absorption from the intestine into the lymphatic system and then to the liver where it is converted into a form that the body can use. Vitamin K is stored in the liver, brain, heart, pancreas, and bone.

Sources

It is manufactured by intestinal bacteria; food sources include dark green leafy vegetables such as collards, turnip greens, spinach, and kale. For people who are not big fans of leafy vegetable, other good sources are broccoli, soybeans, carrot juice and edamame.

Deficiency State

Deficiency is caused by diseases that reduce fat absorption or by using broad-spectrum medications that kill intestinal bacteria. Symptoms include prolonged bleeding and increased clotting time, which could result in hemorrhaging.

Excess State

High doses of vitamin K can interfere with anticoagulants.

Recommended Dietary Allowance

Recommended intake is an RDA of 90 to 120 mcg/day.

Table 5-3 lists the vitamins and their deficiency states.

As a dental health care provider, it is important to know the oral considerations of vitamin deficiencies. Table 5-4 outlines oral deficiency symptoms.

COUNSELING DENTAL PATIENTS ABOUT VITAMINS

Vitamins are associated with many functions that can affect the oral tissues. It is important to recognize when a patient may have a deficiency or an excess state that contributes to oral pathology. Inquiring about nutrition and supplementation lends

Table 5-3	Deficiency States of Vitamins
Vitamin	**Deficiency**
A	Xerophthalmia—night blindness, dry eyes
B_1	Beriberi
B_2	Ariboflavinosis
B_3	Pellagra
B_6	Microcytic anemia—small RBC
B_9	Neural tube defects of fetus
B_{12}	Pernicious anemia
C	Scurvy
D	Rickets—children; osteomalacia—adults
E	Hemolytic anemia—RBC breakage
K	Hemorrhage—failure of blood to clot

Table 5-4	Oral Deficiency Symptoms
Vitamin	**Oral Deficiency Symptoms**
A	Xerostomia
	Oral leukoplakia
	Hyperkeratosis
	Hyperplastic gingival tissue
B	Red swollen lips with vertical fissures and cheilosis
	Burning, smooth, red tongue, which may be ulcerated, geographic, with atrophied papillae
	Red, ulcerated, burning gingival tissues
C	Red-purplish, swollen, bleeding gums
	Loose teeth
	Slow healing
D	Failure of bone wounds to heal
	Enamel hypocalcification
	Loss of alveolar bone
	Thinning of trabeculation
E	No known deficiency symptoms
K	Failure of wounds to stop bleeding

additional information about the patient that will help the practitioner individualize a treatment plan to best address the patient's conditions.

The following is a list of information from the patient that may require follow-up to determine vitamin sufficiency:

- Chronic dieter
- Denture patient
- Early childhood caries or recurrent caries
- Periodontal disease
- Oral lesions
- Polypharmacy and xerostomia

The oral health practitioner should feel comfortable to refer patients with other health conditions that are noted during the oral examination to a doctor, pharmacist, or registered dietitian.[6]

CHAPTER REVIEW

PRACTICE FOR PATIENTS

A 26-year-old female graduate student presents for dental hygiene treatment. She shares that she is working on her dissertation and spends long hours on the task. The patient has a negative medical history, taking no medications, and without a history of any systemic conditions. She has not seen a physician for 6 years or a dentist for 8 years when an oral surgeon removed her third molars.

The patient's extraoral exam reveals cheilitis at the angles of the mouth. An intraoral exam reveals swollen, red gingivae and extremely dry mouth. Her tongue is red with degenerated papillae on the surface of the tongue.

Periodontal examination reveals generalized severe gingivitis with very little plaque and calculus. Pocket depths reflect pseudopocketing. Bleeding and exudate are present in several areas.

1. What follow-up questions should the hygienist ask this patient?
2. Are there additional bits of information that would be helpful in determining the best treatment for the patient?
3. Recommend nutritional counseling that may be beneficial. What vitamin deficiencies might the hygienist anticipate with the patient's assessment results?

RELATE TO YOU

1. Vitamins should dissolve in the stomach within 30 minutes to make them available to the body when they pass to the small intestines. If they do not dissolve with help from hydrochloric acid in the stomach within this time, they can pass through to the intestines whole and will not be available for use by the body. Find out if your vitamin supplement will pass this test; cover your vitamin supplement with vinegar and check back in 30 minutes. If it has not dissolved, it is not worth taking! "Freshness" dates matter when it comes to vitamins.

2. Compare a generic brand of vitamins to a more expensive trade name brand for vitamin content. Place the labels side by side, and determine if the bottles contain the same number and percentage of vitamins. Speculate on the differences and how effective each vitamin may be.

REFERENCES

1. Dietary Supplement Label Database. May 2016. Retrieved from http://www.dsld.nlm.nih.gov/dsld/
2. How to boost your Immune system. June 2016. Retrieved from http://www.health.harvard.edu/staying-healthy/how-to-boost-your-immune-system
3. Hung H-C, Colditz G, Joshipura KJ. The association between tooth loss and the self-reported intake of selected CVD-related nutrients and foods among US women. *Community Dent Oral Epidemiol* 2005;33:167–173.
4. Macaluso M, Mariano L. *Vitamins as an adjunct to traditional periodontal therapy.* Accessed February 2014. Retrieved from https://adha.cdeworld.com/courses/20176-Vitamins_as_an_Adjunct_to_Traditional_Periodontal_Therapy
5. Touger-Decker R. Dietary supplements and oral health: should the dentist ask? *Quintessence Int* 2005;36(4):286292.
6. Micronutrients and mental energy: Topic of the month. (2012, July). Retrieved from http://www.nutri-facts.org/en_US/news/micronutrients-and-mental-energy.html/p_tag/nutrifacts/news/inspiration/p_tag/nutrifacts/news/topic-of-the-month/p_tag/nutrifacts/news/
7. Vitamins. August 2016. Retrieved from https://medlineplus.gov/vitamins.html
8. Chun, O., Frei, B., Gardner, C., Alekel, D. L., Killen, J. Antioxidants: In depth. May 2016. Retrieved from https://nccih.nih.gov/health/antioxidants/introduction.htm
9. Bansal M, Vashisth S, Gupta N, et al. Antioxidants—its preventive role in oral cancer. *Indian J Dent Sci* 2012;4(3):103–105. Retrieved from www.ijds.in/functions.php?fuse=23&SrNo=16&CurrentIssue=No&IssueVol=Vol.4&IssueNumber=Issue 3&ArticleID=300
10. Chun O, Frei B, Gardner C, et al. Antioxidants and health: an introduction. *NIH National Center for Complementary and Integrative Health.* U.S. Department of Health and Human Services. November 2013. Retrieved from https://www.nlm.nih.gov/medlineplus/antioxidants.html

11. Thompson GR. Absorption of fat-soluble vitamins and sterols. *J Clin Pathol (R Coll Pathol)* 1971;5:85–89.

12. Therapeutic Research Center. Pantothenic acid (vitamin B_5). *MedlinePlus.* U.S. National Library of Medicine. August 19, 2015. Retrieved from https://www.nlm.nih.gov/medlineplus/druginfo/natural/853.html

13. Paganii-Hill A, Kavas CH, Corrda MM. Antioxidant vitamin intake and mortality. *Am J Epidemiol* 2014;181(2):120–126.

14. Bradley R, Thompson P, White JD, et al. Coenzyme Q10 (CoQ10): what you need to know. *NIH National Center for Complementary and Integrative Health.* U.S. Department of Health and Human Services. March 2015. Retrieved from https://nccih.nih.gov/.../Get_The_Facts_Coenzyme_Q10_03-24-2015.pdf

15. Tallon MJ. The rise…and rise of Co-Q10. *Funct Ingred* 2008;(72):24.

16. What is a processed food? September 2010. Retrieved February, from www.foodinsight.org/sites/default/files/what-is-a-processed-food.pdf

17. Food Processing and Nutrition. September 2012. Retrieved from https://www.betterhealth.vic.gov.au/health/healthyliving/food-processing-and-nutrition

18. NAS, Food and Nutrition Board, Institute of Medicine. *Dietary Reference Intakes for Thiamin, Riboflavin, Niacin, Vitamin B6, Folate, Vitamin B12, Pantothenic Acid, Biotin, and Choline.* Washington, DC: National Academy Press; 1998:357–358, 365–366. Available at: http://222.nap.edu/catalog/6015.html. March 2, 2010

19. Ulbricht C, Parm D. The top five nutritional deficiencies in the United States. *Altern Complement Ther* 2013;19(3):119–122.

20. Zhang M, Li P, Zhu Y, et al. Higher visceral fat area increases the risk of vitamin D insufficiency and deficiency in Chinese adults. *Nutr Metab* 2015;12(50).

WEB RESOURCES

National Institutes of Health, Office of Dietary Supplements https://ods.od.nih.gov/

DentalCare.com. Informed Professionals. Healthier Patients—Nutrition & Oral Health: Eating Well for a Healthy Mouth http://www.dentalcare.com/en-US/dental-education/continuing-education/ce301/ce301.aspx?ModuleName=coursecontent&PartID=6&SectionID=4

Access Magazine of the ADHA—Guideline on Caries-risk Assessment and Management for Infants, Children, and Adolescents http://www.aapd.org/media/Policies_Guidelines/G_CariesRiskAssessment.pdf

Special Care Dentistry Association—Pharmacologic Management of the Geriatric Patient http://www.scdaonline.org/resource/resmgr/2013_meeting_presentations/pharmacologic_management_of_.doc?hhSearchTerms=%22vitamins%22

6

Minerals

Learning Objectives

- List seven major minerals
- Define the difference between a major and trace mineral
- State five functions of minerals in the body
- Discuss the function of a sodium pump and name the minerals involved in the process
- Outline the cycle of minerals in the ecosystem
- Outline the digestive process of minerals
- Using a chart, identify mineral excess and deficiency as well as roles, recommended dietary allowance (RDA), and sources

> You can trace every sickness, every disease and every ailment to a mineral deficiency.
>
> *Linus Pauling, Two-time Nobel Prize Laureate*

Key Terms

Acid–Base Balance
Active Transport
Bioavailability
Cretinism
Electrolytes
Extracellular
Goiter
Heme Iron
Hemochromatosis
Homeostasis

Intracellular
Ionic Molecule
Macromineral
Major Mineral
Micronutrients
Nonheme Iron
Phytochemicals
Semipermeable Membrane
Trace Mineral

INTRODUCTION

Minerals are all around us in the forms of rocks and soil. Minerals can form beautiful crystals that reflect light, and they are key for the formation of beautiful, healthy tissues in the human body. There are 22 minerals listed in this chapter that are known to be needed for a healthy body and several additional trace minerals that are considered to contribute to health as well, although their specific functions have not yet been well defined.

Most people can get all the minerals needed through a varied daily food intake. However, research indicates there are a few minerals that are deficient in US diets. The deficiencies stem from inadequate nutrient-rich foods in the diet and fad diets. More importantly, deficiencies are found in people who have digestive tract or other systemic disorders, take prescription and OTC medications, or have extremely poor eating habits.[1] Age, gender, and race also play a role in mineral and vitamin deficiency. For example, iron deficiency is indicated to be as high as 13% in certain age groups in the United States. Deficiencies are also more cause for concern in elderly people who have systemic conditions that require medication.[2,3] Remarkably, people in the United States tend to ingest a lot of food, but may not be getting the nutrients they need.

In combination with vitamins, minerals make up a group of *essential* molecules needed for optimal health. Together, noncaloric vitamins and minerals are called **micronutrients** because they are required in such small quantities to facilitate body processes. Vitamins and minerals frequently are combined in daily dietary supplements because their functions are closely intertwined. However, minerals differ from vitamins in several significant ways.

Minerals, in their ionic forms, are available for absorption in the stomach and intestine from food and water, which, conveniently, provide the solvents in which the ions can be dissolved. Minerals can be found in body fluids, cells, and highly mineralized tissues of the body such as bones. We must remember that body tissues, for instance blood, other connective tissues, and even bone are not inert, but are constantly changing and require minerals every day to replace or remodel their structure. Minerals are

- Essential
- Inorganic
- Noncaloric
- Ionic metals, except for fluoride, iodide, and chloride, which are nonmetals
- Function in tandem with many vitamins

CATEGORIES OF MINERALS

There are two categories of minerals: major and trace. The amounts the body needs define in which category the mineral is placed. **Major minerals** are needed in quantities greater than 100 mg/day and are also called macrominerals. Trace minerals are needed in quantities less than 100 mg/day. It is important to note that major minerals are not more important to good health than trace minerals, they are just more abundant in the body.[3] Following are the seven major minerals:

1. Calcium
2. Chloride
3. Magnesium
4. Phosphorus
5. Potassium
6. Sodium
7. Sulfur

More than 30 trace minerals have been identified as essential to life. Some of the more common trace minerals are as follows:

1. Chromium
2. Cobalt
3. Copper
4. Fluoride
5. Iodide
6. Iron
7. Lithium
8. Manganese
9. Molybdenum
10. Nickel
11. Selenium
12. Silicon
13. Tin
14. Vanadium
15. Zinc

PRIMARY ROLES OF MINERALS IN THE BODY

As with vitamins, the body needs minerals for many metabolic and structural functions. Making up a relatively small portion of the body's mass, minerals participate in numerous reactions that result in the synthesis of body tissues and the maintenance of system functions. Minerals assist the body in the following ways:

- Converting glucose, proteins, and fats to energy and improving utilization of energy from food by cells: formation of adenosine triphosphate ($ADP + P \rightarrow ATP$) from these macronutrients

- Synthesizing or activating enzymes for all kinds of functions in the body
- Forming hormones such as insulin and parathyroid hormone
- Participating in the formation of vitamins from precursor molecules
- Forming red and white blood cells and recycling iron from hemoglobin when blood cells are destroyed
- Participating in growth and development of the brain
- Participating with the immune system (it is unclear exactly how this function occurs, but more researchers are convinced that minerals play a role)
- Participating in muscle contraction (including heart muscle) and neural transmission
- Controlling water balance inside and outside our cells
  - Fluid compartments are either **intracellular** (within a cell) or **extracellular** (outside the cell membrane).
  - Fluid outside the cells transports nutrients to cells and wastes to sites for excretion.
  - Water is constantly passing in and out of cell membranes with the help of electrically charged minerals such as sodium, potassium, and chloride ions. The diffusion of particles through the semipermeable membranes of cells maintains **homeostasis**, a healthy equilibrium within body tissues.
- Forming distinctive connective tissues such as blood, bone, fibers, and cartilage
- Functioning as antioxidants with select vitamins[1]

MINERALS IN THE ECOSYSTEM

All of the food groups contain foods that are rich in minerals. A varied diet with selections from dairy, meat, fruits, vegetables, and whole grains will ensure an adequate intake of minerals. Though minerals are ingested through our diets, the quality of the food varies with the soil and environment in which it was produced. According to the USDA (U.S. Department of Agriculture), this is one of the features that complicate food research.[4]

Minerals are found in the air, oceans, lakes, and rivers as well as in the soil where our food is grown. They enter the food chain by way of plants absorbing them from the soil and water. Then, animals eat the plants. To complete the cycle, decaying plants and animals return minerals to the soil. The minerals end up on our table in the food we eat and the beverages we drink. See Figure 6-1 Mineral cycle.

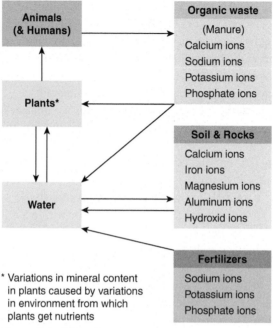

* Variations in mineral content
  in plants caused by variations
  in environment from which
  plants get nutrients

Figure 6-1   Mineral cycle.

ABSORPTION, DISTRIBUTION, AND DIGESTION

Minerals are present in the foods that are consumed. The greater the variety of foods, the greater the variety of minerals that can be taken from those foods. Minerals are released from the food and absorbed into the body from the intestine in their ionic form. Minerals are not digested as food is; instead, minerals are released from food in the small intestine and absorbed into the bloodstream, which distributes them to areas where they are needed. Some minerals have the capacity to be stored, but most are excreted from the body by the kidney when they are in excess.[3]

BIOAVAILABILITY

Bioavailability means that a mineral is available for the body to use for metabolic functions. Bioavailability involves absorption and transport of the mineral in the body as well as its transformation into a form that is usable by cells. The body must be efficient in balancing minerals because excess of one can cause an imbalance of another, leading to dysfunction. Increasing intake of one mineral can affect how others get absorbed as they compete with each other for bioavailability. For example, calcium will bind excess sodium ions, and both are excreted from the kidney resulting in a calcium deficiency. Too much phosphorus decreases the absorption of magnesium resulting in a deficiency. These sorts of imbalances are usually the result of supplements and not food intake.[3]

Phytochemicals known as antioxidants, flavonoids, and phytonutrients are found in fruits and vegetables. A small number of research studies show that excessive amounts of phytochemicals called phytates or oxalates can bind with minerals and prevent absorption or, even worse, cause mineralizations such as kidney stones. With a balanced diet, the contribution of fruits and vegetables with phytochemicals is unlikely to be large enough to cause the problems. Indeed, the benefits of fruits and vegetables far outweigh the risks for poor absorption.[5] The following is a list of phytochemicals and foods in which they are found[6]:

- Lycopene—kale, broccoli, tomatoes, red peppers, watermelon
- Lutein—collard greens, spinach, Brussels sprouts, artichokes
- Resveratrol—red wine, peanuts, grapes
- Anthocyanins—blueberries, blackberries, plums, cranberries, raspberries
- Isoflavones—soybeans

MINERAL IONS

If an electron is added or removed from a neutral atom, it forms an ion. Minerals can be positively charged ions (+) when an electron is removed or negatively charged ions (−) when an electron is added to their atom. An **ionic molecule** is made of a combination of positive and negative ions to achieve a neutral state; however, these molecules easily separate into their component ions when dissolved in a solvent such as water. Nonmetal minerals appear in the ionic form, switching the "ine" suffix to "ide." Examples are fluorine becoming fluoride, iodine becoming iodide, and chlorine becoming chloride. Metal ions team up with nonmetal ions, forming ionic compounds in food. A good example is sodium ion (Na^+) and chloride (Cl^-) making salt (NaCl). You may see the minerals named in textbooks as either the element or ion, but for the purpose of this text, they will be referred to as the "ion."

MINERAL DEFICIENCY

A carefully chosen diet will provide an abundance of all minerals needed for daily metabolism, making supplements unnecessary. Occasionally, deficiencies do exist because of diets that restrict or eliminate foods rich in minerals or the vitamins needed to facilitate the absorption or activation of the mineral. Specific groups are particularly at risk for mineral deficiencies:

- Lactose-intolerant people who must eliminate calcium-rich dairy products from their diets, creating a deficiency in calcium.

- People with anorexia nervosa who are on severe calorie-restricted diets eventually develop a deficiency in potassium.
- Children and young women of childbearing age may be deficient in iron.
- Young women, aged 20 to 39, have higher risk of iodine deficiency.
- Men or women taking certain medications such as diuretics that can lead to magnesium and potassium deficiency.[17]
- Strict vegetarians or vegans who eliminate all forms of animal products and who are not efficient in combining proteins may develop a deficiency in zinc.
- Severe alcoholics who choose drinking alcohol over eating will develop a deficiency in magnesium over time.[26]

There is a rising concern about changes in eating habits and the food preferences that have developed in recent years and the unintentional mineral deficiencies that can occur. For instance, calcium deficiency has been a concern in Asian countries for years because of the genetic predisposition to lactose intolerance and the limited consumption of dairy products. A food preference for anchovies has balanced the deficit because the small fish contain high levels of calcium. However, in recent years, the anchovies are being cleaned and the internal organs removed prior to marketing. The resulting reduction in calcium content of the fish creates potential for mineral deficiency in the population.[8]

Not to be overly concerned, most minerals are stable in foods and are resistant to the effects of heating and freezing used in preserving and preparing food. Decreases in chromium may occur when grains are processed; fortification and enrichment are often used to replace the loss.[9]

A deficiency in each of these minerals will manifest their own set of symptoms (see Specific Minerals for a list of deficiency symptoms). The following are common mineral deficiencies[2,10]:

- Calcium
- Zinc
- Iron
- Magnesium
- Iodide

MINERAL EXCESS

Mineral excess is rare in people consuming a varied diet. Supplementation is typically the cause of mineral excess. In fact, mineral excess is not all that common even with supplementation because the kidney filters excesses into the urine. Nonetheless, ingesting an excess of minerals can have a toxic effect on the body.

One such excess is sodium from salt. The sodium ion has several critical functions in the body: transmission of nerve impulses, contraction of muscle cells, and fluid balance. On the other hand, excess sodium can increase the amount of fluid in blood vessels and contribute to high blood pressure in susceptible people. Alternatives to foods with high salt content are advised so that people can cut down on sodium intake.

Approximately 50% of the US population takes some form of a mineral supplement, usually in a multiple vitamin. A surprising majority of Americans believe that vitamins and minerals are effective in treating or preventing certain chronic diseases. That the typical diet lacks sufficient minerals is a popularly held belief, and despite scientific evidence that indicates otherwise, many people continue to purchase supplemental multiple vitamins and minerals.[11,12] In fact, supermarkets with in-store pharmacies have noted a new marketing strategy in cross-marketing "heart-healthy" products with prescriptions! Tagging along are supplements for people with gastrointestinal reflux, menopause, diabetes, and arthritis![12]

Substantial amount of the information about individual minerals that follows is taken from the National Institutes of Health Office of Dietary Supplements at: www.ods.od.nih.gov, MedlinePlus at: https://www.nlm.nih.gov/medlineplus/druginformation.html, Merck Manuals at: http://www.merckmanuals.com/home/disorders-of-nutrition/overview-of-nutrition/vitamins-and-minerals, Linus Pauling Institute at: http://lpi.oregonstate.edu/mic.

MINERALS THAT FUNCTION AS ELECTROLYTES

Several of the macrominerals participate in major regulation activities in the body as electrolytes. These minerals assist in the regulation of neural transmission, muscle cell contraction, acid–base balance of the blood, and water balance inside and outside cells.

Active transport of electrolytes occurs as ionic particles move from one side of a semipermeable membrane to another and requires the cell to expend energy in the form of ATP. A semipermeable membrane, as human cells are designated, permits some substances such as mineral ions, to pass through the membrane, while others cannot. The *sodium–potassium pump* in the human body works by movement of sodium, potassium, and calcium ions across the cell membrane to create electrical changes in the surface of the membrane for the transmission of messages along the membrane. As the charges inside and outside of the cell membrane are changed and then equalized, a "wave-like" message is sent from one cell to the next. Neurons (nerve cells) and muscle cells work in this way.[13]

Acid–base balance is also an electrolyte function that occurs in the blood. Precision control of the acidity and alkalinity of the blood is required for life. Variances in pH of the blood are poorly tolerated by the human body. When intake of minerals that contribute to acidity are present or failure to eliminate those minerals occur, the blood becomes acidic (called *acidosis*). On the contrary, when low intake of the minerals is present or excess elimination of the minerals occurs, the blood becomes basic or alkaline (called *alkalosis*). Both events are life threatening.

Following is a list of minerals that are considered electrolytes.[14]

- Sodium
- Potassium
- Chloride
- Calcium (see Minerals Needed for Tissue Synthesis.)
- Magnesium (see Minerals Needed for Energy Metabolism.)
- Phosphorus (see Minerals Needed for Energy Metabolism.)

Sodium (Na⁺)

Function

Sodium is a mineral that is abundant on earth. It can be found on the surface of almost any structure, living or nonliving. As one of the principle components of table salt, it is used liberally as a food additive for flavoring, as a preservative, and in making baking soda. It is present in extracellular fluid to regulate fluid balance and plays an important role in maintenance of blood volume and pressure. In addition, sodium plays a role in the conduction of nerve impulses and muscle contraction as described in the previous section on electrolytes.

Sources

Sodium is available from many food sources. It is rare that a person would need to seek additional sodium in the diet for it occurs naturally in milk, cheese, beets, celery, beef, and pork. Even more abundant sources are processed food with added salt for flavor or preservation.[15]

The American Heart Association has identified the "Salty Six" foods that add the most sodium to your diet (Https://sodiumbreakup.heart.org/salty-six-surprising-foods-add-sodium-diets/):

- Breads and rolls
- Cold cuts and cured meats
- Pizza
- Poultry products
- Canned soup
- Fast food and deli sandwiches

A popular idea is that sea salt contains less sodium than does table salt. The actual content of the salt crystals in both cases is about 40% sodium. The crystal size of sea salt, and kosher salt for that matter, is much larger than the crystal size of table salt, so fewer crystals of the sea salt fit on a spoon. In that case, you may be using less sodium even though the molecular content of the two types are the same.[16]

Absorption

Absorption of sodium occurs in the small intestine along with its frequent ionic partner, chloride. It also assists in the absorption of amino acids, glucose, and water.

Recommended Dietary Allowance

The RDA is considerably less than most US resident use daily at 1.2 to 1.5 g/day. That amount would fit in the palm of your hand. In estimating the amount of sodium in the daily diet, you should consider sodium added during processing and preparation of food as well as the natural content of sodium in the food.

Figure 6-2 Table salt versus sea salt illustrates a comparison of table salt and sea salt.

Deficiency and Excess

Deficiency state is called *hyponatremia*, in which the level of sodium in the blood is too low. Generally, this is a rare state associated with specific conditions (www. merckmanuals.com):

- Consumption of too many fluids
- Kidney failure
- Heart failure
- Cirrhosis
- Use of diuretic medications
- Prolonged endurance exercise
- Several other less common conditions

Figure 6-2 Table salt versus sea salt.

Disease of excess is *hypernatremia*, or high levels of sodium in the blood. Excess sodium intake is by far the more common (www.merckmanuals.com). There are several studies that strongly support the connection between high blood pressure and sodium intake. The specific conditions associated with excess are

- Dehydration
- Diabetes with high blood sugar levels
- Diabetes insipidus
- Kidney disorders
- Adrenal gland disorders

Hypernatremia is most often seen in elderly people.

Both hypernatremia and hyponatremia present with mental confusion, muscle twitching and seizures, coma, and death if not promptly treated.

Potassium (K⁺)

Function

Potassium plays multiple roles in the maintenance of the human body. Potassium is an electrolyte that participates in fluid balance in the extracellular fluids and plasma. It is essential for contraction of muscle cells including heart muscle and contributes to bone health in its coordinated action with magnesium to prevent calcium loss from bones. The following is a list of the functions of potassium in the body[17]:

- Build proteins and muscle tissue
- Use carbohydrates to produce energy for cell use
- Control electrical stimulation of the heart muscle
- Control acid–base balance
- Maintain bone mineralization and body growth

Source

Potassium is found in milk products, bananas, tomatoes, oranges, melons, sweet potatoes, and raisins. It can also be found in fortified and processed foods.[7,17]

Deficiency and Excess

Deficiency of potassium is *hypokalemia*, and it is rare except in dehydration or in association with some medications used to treat high blood pressure. Diuretic medications stimulate the kidney to remove excess water from the blood, and in doing so, potassium is also lost.

Conditions that may cause hypokalemia are[17,19]

- Kidney disease
- Uncontrolled diabetes
- Diarrhea and vomiting
- Excessive alcohol use
- Excessive laxative use
- Excessive sweating
- Some medications: antibiotics, diuretics
- Eating disorders: bulimia

Symptoms of deficiency include the following[17,19]:

- Heart palpitations
- Constipation
- Fatigue and muscle weakness
- Tingling and numbness

In severe cases of deficiency, cardiac arrest or paralysis may occur.
Hyperkalemia is the term for excess potassium that can cause the following symptoms[17]:

- Fatigue and muscle weakness
- Paralysis
- Cardiac arrhythmias: abnormal heart contractions

Hyperkalemia is a life-threatening disorder.

The following Food for Thought explains the importance of adequate potassium when taking diuretic medication.

FOOD FOR THOUGHT   **MORE ABOUT DIURETICS**

- Diuretic medications are used to lower blood pressure by removing sodium, chloride, and water from the blood at the kidney.
- Less water in the blood means lower pressure on the walls of the blood vessels.
- Potassium is also removed during the process in the kidney when most diuretics are used.
- Common diuretic medications: thiazide and loop diuretics both can result in hypokalemia.
- Potassium-sparing diuretics do not contribute to hypokalemia.
- Diuretics are also used to reduce several conditions presenting as edema (particularly in the lungs, heart failure, and liver cirrhosis).

Recommended Dietary Allowance

There is no RDA for potassium, though 3.5 g/day is a generally accepted recommendation for healthy adults.[17]

Chloride (Cl⁻)

Function

Chloride is the partner to sodium in table salt. Together they work in extracellular fluid to maintain the body's fluid balance. Chloride is also a component of a strong acid, hydrochloric acid, which is produced by the stomach where it helps to eliminate some bacteria from consumed food (preventing food poisoning!). Hydrochloric acid plays an important role in gastric juice, which denaturizes proteins for digestion and prepares other nutrients for absorption in the intestine.

Source

Sources include table salt, meat, fish, eggs, and processed foods.

Absorption

Chloride is absorbed from the small intestine with sodium, amino acids, glucose, and water. It is also reabsorbed into the bloodstream from the kidney during normal operation.

Recommended Dietary Allowance

The RDA for chloride is 1 g/day and chloride is mostly consumed as table salt. Recommendations for people over 70 years old are at the lower end.

Deficiency

Deficiency is rare because of its abundance in processed foods.

MINERALS FOR ENERGY METABOLISM

The following five minerals play a role in energy metabolism:

- Phosphorus
- Magnesium
- Manganese
- Iodine
- Chromium

Phosphorus (P as PO_4^{3-})

Function

Phosphorus assists with the formation of teeth and bones, and eighty percent of the phosphorus in the body is stored. It also acts as component in energy metabolism during the reduction of ATP to release energy. Phosphorus is found in every cell in the body in the cell membranes, DNA and RNA. It is essential for protein synthesis and participates in muscle contraction.

Absorption

Phosphorus is easily absorbed in the digestive tract. Some research conducted in the early 2000's indicated that the absorption of phosphorus may be linked to calcium and that bone density was reduced when phosphorus was in excess in the ratio between phosphorus and calcium. Since then, the ratio has been strongly questioned by the research, and bone density seems to be good even when the ratio is skewed toward phosphorus. The debate goes on.[1,24]

Source

Phosphorus occurs most often in nature in an ionic form called phosphate, in which it is combined with oxygen to form a relatively stable ion. Food sources for phosphate are abundant, but the best sources are dairy foods, meat, and fish. Vegetarians can get a moderately good amount of phosphate from cereals, nuts, and legumes. Soda drinks are also high in phosphate.[1,7,20]

Deficiency and Excess

Deficiency or *hypophosphatemia* can happen when a person has insufficient phosphorus for an extended time. Causes for deficiency include the following:

- Hyperparathyroidism
- Chronic diarrhea
- Use of certain diuretics over an extended period of time
- Consuming antacids that contain aluminum over an extended period of time
- Taking theophylline, a drug used to treat asthma
- Severe malnutrition
- Certain diabetic conditions
- Severe alcoholism
- Severe burns[22]

Symptoms of hypophosphatemia:

- Muscle weakness
- Bone pain and fracture
- Loss of appetite
- Coma and death

Historically, it was recorded that concentration camp survivors with low phosphate levels due to their starvation while imprisoned died after their rescue when they began eating a normal diet again. The return to normal eating caused a sudden, dramatic reduction in phosphate levels resulting in severe hypophosphatemia called "refeeding syndrome."[22]

Hyperphosphatemia is the rare condition when phosphate is in excess in the body. It typically only occurs in people undergoing dialysis, which is not effective in removing phosphate from the blood. The phosphate then builds up, and the body has no way of ridding itself of the excess. Drugs to alleviate the problem will bind the phosphate to prevent its absorption and promote its excretion.[23,24]

Other conditions that may create hyperphosphatemia are:

- Inadequate production of or lack of response to parathyroid hormone
- Crushing injury (such as a car crash)
- Massive infections
- Excessive supplementation of phosphate

There are few symptoms associated with excessive phosphate in the blood. However, the combination of calcium and phosphate may cause crystals to form in walls of arteries or the skin.[24]

Recommended Dietary Allowance

RDA is around 700 mg/day for healthy adults.[9]

Magnesium (Mg^{2+})

Function

Magnesium is an ionic mineral with a positive charge that is essential for mineralization of bones and teeth where as much as sixty percent of magnesium in the body is stored. The remainder can be found in soft tissues and in extracellular fluid. Magnesium also has critical roles in neural transmission, muscle contraction, conversion of food to energy, protein synthesis particularly enzymes, and regulating blood pressure and heart rhythm.[25] Research indicates that magnesium may also play a role in improving sleep quality.[26]

Sources

Food sources of magnesium are numerous and varied. Green leafy vegetables such as spinach are especially good sources because the green color comes from a chemical, chlorophyll, that contains magnesium in its structure. Other sources include almonds and cashews, potatoes, and whole grains. Oh, and yes, chocolate![17,26]

Absorption

The rate of absorption of magnesium is dependent upon the form the ion takes. Magnesium compounds that dissolve well in water are most easily absorbed in the intestine. In addition, the presence of large amounts of zinc ion inhibits magnesium absorption. People with gastrointestinal absorption disorders will have trouble absorbing magnesium as well.

Deficiency and Excess

The deficiency of magnesium in the blood is called *hypomagnesia*. Very little magnesium is found in blood; most is harbored in bone and teeth; however, adequate levels are required to maintain normal muscle and nerve functions. More often than any other reason, magnesium levels are low because of inadequate consumption associated with starving (anorexia), a malabsorption syndrome, or kidney and intestinal dysfunction.

Hypomagnesemia may occur as a result of the following[27]:

- Diarrhea
- Chronic alcohol abuse
- Excessive excretion of some hormones
- Insulin resistance in diabetics
- Drugs that increase urination: diuretics, some antifungal medication, some anticancer drugs

Signs of hypomagnesemia include the following:

- Nausea and vomiting.
- Weakness and drowsiness.
- Personality changes.
- Muscle tremor.
- In severe cases, seizures may occur.

The excess magnesium in the blood is called *hypermagnesemia*. It is a rare condition and is usually only associated with kidney failure; however, it is possible to induce the condition with disproportionate use of laxatives or antacids that have magnesium as an ingredient. High levels of circulating magnesium are very serious and can result in removal of calcium from bone,[7] low blood pressure, difficulty breathing, and cardiac arrest.[28]

Recommended Dietary Allowance

Some controversy exists about the RDA for magnesium. The RDA is established at 320 mg/day for women and 420 mg/day for men; however, in 2007, a much lower RDA was suggested at 237 mg/day for women.[26] Either way, many women have an intake between 222 and 150 mg/day, which is below recommendations. Elders and teens are also groups that may not be getting enough magnesium; their requirements are slightly higher than those for healthy adults.[18,25]

Manganese (Mn)

Function

Manganese is needed for many enzyme reactions. It aids in the synthesis and activation of many enzymatic processes. They include the metabolism of carbohydrates, the production of glucose from noncarbohydrate sources (such as protein), the detoxification of by-products from the metabolism of protein (ammonia especially), and the production of neural transmission substances. Manganese is also a component of enzymes required for the formation of bone and cartilage, and the collagen fibers needed for wound repair.

Source

Food sources are raisin bran cereal, brown rice, pineapple, pecans, and instant oatmeal. Green tea is also a good source of manganese.

Absorption

Manganese has limited absorption into the body. Less than 10% of the mineral that is consumed is absorbed. Research demonstrates that there is an inverse relationship between iron absorption and manganese absorption; when one is increased, the other decreases. The risk of toxicity rises when either mineral is deficient or in excess.

Medications containing magnesium such as antacids and laxative or tetracycline (an antibiotic) can decrease manganese absorption as well.

Deficiency and Excess

Deficiency in manganese is associated with poor reproduction rates, growth retardation, skeletal abnormalities, and glucose intolerance.

Excess has been noted in people who are environmentally exposed to high levels of manganese that is inhaled, such as welders. Also at increased risk for manganese toxicity are people who have chronic liver disease, newborn babies and children, and people who have iron deficiency. The following are symptoms of manganese toxicity:

- Parkinson's-like symptoms
- Tremors
- Difficulty walking
- Facial muscle spasms
- Psychiatric symptoms: irritability, hallucinations, aggressive behavior[29]

Recommended Dietary Allowance

Most people will be able to get all the manganese they need from their daily diet. The RDA is between 2.3 mg/day for men and 1.8 mg/day for women.

Iodide (I⁻)

Function

Iodide is the negative ion formed when elemental iodine interacts with a metallic ion. Iodide is part of the two thyroid hormones that regulate protein synthesis and enzyme activities. It also is believed to participate in the immune system functions. Iodide deficiency is a problem in pregnant women who risk giving birth to babies with mental impairment because of the deficiency. The exact role that iodide plays in regard to fetal development is not completely understood.[30]

Source

Sources of iodide are plentiful since the development of iodized salt that is used in over 70 countries, including the US. Natural food sources of iodide are plentiful such as cod, yogurt, reduced fat milk, and enriched bread.[7]

Absorption

Iodide is easily absorbed from both the stomach and intestine in its ionic form. The thyroid gland grabs the iodide it needs, and the rest is filtered and excreted in urine.

Deficiency and Excess

Iodide deficiency has dramatic consequences on growth and development of fetus and infant when it occurs during pregnancy. Consequences in the fetus and the newborn are irreversible including the following:

- Miscarriage and stillbirth
- Neurological abnormalities and mental deficits

Figure 6-3 Goiter.

- Growth retardation
- Deafness
- Poor muscle coordination and physical abnormalities
- Attention deficit disorders
- **Cretinism**: severe iodide deficiency in a developing fetus

An iodide deficiency in adults and children may also manifest as a **goiter**, which appears as an enlarged thyroid gland. Symptoms are related to decreased thyroid gland function—*hypothyroidism*: weight gain, dry skin and hair, low blood pressure, intolerance of cold, and lethargy.

See Figure 6-3 Goiter for an illustration of thyroid enlargement.

Interestingly, excessive intake of iodide can result in similar symptoms that occur with deficiency including hypothyroidism and goiter because of the inhibition of thyroid hormone production. In contrast, in some cases, excess iodide can cause *hyperthyroidism*, thyroiditis, and potentially thyroid cancer. More acute iodide excesses produce symptoms of burning mouth and stomach, fever, nausea and vomiting, pain, and diarrhea, followed by reduced heart rate and coma.

Recommended Dietary Allowance

RDA is approximately 150 mcg/day for healthy adults.

Chromium (Cr^{3+})

Function

Chromium in its two ionic forms may be a biological asset (Cr^{3+}) or a toxic industrial pollutant (Cr^{6+}). The biological ion is essential for the mobilization of glucose by enhancing the function of insulin on cells. Chromium has been indicated to participate in the metabolism of carbohydrates, fats, and proteins for energy.

Source

In the diet, chromium is found in meat and whole grains, broccoli, and grape juice. One very good source of chromium is red wine! Enjoy your chromium.

Absorption

Very little chromium is absorbed from the intestine except in the presence of vitamin C and niacin, which seem to enhance absorption of the mineral. Any excess mineral that enters the bloodstream is stored in the liver, bone, and other soft tissues.

Deficiency and Excess

Deficiency in chromium may be created by diets high in simple carbohydrate, which causes chromium to be excreted. This might be a precursor to type II diabetes. Deficiencies have also been noted in people who are experiencing heavy exercise, infection, and stress. Special care must be given to avoid chromium deficiency during pregnancy and lactation as these women are especially susceptible.

Excess state of chromium is rare. However, medications can alter the absorption of chromium and result in either a deficiency or excess of the mineral. Examples include:

- Reduce absorption—lower chromium levels
  - Medications that treat gastrointestinal reflux
  - Antacids
  - Corticosteroids
- Increase absorption—raise chromium levels
  - Ibuprofen and aspirin
  - Insulin
  - Corticosteroids
  - Certain high blood pressure medications (beta-blockers)

Recommended Dietary Allowance

RDA for chromium differs for men and women. For men, 35 mcg/day is recommended and for women 25 mcg/day for healthy adults.

MINERALS NEEDED FOR TISSUE SYNTHESIS

The following five minerals play a role in tissue synthesis:

- Calcium
- Fluoride
- Zinc
- Phosphorous (see Minerals Needed for Energy Metabolism)
- Magnesium (see Minerals Needed for Energy Metabolism)

Calcium (Ca^{2+})

Function

Calcium is the most abundant mineral in the body, and the majority is in teeth and bones. The remaining small percentage found in blood and soft tissue plays roles in essential functions:

- Contributing to muscle contraction—especially constriction and dilation of blood vessels impacting blood pressure[25]
- Conducting neural signals and hormone production
- Synthesizing blood-clotting proteins
- Maintaining normal heart rhythm
- Participating in production of parathyroid hormone

These physiologic needs of calcium are so vital to survival that if calcium levels fall, the body will take calcium from bone to support these functions, at the expense of bone density. Throughout life, bone is constantly being remodeled through the circulation of calcium and other constituent minerals in bone (also called "turnover," a process in which new bone is made and existing bone minerals are recycled back into the blood).

See Figure 6-4 Bone mass in relation to age.

Absorption

Calcium is absorbed from the intestine into the bloodstream. However, calcium absorption is impacted by other factors, such as:

- Amount consumed at one time—megadoses of calcium will not be absorbed in amounts greater than about 500 mg.
- Increasing age, especially in women.
- Presence of phytic or oxalic acids in foods eaten at the same time as calcium-laden foods inhibits calcium absorption (examples of foods with these acids are greens, sweet potatoes, rhubarb, whole grains, beans, and nuts).

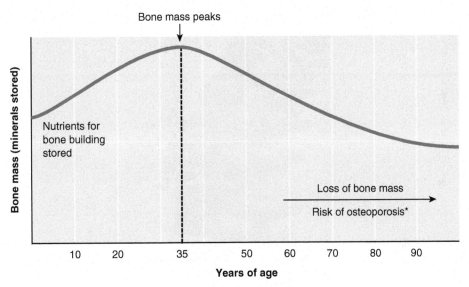

* With loss of minerals in bone, risk of osteoporosis increases

Figure 6-4   Bone mass in relation to age.

- High sodium intake interferes with calcium absorption.
- Consuming large amounts of alcohol.

On the contrary, calcium absorption can be enhanced with consuming vitamin D and proteins with the calcium-laden foods.

Source

The best food sources are dairy products such as yogurt, various cheeses, and milk. Sardines and fortified versions of soymilk, almond milk, and orange juice are very good choices as well.

Deficiency and Excess

Hypocalcemia is the term for calcium deficiency. It occurs primarily in people who have specific medical conditions (kidney disease, surgical removal of the stomach or intestine) and people who require diuretic medications. Conditions that occur because of hypocalcemia are as follows:

- Osteomalacia—calcium deficiency during growth years where bone mineralization is reduced
- Osteopenia (insufficient calcium in the blood) and subsequent osteoporosis (loss of minerals—calcium from the bones)

Figure 6-5   Osteoporosis.

• Rickets (when accompanied by vitamin D deficiency occurs in children where bones will "flex" under the upper body mass of the child creating the appearance of bowed legs)

See Figure 6-5—Osteoporosis.

Hypercalcemia means high levels of calcium in the blood. The disorder is often caused by parathyroid gland dysfunction and results in excessive fluid loss through urination. It can be life threatening, but is usually caught via routine blood tests.[31]

Ongoing studies relative to excessive intake of calcium or megadosing calcium supplements have resulted in interesting preliminary findings. For instance, some evidence indicates that megadoses of calcium supplements may contribute to cardiovascular disease such as intravascular blood clots and calcifications; however, dietary calcium seems to cause a decrease in blood pressure. Numerous studies have been made, and more are indicated to determine the absolute validity of these findings.

Recommended Dietary Allowance

The RDA for calcium is 1.0 g/day for healthy adults. The RDA for women over 50 goes to 1.2 g/day.

Fluoride (F⁻)

Fluoride is a nonmetal that is most often found as the negative ion in an ionic bond with a metallic mineral. In bones and teeth, it is present as calcium fluoride, a component of the hydroxyapatite crystals. In water supplies, it may be found as a component of a number of different ionic molecules. In ocean water, it is present as sodium fluoride.[32]

Function

Fluoride increases retention of calcium in teeth and bones. If consumed by the pregnant woman or infant, it becomes incorporated into the developing tooth structure. The hydroxyl ion in the tooth combines with the fluoride ion to form fluorohydroxyapatite, which makes the structure less soluble and more resistant to demineralization.

Source

Fluoride is present in many groundwater sources around the world. There are belts of mineral deposits with high concentrations of fluoride in Africa, Asia and China, and the Middle East. Although less common, there are similar belts in the United States. Fluoride is also added to community water supplies where natural groundwater does not have the ion.

Food sources of fluoride include any foods prepared in fluoridated water, tea, and gelatin. Not to worry! The best way to make sure you have the minerals you need is to eat a balanced diet of a variety of foods! Importantly, please note that breast milk typically does not contain fluoride, though infant formula often does.[32]

Deficiency and Excess

A fluoride deficiency correlates with increased incidence of dental caries and bone fractures in the elderly.[33] A small excess of fluoride during tooth development can manifest as dental fluorosis, a pitting of the enamel known as mottled enamel.[33] Amounts of fluoride in excess of eight times the recommended dosage are known to produce crippling skeletal deformities.[33]

Recommended Dietary Allowance

There is no RDA. However, research indicates that varying amounts of fluoride during different life periods will help with maintaining teeth and bones in optimal health. Below are recommendations from the Food and Nutrition Board at the Institute of Medicine:

- Infants
  - 0 to 6 months: 0.01 mg/day
  - 7 to 12 months: 0.5 mg/day

- Children
  - 1 to 3 years: 0.7 mg/day
  - 4 to 8 years: 1.0 mg/day
  - 9 to 13 years: 2.0 mg/day
- Adolescents and Adults
  - Males, 14 to 18 years: 3.0 mg/day
  - Males, over 18 years: 4.0 mg/day
  - Females, over 14 years: 3.0 mg/day

Zinc (Zn)

Function

Zinc is widely used in the body for many essential functions. It is involved in the actions of over 100 different enzymes and plays important, though not well-understood, roles in immune function and wound healing. Zinc supports growth and development through its role in synthesis of proteins and DNA and cell division. Zinc in combination with the function of copper appears to have a role in eye health as well.

Source

Red meat, shellfish, and poultry hold the most zinc, with plant sources holding much less. Zinc is also available in many over-the-counter cold remedies, not to mention supplements.

Patients should be counseled about the use of denture adhesives that contain zinc because excess exposure to the mineral has been reported.

Absorption

Zinc and copper compete for absorption in the small intestine. In the presence of excess zinc, copper deficiency may occur. Absorption is decreased in people who consume large amounts of alcohol. Absorption is altered by any form of malabsorption syndrome such as Crohn's disease or colitis.

Deficiency and Excess

A deficiency in zinc can cause anorexia (loss of appetite), slow tissue repair, eye and skin lesions, slow growth, and a loss of taste and smell. Of special concern for deficiency are lactating mothers and their infants who are strictly breast-fed, as zinc is rapidly depleted from maternal stores. Additionally, vegetarians who do not eat any animal product are of concern, for zinc is not found in plants in large amounts.

An excess of zinc can interfere with copper absorption, alter iron function and immune system activities, and reduce HDL levels.

Zinc interacts with medications in several ways. For instance, tetracycline antibiotics inhibit the absorption of zinc and of the antibiotic itself.

Recommended Dietary Allowance

RDA ranges from 8 to 9 mg/day for women and 11 mg/day for men.

MINERALS NEEDED FOR RED BLOOD CELL SYNTHESIS

The following two minerals are needed for red blood synthesis:

- Iron
- Copper

Iron (Fe^{2+} and Fe^{3+})

Function

The majority of iron in the body is found in the blood as a component of hemoglobin, the protein that binds oxygen for transport. The rest, about 20% of the iron in the body, is stored in bone marrow, the liver, the spleen, and muscles to act as a reserve in times of iron depletion. Aside from transportation of oxygen, iron functions in synthesis of proteins in hormones and connective tissue; each of these are significant factors in growth and development.

Absorption

Iron absorption occurs in the intestine and is generally not excreted in significant amounts once it enters the body. Its absorption is regulated by hormones. Absorption can be hampered by the presence of phytochemicals and enhanced by the presence of vitamin C in the food stuffs that are present in the digestive tract with the iron.

Source

The source of iron in the diet makes a difference in its bioavailability. More iron is absorbed from animals (40%) than plants (10%). Iron from animal sources is called **heme iron** and from plant sources is called **nonheme**. Bioavailability of nonheme iron is enhanced by consumption of foods rich in vitamin C at the same time as the food rich in nonheme iron.

- Heme iron food sources include meat, fish, and poultry.
- Nonheme iron is found in white beans, lentils, leafy greens, and chocolate.

Vitamin C helps with absorption of iron. Drinking orange juice or including other foods rich in vitamin C can enhance the uptake of iron from the meal.

Deficiency and Excess

Other than bleeding, iron stores are not readily depleted—including menstruation, bleeding ulcer, or severe wounds. In the United States, iron deficiency is most likely in "food-insecure" households where children, women of childbearing age, and the elderly are most significantly affected. Along with poor diet, iron deficiency may be caused by malabsorption syndromes and intestinal parasites. Iron deficiency anemia is one of the most prevalent world nutritional problems.

Anemia is detected through a blood test that shows hemoglobin levels less than needed to supply the oxygen demands of the body. There will be a decrease in the number of red blood cells and low plasma levels. Symptoms of anemia are as follows:

- Pallor of mucous membranes
- Angular cheilosis
- Lethargy and apathy and impaired work performance
- Short attention span
- Impaired immune function
- Impaired temperature regulation

Iron is the most toxic mineral in the diet because the body has the capacity to store it. Excess absorption occurs with overconsumption of vitamin C. **Hemochromatosis** is a hereditary disease where there is increased iron absorption from the small intestines.

Recommended Dietary Allowance

RDA is 8 mg/day for men and 18 mg/day for premenopausal women. The RDA for postmenopausal women is reduced to 8 mg/day.[9]

Copper (Cu^{2+} and Cu^{3+})

Function

Copper aids the absorption of iron and, with iron, works to synthesize hemoglobin. On the other hand, copper competes with zinc for absorption at the intestinal sites. Copper regulates energy production and formation of red blood cells, bone, and connective tissues. Copper also functions as an antioxidant in cells.

Source

Food sources include shellfish, organ meats, whole grains, nuts, and beans. Vegetarians can also get copper from plant foods such as leafy greens, dried fruits, cocoa, and black pepper.[1,34]

Deficiency and Excess

Deficiencies are rare, but people at risk are those with malabsorption disorders such as celiac disease, Crohn's disease, and sprue. Those who have had bariatric surgery must be cautious to meet dietary needs of vitamins and minerals because of limited absorption capabilities. Symptoms of copper deficiency include:

- Anemia with a decrease in white blood cells
- Muscle weakness and fatigue
- Osteoporosis[34,35]

Excess of copper is toxic, and the mineral will deposit in liver and brain leading to hepatitis and brain disorders.[35] Symptoms of excess copper ingestion are

- Nausea, vomiting, and diarrhea
- Hemolytic anemia (rupture of red blood cells)
- Kidney damage, which prevents urine formation
- Death[35]

Recommended Dietary Allowance

The RDA is 900 mcg/day for healthy adults.

ANTIOXIDANTS

The following two minerals work in tandem with vitamins A, C, and E to serve as antioxidants:

- Selenium
- Sulfur

Selenium (Se^{2-})

Function

Selenium is a nonmetallic trace mineral that participates in reproduction, thyroid hormone metabolism, DNA synthesis, and with vitamin E as an antioxidant.

Absorption

Once absorbed, selenium travels through the bloodstream to skeletal muscle and the thyroid for storage. From that site, it will be converted into the active forms needed by the body.

Source

Food sources depend on the abundance of selenium in soil and animals that eat plants grown in the soil. Because of this, it is geographically higher in some areas than others. Foods containing selenium are grains, vegetables, and meats. Brazil nuts have the highest food content of selenium at approximately 544 mcg/serving!

Deficiency and Excess

A selenium deficiency can cause cardiac weakness, an unusual form of osteoarthritis, and it may cause an iodide deficiency to get worse. High risk for selenium deficiency occurs in Asian countries where the soil has low concentrations of selenium, people on dialysis, and people with HIV.

An excess can cause hair loss, fatigue, and vomiting. Sudden excessive doses cause serious symptoms resulting in respiratory distress, heart attack, and neurological problems.

Recommended Dietary Allowance

RDA is 55 mcg/day for health adults.

Sulfur (S)

Function

Sulfur is part of the vitamins biotin and thiamin. It is also found in enzymes that are part of the body's drug-detoxifying pathway. Sulfur is needed for liver function and also to maintain the acid–base balance of body fluid.

Source

Food sources include meat, poultry, fish, and legumes; it is also found in food preservatives.

Recommended Dietary Allowance

There is no RDA for sulfur.

Deficiency and Excess

There are no known deficiency or toxicity states.

RELATE TO PATIENTS

Consider the following when counseling patients:

- Use the same caution in purchasing mineral supplements as with vitamins.
- Excessive use of processed food may lead to:
  - Deficiencies of calcium, iron, and zinc
  - Absorption difficulties between minerals, vitamins, and other nutrients
  - Imbalances in nutrients within the body
  - Excess of sodium and chloride and other minerals
- When preparing food:
  - Although minerals are not destroyed by heat, boiling and stewing cause leaching into surrounding fluid. Use this fluid to prepare rice, mashed potatoes, pasta, and so on.
  - Steaming and stir frying retain minerals.
  - Be frugal when adding salt to a prepared meal.
  - Cast-iron cookware adds absorbable iron, especially when cooking acidic foods such as tomatoes.

CHAPTER REVIEW

PRACTICE FOR PATIENTS

Patient #1

A 67-year-old male presents for dental hygiene treatment. Following assessments, the hygienist in consultation with the dentist determines that the patient has generalized moderate periodontitis and localized severe periodontitis in the mandibular anterior. Accompanying deep pocket depths is significant inflammation of all of the tissues. Bleeding on probing is generalized. The patient also exhibits bruised areas on the buccal mucosa and tongue, which he explains occur sometimes when he chews crunchy foods.

The patient explains that he is currently on metoprolol, metformin, warfarin, and 81-mg aspirin for his conditions, which include atrial fibrillation, hypertension, and prediabetes. When questioned further, the patient states that he takes fish oil and garlic to help control his blood pressure and ginseng for memory enhancement.

1. What concerns do you have about his medications and the potential for bleeding with the debridement procedures?
2. What information will you give this patient about the supplements he is taking? What recommendations might you consider?
3. What recommendations for treatment modifications might you suggest to the dentist in planning his dental hygiene treatment? Other treatments that the dentist might propose?

 RELATE TO YOU

1. Place the labels from the box, package, can, or bottle of your favorite processed foods in front of you. Read the list of ingredients and locate as many minerals as you can. Write down all the minerals that are more than half the daily recommended allowance.
2. Check the label of your daily multivitamin/mineral supplement to determine which minerals and their percentage of RDA it contains. Add the percentage of the minerals in the supplement with the percentage contained in your favorite processed foods to determine your daily consumption.
3. Which minerals are you consuming in excess?
4. Which minerals are deficient in your diet?

REFERENCES

1. Vitamins and minerals—others. (February 18, 2015). Retrieved from http://www.nhs.uk/Conditions/vitamins-minerals/Pages/Vitamins-minerals.aspx
2. CDC's second nutrition report: Frequently asked questions. (March 27, 2012). Retrieved from http://www.cdc.gov/nutritionreport/faq.html
3. Vitamins and minerals: Are you getting what you need? (2015). Retrieved from http://www.helpguide.org/harvard/vitamins-and-minerals.htm
4. Nakata P, Grusak M. (March 31, 2014). Research Project: Absorption and metabolism of essential mineral nutrients in children. Retrieved from http://www.ars.usda.gov/research/projects/projects.htm?accn_no=416463

5. Weil A. (July 19, 2010). Are phytates good or bad? Retrieved from http://www.drweil.com/drw/u/QAA400758/Are-Phytates-Bad-or-Good.html

6. What are phytonutrients? (2016). Retrieved from http://www.fruitsandveggiesmorematters.org/what-are-phytochemicals

7. Fitness and nutrition. (June 17, 2008). Retrieved from http://womenshealth.gov/fitness-nutrition/nutrition-basics/minerals.html

8. Henry CJ, Bi X, Lim J, et al. Mineral decline due to modernization of food habits. *Food Chem* 2015;190:194–196. Retrieved from http://www.ncbi.nlm.nih.gov/pubmed/26212960

9. Dahl WJ, Turner RE. (April 2015). Facts about minerals. Retrieved from http://edis.ifas.ufl.edu/fy891

10. Ulbricht C. Top five nutritional deficiencies in the United States. *Altern Complement Ther* 2013;19(3):119–122.

11. Guallar E, Stranges S, Mulrow C, et al. Enough is enough: stop wasting money on vitamin and mineral supplements. *Ann Intern Med* 2013;159(12):850–852.

12. Sloan A. Why people use vitamin and mineral supplements. *Nutr Today* 2007;42(2):55–62.

13. Higdon J. (November 2008). Sodium (chloride). Retrieved from http://lpi.oregonstate.edu/mic/minerals/sodium

14. Lewis JL III. (2016). Overview of acid–base balance. Retrieved from http://www.merckmanuals.com/home/hormonal-and-metabolic-disorders/acid-base-balance/overview-of-acid-base-balance

15. Sodium and food sources. (February 29, 2016). Retrieved from http://www.cdc.gov/salt/food.htm

16. Sea salt vs table salt. (June 2014). Retrieved from http://sodiumbreakup.heart.org/wp-content/uploads/2014/06/SeaSaltTableSalt.jpg

17. Chen MA. (May 13, 2014). Potassium in diet. Retrieved from www.nlm.nih.gov/medlineplus/ency/article/002413.htm

18. Gavin ML. (July 2014). Minerals. Retrieved from http://kidshealth.org/en/teens/mineral-chart.html

19. Low potassium (hypokalemia). (July 8, 2014). Retrieved from http://www.mayoclinic.org/symptoms/low-potassium/basics/causes/SYM-20050632

20. Johnson LE. (2016). Overview of minerals. Retrieved from http://www.merckmanuals.com/home/disorders-of-nutrition/minerals/overview-of-minerals?qt=

21. High potassium (hyperkalemia). (November 25, 2014). Retrieved from http://www.mayoclinic.org/symptoms/hyperkalemia/basics/definition/SYM-20050776?p=1

22. Lewis JL III. (2016). Hypophosphatemia (low level of phosphate in blood). Retrieved from http://www.merckmanuals.com/home/hormonal-and-metabolic-disorders/electrolyte-balance/hypophosphatemia-(low-level-of-phosphate-in-the-blood)

23. Lanthanum. (May 15, 2014). Retrieved from https://www.nlm.nih.gov/medlineplus/druginfo/meds/a605015.html

24. Lewis JL. (2016). Hyperphosphatemia (high level of phosphate in blood). Retrieved from http://www.merckmanuals.com/home/hormonal-and-metabolic-disorders/electrolyte-balance/hyperphosphatemia-(high-level-of-phosphate-in-the-blood)

25. Key minerals to help control blood pressure. (August 1, 2015). Retrieved from http://www.health.harvard.edu/heart-health/key-minerals-to-help-control-blood-pressure

26. Nielsen F. (July 9, 2007). Do you have trouble sleeping? More magnesium might help. Retrieved from http://www.ars.usda.gov/News/docs.htm?docid=15617

27. Lewis JL III. (2016). Hypomagnesemia (low level of magnesium in the blood). Retrieved from http://www.merckmanuals.com/home/SearchResults?query=hypomagnesemia

28. Lewis JL III. (2016). Hypermagnesemia (high level of magnesium in the blood). Retrieved from http://www.merckmanuals.com/home/hormonal-and-metabolic-disorders/electrolyte-balance/hypermagnesemia-(high-level-of-magnesium-in-the-blood)

29. Higdon J, Drake VJE. (March 2010). Manganese. Retrieved from http://lpi.oregonstate.edu/mic/minerals/manganese

30. Micronutrient facts. (March 31, 2015). Retrieved from http://www.cdc.gov/immpact/micronutrients/index.html

31. Lewis JL III. (2016). Hypercalcemia (high level of calcium in the blood). Retrieved from https://www.merckmanuals.com/home/hormonal-and-metabolic-disorders/electrolyte-balance/hypercalcemia-(high-level-of-calcium-in-the-blood)

32. Wax E. (March 2, 2016). Fluoride in diet. Retrieved from https://www.nlm.nih.gov/medlineplus/ency/article/002420.htm

33. Water sanitation and health. (2001). Retrieved from http://www.who.int/water_sanitation_health/naturalhazards/en/index2.html

34. Wax E. (February 2, 2015). Copper in diet. Retrieved from https://www.nlm.nih.gov/medlineplus/ency/article/002419.htm

35. Johnson LE. (2016). Copper. Retrieved from https://www.merckmanuals.com/professional/nutritional-disorders/mineral-deficiency-and-toxicity/copper

WEB RESOURCES

American Heart Association http://www.heart.org/HEARTORG/HealthyLiving/HealthyEating/Nutrition/Nutrition_UCM_310436_SubHomePage.jsp

US National Library of Medicine https://www.nlm.nih.gov/medlineplus/minerals.html

National Center for Complementary and Integrative Health https://nccih.nih.gov/health/vitamins

Oregon State University Linus Pauling Institute http://lpi.oregonstate.edu/mic/minerals

Centers for Disease Control and Prevention http://www.cdc.gov/nutritionreport/

US Anti-Doping Agency http://www.usada.org/resources/nutrition/

SUGGESTED READING

United States Department of Agriculture Agricultural Research Service https://ndb.nal.usda.gov/ndb/nutrients/

Oregon State University Linus Pauling Institute http://lpi.oregonstate.edu/mic

Harvard Health Publications, Harvard Medical School http://www.health.harvard.edu/topics/healthy-eating

Water

> When the well is dry, we will know the worth of water.
>
> *Benjamin Franklin—*
> *Founding Father*

Learning Objectives

- Give an example of how the body attains homeostasis
- List important ways that water benefits the body
- Explain how water acts as a solvent during metabolic processes
- Discuss why the female body contains less water than does the male body
- Explain how we meet our daily need for water and the importance of meeting that need
- State the recommended daily intake for water and list sources
- Differentiate between water intoxication and water imbalance
- List symptoms of water dehydration
- Discuss the difference between hard and soft water
- Explain which water is best for drinking—tap, bottled, spring, or distilled

Key Terms

Antidiuretic Hormone (ADH)
Dehydration
Diuretic
Euhydration
Homeostasis

Hyperthermia
Hyponatremia
Potable
Solute
Vasopressin

INTRODUCTION

Water constantly recirculates but cannot be created, which means the amount on planet Earth is the same that was present at creation. Taken literally, this means it is possible you are drinking the same water as dinosaurs (www.epa.gov).

Water is second in importance after oxygen for sustaining life. You can survive about 28 days without food but find yourself fighting for life after 3 days of water deprivation. Although water covers 326 million cubic miles of the earth's surface, less than 1% is available for drinking. Ninety-nine percent of the earth's water is frozen in ice caps and icebergs or is oceanic salt water. The water your body *can* use is found in aquifers, rivers, and fresh water lakes. See Figure 7-1 for available drinking water on earth. Most of your daily replenishment is provided through daily allotment of food, drink, and that which is created during metabolic processes.

Just as water is abundant on earth, so it is in body tissues. Water is *everywhere* in the human body, with total composition being roughly 45% to 70% as illustrated in Figure 7-2. Your body's water content is more than the combined remaining hard structures. The range may seem large, but is dependent on fat content. The larger the amount of adipose tissue, the less percentage water composition. This means someone who carries around more adipose tissue would be at the lower end of the water composition range, and a body that is very lean would be at the high end of range. Women have a lower percentage of water than do men because they usually have more subcutaneous fat deposits

> *Even though your body can metabolically generate water, it is not enough to sustain you beyond a few days. Daily rehydration is vital for life.*

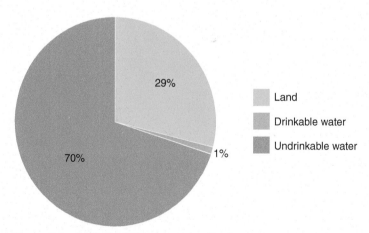

Figure 7-1   Available drinking water on Earth.

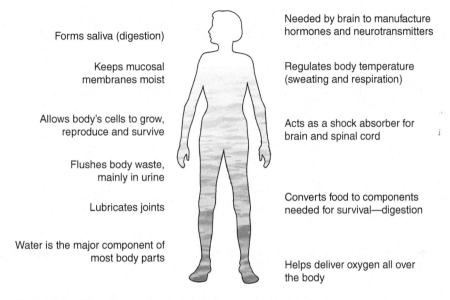

Forms saliva (digestion)

Keeps mucosal
membranes moist

Allows body's cells to grow,
reproduce and survive

Flushes body waste,
mainly in urine

Lubricates joints

Water is the major component of
most body parts

Needed by brain to manufacture
hormones and neurotransmitters

Regulates body temperature
(sweating and respiration)

Acts as a shock absorber for
brain and spinal cord

Converts food to components
needed for survival—digestion

Helps deliver oxygen all over
the body

Figure 7-2   What does water do for you.

(seen as cellulite). Table 7-1 estimates water content of body structures. For a visual of your body's total water content, picture 10- or 12-gallon containers lined up. That is how much water you carry around. You would think if we are made up of that much water we would slosh when we walked. We don't because most of our water is within every body cell, neatly encased by cell walls and membranes.

Table 7-1	Tissue Water Weight

The following are estimates of percentage of water weight of body organs:
Brain 90%
Lungs 90%
Blood 80%
Muscle 80%
Skin 80%
Organs 80%
Fat depots 25%
Bones 22%

MAJOR ROLE OF WATER IN THE HUMAN BODY

- Maintains homeostasis
- Removes and dilutes toxic waste
- Serves as a major transport system
- Regulates body temperature
- Protects delicate body tissues

Water Maintains Homeostasis

The main role of nutritive water is to maintain homeostasis (required level of water to remain stable) so your body can perform necessary chemical reactions. These functions require a delicate balance of fluid within the cells (accounts for two thirds of your body's water content) and outside and between cells (blood plasma and lymph). Figure 7-3 illustrates the flow of water between the two compartments. Water constantly passes in and out through cell membranes with the help of the electrically charged minerals: sodium, potassium, and chloride. This is sometimes referred to as *pumping action* that maintains water balance within and between our cells. Figure 7-4 lists additional contents of intracellular and extracellular fluid.

Orchestration of making adjustments to maintain the correct amount of fluid within and outside your cells is assisted by hormones and nerves. Body mechanisms that modulate the amount of fluid are exact to within a few hundred millimeters.[1] When water level is *low*, **extra**cellular ionic concentration *increases*. Water is drawn

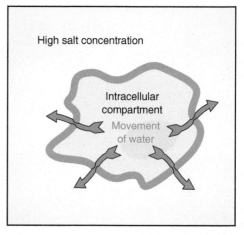

Figure 7-3   Flow of water.

Figure 7-4 Contents of intracellular and extracellular compartments.

from the intracellular compartment causing cells to collapse. Brain sensors pick up on this movement and send a message to the kidneys to concentrate and conserve urine output. The hormone that controls this process is called **vasopressin**, also known as **antidiuretic hormone (ADH)**.

When water level is *high*, the process works in reverse. More fluid flows **intra-cellularly**: cells puff up, sensors limit your drinking, and kidneys are on full alert to excrete urine. Health of your kidneys is vital for maintaining homeostasis. Providing a good amount of clean drinking water every day is a must. Diets that are high in salt, sugar, or artificial colorants and sweeteners (prepackaged, sodas, and fast food) put added stress on this vital organ.

Water Removes Toxic Waste

Water removes toxic waste such as dissolved flavoring compounds in food and *noxious substances* (poisonous) that are accidentally ingested. Your body must remove the waste, even in the absence of fluid intake, to keep from becoming ill or poisoned. Water removes toxic waste through various mechanisms.

- Two thirds leaves as urine. Kidneys help accomplish this by producing a minimum of one pint of urine each day.
- One third evaporates through the lungs and skin. You lose approximately 2.5 cups of fluid from normal perspiration and up to 3 gallons or more if exercising for an extended period in a hot climate.

It is *necessary* to drink pure water each day to provide your body with the ability to remove toxins and waste. Think of washing dirt from hands. You would not wash them in soda, juice, or milk as they would all leave more residue to clean.

Water Serves as a Major Transport System

Since both blood and lymph fluid are primarily water, maintaining an adequate level is necessary to complete their job. Blood and lymph systems are the body's roadway for delivering needed supplies to every body cell. Blood/plasma delivers oxygen, carbon dioxide, hormones, and nutrients. Lymph fluid delivers protein and infection-fighting white blood cells.

- Blood is 55% plasma; plasma is 92% water.
- Lymph fluid is 95% water.

Water Regulates Body Temperature

Maintaining normal body temperature is a dynamic relationship between heat production and heat loss. Your body's main mechanism for staying cool is by evaporating water through skin (sweat). The amount of sweat produced is dependent on level of physical activity and transient climate. More sweat would be produced running a marathon in a desert than walking through Central Park on a spring day.

If water lost through sweat is not replaced, you would be in a state of **hypohydration**, and your body's temperature would rise. Excessive sweating will result in loss of electrolytes and reduction of plasma volume. When this happens, your body reduces sweat output causing an increase in body temperature. This increase in temperature is called **hyperthermia**, which is a very dangerous predicament. Immediate rehydration is necessary to avoid heat exhaustion or heat stroke. Bringing the body back to **euhydration** (normal water levels) is necessary to maintain efficient body function.

Because the body uses water as a coolant, any condition that increases body temperature, such as physical activity or fever, increases the need for water.

Water Protects Delicate Body Tissues

Water is a component in biological fluids that cushion and protect body tissue. Some self-explanatory examples are

- Synovial fluid in joints
- Vitreous fluid in eyes
- Cerebrospinal fluid
- Mucus in the gastrointestinal and respiratory tracts

RECOMMENDED DAILY INTAKE

Required daily water intake is not a one size fits all. Individual water needs vary from person to person: amount and intensity of exercise, living environment, presence of chronic illness, pregnancy, or breast-feeding all weigh in on what is the right amount for you. Levels of hydration can vary throughout the day, so continually moderating your intake is necessary for optimum cognitive performance.[2] Every day, you lose an average of 10 cups of water through a combination of breathing, urination, and feces elimination. This amount must be replaced daily or the body will be in a state of **dehydration**. At the very least, humans need a little over one quart of water each day just to replenish unavoidable losses in urine, feces, sweat, and expired air. Eight 8-oz. glasses of water per day for the average *inactive* man or woman has been recommended, although the number 8 is not science based. According to a 2008 review of the literature, there is no supporting evidence for recommending "8 × 8" for everyone.[3] Your best bet is to pay attention to your innate wisdom. If you are thirsty, drink water. You can always check the color of your urine to determine if you are drinking enough: light yellow means right on target; dark yellow signals dehydration.

If you suddenly increase your intake of water, you will temporarily increase your frequency of urination. Over time, the body will eventually accommodate the increased water intake without any noticeable side effects.

Sources of Dietary Water

We meet our daily water needs through food and beverages and water created from metabolic processes.

- *Two thirds* comes from drinking water and beverages, including coffee, tea, and colas. Although caffeine has a **diuretic** effect, when consumed in moderation, it does contribute to daily fluid requirements.[4]

- *One third* comes from food. Most food offers the benefit of some water—even the driest cracker contains almost 3% of water. Fatty foods and those with high sucrose content provide very little water. Soup, salad, fruits, and vegetables are good sources of water. See Table 7-2 for water content of common foods.
- A little over *one cup* of water is released as the body metabolizes carbohydrates, proteins, and lipids.

Table 7-2	Percentage of Water in Common Foods
Food	**Water (%)**
Lettuce	98
Celery	96
Watermelon	92
Carrots	90
Milk	88
Oranges	87
Pears	85
Broccoli	85
Apples	84
Peaches	83
Blueberries	80
Beans	79
Eggs	75
Bread	37
Margarine	15
Nuts	5
Crackers	3

WATER INTOXICATION (HYPONATREMIA)— TOO MUCH

Hyponatremia (toxic water overdose) is *uncommon*, but does occur. It usually happens when you inadvertently drink too much water after exercising or finish off the glass or bottle too quickly. The kidneys are not able to eliminate water fast enough, and the water overload dilutes sodium levels. When sodium levels are low and water levels are too high, the water gets pulled into all your cells. This can lead to swelling inside the brain, which would require immediate attention.

Symptoms include headache, nausea, and uncoordinated movements with possible progression to unconsciousness, bloating, low body temperature, and seizures. The change in osmotic pressure as water flows from extracellular fluid into cells can put pressure on the brain, which can lead to seizures or death.

Even if your water level is normal (euhydration), any substance or state that alters sodium levels in the blood can create a state of hyponatremia: diarrhea and severe vomiting, kidney disease, cirrhosis of the liver, heart failure, and diuretic medications.

WATER DEFICIENCY (DEHYDRATION)—TOO LITTLE

Your body's innate wisdom will let you know when water stores are depleted and it is time to replenish. Thirst is the first sign of dehydration. Other initial physiologic effects are lowered physical and cognitive function and headache. As the condition worsens, you will begin to experience heartburn, stomach cramps, low back pain, or fatigue. If you do not immediately rehydrate, the condition progresses rapidly to exhaustion, delirium, and in the most extreme case, death. If you experience severe dehydration and too much time lapses before restoring water balance, your kidneys may have permanent damage.

Those who experience mild dehydration symptoms on a daily basis should keep in mind that certain foods are more dehydrating than others. Caffeinated beverages affect your hormones that regulate the body's fluid balance, causing water loss through urine production. Sugar and salt in fruit juices, soups, and soft drinks increase the concentration of solutes in blood. The body's first response is to pull fluid from the cells into the bloodstream to dilute the sugar and salt. Keeping these foods to a minimum in the diet and/or increasing dietary water intake will maintain better euhydration.

Thirst sensation diminishes as you age. The ability to conserve water is also reduced as you age, leading to frequent mild dehydration. This biologic change puts the elderly at higher risk for stroke.[5] Infants and children are also at risk of dehydration because their bodies contain more water per pound than do the bodies of adults. Need for hydration is greater for infants and small children.

Dehydration symptoms are as follows:

- thirst
- dark-yellow urine
- difficulty concentrating
- cognitive deterioration[2,6,7]
- slight headache[1,8]

FOOD FOR THOUGHT — PAY ATTENTION TO YOUR SENSE OF THIRST

- You eat pizza and find yourself feeling thirsty.
- Sodium from highly salted food accumulates in the extracellular fluid and pulls water from your cells.
- Sensors in the cells signal your brain of the danger in cellular dehydration and you become thirsty.
- You drink until you no longer feel thirsty.
- By drinking more than the cells need, your body will signal the kidneys to make more urine by filtering the excess fluid out of the blood.

The ability of the salt to attract water is the reason why it has been used to clean wounds and preserve meats. It kills bacteria by dehydrating them.

POTABLE WATER

Potable water is that which is fit to drink. The purest, healthiest, and tastiest water may be right from your tap. Depending on your municipality, tap water may be considered soft or hard. This will depend on the depth of well or water source and its natural mineral content. Since most water sources come from underground, it is important to have your water periodically tested.

Rainwater and irrigation leach pesticides, herbicides, and fertilizers into the water supply.

FOOD FOR THOUGHT — WHAT IS THE DIFFERENCE BETWEEN SOFT AND HARD WATER?

Soft Water
- Has a low mineral content
- Comes from sources *deep* in the ground
- Produces good soapsuds
- Pipes remain clean

Hard Water
- Usually high in calcium and magnesium
- Comes from *shallow* sources
- Reduces the sudsing action
- Produces mineral deposits in pipes, tubs, and sinks, and on clothes and dishware

STORING WATER

Sometimes it is necessary to store water for future use. If you live in a geographic area that requires storing days or months-worth of water, replenish holding containers with new water every few weeks so that bacteria do not grow.[9] Water is best stored in a bleach-sterilized container or one that was soaked in a baking soda solution. Glass containers are superior because plastic containers may leach harmful chemicals into the water when exposed to extreme temperatures.

BOTTLED WATER

The U.S. International Bottled Water Association expects profits to surpass 13 billion in 2015. More people are buying bottled water than ever imagined 20 years ago, with sales increasing exponentially each year. More than 700 brands of water are offered worldwide. Most bottled *drinking* water is simply municipal tap water that has been processed for purification and taste. Bottled water is not necessarily safer than tap water. Although bottled water plants are inspected by the U.S. Food and Drug Administration, budget and staffing constraints place monitoring at a low priority.[10]

The U.S. Food and Drug Administration (FDA) regulates bottled water, whereas the Environmental Protection Agency (EPA) regulates tap water.

With the increase in bottled water consumption, environmentalists encourage you to think of the 1.5 million tons of plastic containers used each year:

- Plastic bottles add to landfill overload (unless recycled)
- Bottling plants tax ground aquifers and streams
- Groundwater reserves are being depleted
- Pumping reduces the flow of streams and lakes, altering the ecosystems
- Transporting 30 billion of bottles around the world increases carbon dioxide emission

As dental professionals, you should be aware that not all bottled water contains fluoride. The only time the amount of fluoride is listed on the label is when it is added. Spring water is the most likely to contain fluoride as it is naturally available in groundwater. The following link is for the FDA Code of Federal Regulations #21 document that lists allowable amounts of chemicals in bottled water. http://www.accessdata.fda.gov/scripts/cdrh/cfdocs/cfcfr/cfrsearch.cfm?fr=165.110.

Bottled water packaged in the United States to which fluoride is added shall not contain fluoride in excess of specified levels and shall be based on the annual average of maximum daily air temperatures at the location where the bottled water is sold at retail.

TAP WATER

The EPA sets safety standards for tap water in the United States, imposing limits on 80 potential contaminants. Although your municipal water supply may meet these limits, it can still make you sick. In 2002, the EPA tested 8,100 of the 55,000 municipal water systems and found that 10% had unsafe levels of lead, which is known to cause permanent neurologic damage. Over a period of 2 years, the EPA issued more than 300,000 violations to water systems around the country for failing to test or treat the water properly. Many municipalities failed to notify the public when known contaminants were at higher-than-safe levels. Even if the contaminants in your tap water meet the minimum requirements, a lot can happen on its way to the tap, such as:

- Pesticide runoff into rivers and streams.
- Reaction between chlorine disinfectant and decaying leaves forms toxic by-products.
- Contamination with lead from old residential pipes.

For more information, read the published document by the U.S. EPA and learn about safe drinking water.

http://water.epa.gov/drink/guide/upload/book_waterontap_full.pdf   Water on Tap: What You Need to Know

Well water that pours from a tap is not regulated by the EPA. Monitoring of contaminants is the responsibility of the owner.

FOOD FOR THOUGHT   BOTTLED VERSUS TAP: WHICH IS BETTER?

Drinking bottled water or tap is no more than personal preference. People choose to drink bottled water for many reasons but improved taste, purity, and convenience predominate. Three main differences between the two sources:

	Type of Disinfection Used	Fluoride Content	Cost
Tap water	Chlorine added at treatment plant	Correct amount of fluorine ion added at treatment plant	$.004/gal
Bottled water	Ozonation and exposure to ultraviolet light to avoid chlorine aftertaste	Most bottled water does not contain fluoride. Spring water may have it if occurring naturally at point of source	$7.50/gal

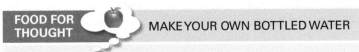

According to the Center for Disease Control, "boiling can be used as a pathogen reduction method that should kill all pathogens."

Make your own bottled water by drawing up a container of tap water, bring to a rolling boil for at least 1 minute; 10 minutes is better. The higher your altitude, the longer you should boil. Leave water uncovered and exposed to the air for 24 hours. Chlorine added to the water supply by the municipality (to disinfect) will dissipate into the air. Or, if you so choose, a filter can be installed for safer drinking water. See Table 7-3 for information on water filters.

Know what is in your water before boiling. Caution: Boiling nitrate- and lead-laced water increases the amount of nitrate and lead.

According to Mayo Clinic, some people have a higher risk of getting ill from contaminates in water. If you are undergoing chemotherapy, are diagnosed with HIV/ADIS, have a transplant or are pregnant, you should probably boil your tap water. One contaminant in particular—cryptosporidium—can cause death for someone with an immunocompromised system. Water treated by distillation and reverse osmosis can protect against it.

DISTILLED WATER AND SPRING WATER

Distilled water is processed to remove all minerals and impurities. It is advisable to keep bottles of distilled water capped when not in use because exposure to air causes impurities to be absorbed by the water. Distilled water is not recommended for drinking; there is speculation that when you drink distilled water, it can attract minerals from your body, depleting them as they are excreted in urine.

Spring water comes from a natural spring and contains minerals indigenous to the area. Trace minerals—calcium, magnesium, potassium, phosphorus, copper, and zinc—are sometimes too small to measure. If you want to bottle your own water from a nearby spring, ozonate or disinfect the water before drinking to minimize the possibility of ingesting dangerous bacterium such as *Giardia*, a microscopic parasite that causes diarrhea.

RELATE TO PATIENTS

The American Dental Association (ADA) recommends that you always inquire about primary and secondary sources of water on health history forms to identify the amount

Table 7-3	Water Filters		
Purification System	**What It Filters**	**What It Cannot Filter**	**Comments**
Carbon filter	Pesticides Chlorine	Inorganic chemicals Lead Biologic contaminants	
Ceramic filter	Rust Dirt Parasites	Organic pollutants Pesticides	
Ozone	Bacteria Viruses Algae Parasites	Heavy metals Minerals Pesticides	
Ultraviolet (UV) light	Bacteria Viruses	Heavy metals Pesticides Contaminants	
Ion exchange		Everything	Softens water
Copper–zinc (KDF)	Copper	Pesticides	Chemical reaction releases ozone that kills bacteria, chlorine, and heavy metals; works like a magnet
	Zinc	Organic contaminants	
Reverse osmosis	90%–80% heavy metals		Wastes 3–8 Ga of water for every gallon purified
	Bacteria Viruses Organic and inorganic chemicals		
Distillation	Bacteria		Uses more electricity than do other systems; produces heat when operating
	Viruses Parasites Pathogens Pesticides Herbicides Organic and inorganic chemicals Heavy metals Radioactive contaminants		Organic chemicals boil at a lower temperature than does water and will rise to mix with water vapor—ends up in drinking water

KDF, kinetic degradation fluxion.

of fluoride ingested in water. ADA supports the labeling of bottled water with the fluoride concentration of the product and means of contact, but support does not mean bottlers will follow their advice.

When determining how much water fluoridation benefit your patient receives, consider the following:

- Home water treatment systems may remove the fluoride in water.
- Bottled water may or may not contain fluoride.

When assessing total water consumption, advise your patient that:

- Beverages such as coffee, tea, soda, and alcohol are considered diuretics and actually deplete water stores. If consuming daily, increase water intake accordingly.
- Fruits and vegetables are the food groups that contain high amounts of water.
- Nuts, meats, grains, and fats have some water content, but much lower than that found in fruits and vegetables.

During initial assessment, determine:

- Moisture of mouth: Check for xerostomia and amount/nature of salivary flow of saliva.
- Level of activity and exercise: Patients should sip water every 15 minutes while exercising.
- Age: The very young and old are at greater risk for dehydration. We lose sense of thirst as we age, and preadolescents sweat less than do teens and adults, so body temperature rises rapidly during exercise
- Weather and climate: Hot, dry climates increase the body's need for water.
- Illness: Fever, diarrhea, and vomiting cause dehydration.
- Pregnancy: Water is needed to support increased blood supply.

Tips for increasing daily water intake are as follows:

- Drink a glass of water with each meal.
- Take a bottle/container of water when leaving for work and drink it in the car, train, or subway.
- Take a drink of water every time you pass a drinking fountain.
- Drink water while you prepare the evening meal.
- Take a water bottle with you when you exercise.
- Gradually increase the amount you drink to allow your bladder to adjust.
- Fill an empty milk container daily with water, and use it to replenish your cup or bottle to keep track of how much you drink.

PRACTICE FOR PATIENTS

Your patient is a 75-year-old female whom you suspect is undernourished. As is typical of septuagenarians, her sense of thirst is diminished. Upon oral examination, her gingival tissues appear anemic, she has chapped lips and dry skin, and her tissues stick to your gloves. You suspect she is dehydrated and is not drinking enough fluids or eating enough foods that are water dense. When you mention your suspicion to your patient, she acts surprised. She states she never feels thirsty so feels there is no need to increase fluid intake. Besides, drinking water makes her gag.

1. How can you explain the phenomenon of not feeling thirsty?
2. If water makes her gag, what other choices does she have for hydration?
3. If not corrected, what harm could come to her oral structures?

 RELATE TO YOU

Assignment #1

Find out if your drinking water is safe. Access the following landing page on the EPA Web site to learn more about your state's drinking water:

http://www3.epa.gov/enviro/facts/sdwis/search.html U.S. EPA Safe Drinking Water Information System

Assignment #2

Compare bottled water available at your grocery store

1. What types of bottled water are available?
2. If drinking water is available, is it bottled from another municipality in your state?

3. Call your city or county water utility and ask to speak with a chemist. Find out if your water is soft or hard. Ask which minerals are in the water and in what proportion.
4. Write a synopsis of the water purification system and the date of the last treatment center inspection.
5. Write an explanation of the benefits of keeping your body hydrated throughout the day.
6. List some situations that could dehydrate the body.
7. List some benefits to the oral cavity of staying hydrated.

REFERENCES

1. Popkin BM, D'Anci KE, Rosenberg IH. Water, hydration and health. *Nutr Rev* 2010;68(8):439–458.
2. Perry CS, Rapinett G, Glaser NS, et al. Hydration status moderates the effects of drinking water on children's cognitive performance. *Appetite* 2015;95:520–527.
3. Valtin H. Drink at least eight glasses of water a day. Really? Is there scientific evidence for 8 × 8? *Am J Physiol Regul Integr Comp Physiol* 2002;2833:R993–R1004.
4. Killer SC, Blannin AK, Jeukendrup AE. No evidence of dehydration with moderate daily coffee intake: a counterbalanced cross-over study in a free-living population. *PLoS One* 2014;9(1):e84154.
5. Frangeskou M, Lopez-Valcarcel B, Serra-Majeem L. Dehydration in the elderly: a review focused on economic burden. *J Nutr Health Aging* 2015;19(6):619–627.
6. Faraco G, Wijasa TS, Park L, et al. Water deprivation induces neurovascular and cognitive dysfunction through vasopressin-induced oxidative stress. *J Cereb Blood Flow Metab* 2014;34(5):853–860.
7. Masento NA, Golightly M, Field DT, et al. Effects of hydration status on cognitive performance and mood. *Br J Nutr* 2014;111(10):1841–1852.
8. Price A, Burls A. Increased water intake to reduce headache: learning from a critical appraisal. *J Eval Clin Pract* 2015;21:1212–1218.
9. Gerla SR, Lloyd MA, Eggett DL, et al. Microbial and chemical safety of non-commercially packaged water stored for emergency use. *J Water Health* 2015;13(3):819–826.
10. Hu Z, Morton LW, Mahler RL. Bottled water: United States consumers and their perceptions of water quality. *Int J Environ Res Public Health* 2011;8(2):565–578.

WEB RESOURCES

International Bottled Water Association www.bottledwater.org
The Public Health and Safety Company (certifies products and writes standards to protect food and water) www.nsf.org
U.S. Environmental Protection Agency www.epa.gov

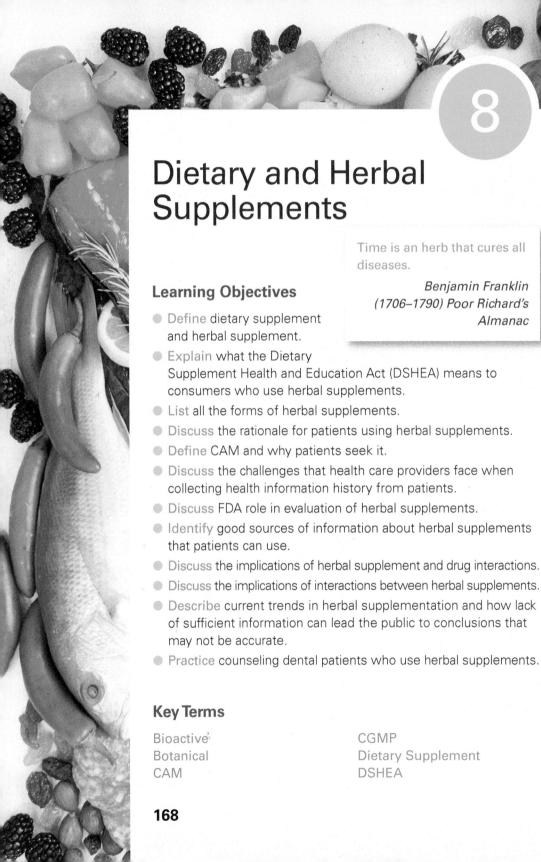

8

Dietary and Herbal Supplements

> Time is an herb that cures all diseases.
>
> *Benjamin Franklin (1706–1790) Poor Richard's Almanac*

Learning Objectives

- Define dietary supplement and herbal supplement.
- Explain what the Dietary Supplement Health and Education Act (DSHEA) means to consumers who use herbal supplements.
- List all the forms of herbal supplements.
- Discuss the rationale for patients using herbal supplements.
- Define CAM and why patients seek it.
- Discuss the challenges that health care providers face when collecting health information history from patients.
- Discuss FDA role in evaluation of herbal supplements.
- Identify good sources of information about herbal supplements that patients can use.
- Discuss the implications of herbal supplement and drug interactions.
- Discuss the implications of interactions between herbal supplements.
- Describe current trends in herbal supplementation and how lack of sufficient information can lead the public to conclusions that may not be accurate.
- Practice counseling dental patients who use herbal supplements.

Key Terms

Bioactive
Botanical
CAM

CGMP
Dietary Supplement
DSHEA

Hepatotoxicity
Herbal Supplement
ODS, Office of Dietary Supplements

Phytocannabinoids
Synergistic

INTRODUCTION

Dietary supplements have a broad definition that includes a variety of materials including vitamins, minerals, herbs, amino acids, and other compounds. Dietary supplements are taken orally in one of several forms: tablets, powders, gel forms, and liquids. The terms **herbal supplement** or **botanical** are used for products that are plants or some part of a plant. This definition includes leaves, flowers, stems, roots, and seeds. A herbal supplement may contain only one herb, or it may consist of several botanical components.[1] Later in the chapter is a discussion of the impact that the inclusion of multiple herbal components in a single supplement may have.

Herbal supplements are apart from the herbs added to foods because supplements are considered substances that are taken separately from food. Herbs used to flavor and enhance the enjoyment of food have long been an asset to the cook and the consumer. Herbs used in cooking can reduce or eliminate other additives in foods, especially salt, and are generally used in smaller amounts and in lower concentration than herbal supplements. However, herbal supplements may have interactions in the person's body with other supplements, medications, or disease conditions, and that is what this chapter is addressing.

RATE OF USAGE OF HERBAL SUPPLEMENTS

In the 2007 National Health Interview Survey (NHIS), it is reported that almost 18% of US adults used a nutritional supplement, other than vitamins or minerals, in the past year.[2] An additional survey of patients attending specialty clinics at Mayo Clinic reported that almost 40% of the patients were taking dietary supplements. Patients in treatment for fibromyalgia were taking supplements at a rate of 52%.[2]

The NHIS survey data also examined the expenditures made for supplements in the United States. When the survey was most recently conducted in 2007, approximately $30 million was spent on dietary supplements. When vitamins and minerals were excluded and herbals alone were considered, the expenditure was almost $15 million.[3] In 2010, the American Botanical Council conducted a survey that claimed an increase in use of herbal supplements by 2% each year since 2000. By 2010, the estimate for expenditures for herbal supplements was $5.2 *billion* in the United States.[4] Clearly, adults are willing to spend considerable sums in pursuit of health, prevention, or nondrug treatment of medical conditions.

Without doubt, any form of supplementation in pregnant and nursing women should be considered only with the consultation with their health care provider. However, the use of supplementation in children and adolescents is also to be considered. In the 2007 NHIS, almost 3 million children and adolescents were using herbal supplements. It is noted that children with chronic medical conditions who required long-term drug therapy and frequent trips to the physician were the mostly likely to be given supplements. Although the herbal supplement usage in children is considerably lower than that in adults, it is still of significance.[5]

Further examination of the NHIS data shows that about 40% of adults use one or more forms of **complementary and alternative medicine (CAM)** (see Chapter 18). CAM includes not only nonvitamin and nonmineral "natural" products but also forms of meditation, deep breathing, massage, and yoga.[3] Estimates for the cost of all CAM are upward of $38 billion a year beyond the cost of traditional medicine and prescription drug therapy. For many, herbal supplementation provides an attractive alternative to traditional medical treatment.[6]

PURPOSES OF HERBAL SUPPLEMENTATION

From the users' point of view, herbal supplementation serves many purposes. First, herbal supplementation is considered a "safe" alternative to traditional drug therapy. It is a form of "self-care" for people who believe that herbs can prevent or treat disease conditions. For many people who take herbal supplements, their intent is to promote wellness and avoid trips to the physician's office.[4,5] In fact, for many, herbal supplements are not considered medication at all and are infrequently reported to physicians on their medical history. Therefore, the interactions between herbal supplements themselves or between the herbal supplement and an OTC or prescription medication goes unrecognized because the patient has failed to fully disclose information to his or her health care provider.[4]

Although there are many reasons people choose to use herbal supplementation, some of the most common are[4]:

- Pain
- Anxiety, insomnia, and headache
- High cholesterol
- Upper respiratory infections, colds, and sore throat, mouth, or gums
- Memory
- Energy

Sources of high-quality scientific information about herbal supplements are available but may not be correctly interpreted by the person seeking information. Certainly, there are many unreliable sources readily available, and it is often difficult to discern what is legitimate and what is not. Historically, many health care providers have been skeptical about herbal supplementation for a number of reasons. First, the scarcity of well-designed research with reproducible results that demonstrate effectiveness of the herbal supplements for the conditions for which they are promoted brings the usefulness of the supplement into question. Secondly, many health care providers lack training and experience in the field of herbal supplements. Finally, concerns about lack of information regarding safety of the herbal supplement cause health care providers to discourage their use, especially in patients who are taking other medications.[4]

FOOD FOR THOUGHT   **TIPS FOR HEALTH CARE PROVIDERS**[4]

- Encourage patients to eat a varied and healthy diet.
- Invite patients to discuss their supplements and rationale for taking them.
- Do the search of the literature to determine safety, effectiveness, and interactions between supplements and medications.
- Educate patients about herbal supplements.
- Help the patient to determine if the supplement is of high quality.
- Monitor the patient's response to the herbal supplement.
- Document and report adverse reactions.

REGULATION OF SUPPLEMENTS

In 1994, Congress passed the Dietary Supplement Health and Education Act, 1994 (DSHEA), which defined and set standards for **dietary supplements**. Dietary supplements are recognized as vitamins, amino acids, minerals, herbs, or botanicals that can be in tablet, capsule, powder, tea, softgel, gelcap, or liquid form. Their purpose is not to replace food as a source of valuable nutrition, but as an addition to the diet for "health promotion and disease prevention."[7] Congress was committed to providing safe supplements that Americans could use with confidence. This act gave authority to the federal government, more specifically the U.S. Food and Drug Administration (FDA), to ensure the safety of supplements and the accuracy of marketing claims.[7] Food for Thought below is a synopsis of the 1994 DSHEA law.

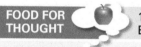

FOOD FOR THOUGHT   1994 DIETARY SUPPLEMENT HEALTH AND EDUCATION ACT[7]

- Product intended to supplement the diet
- Tablet, capsule, powder, softgel, gelcap, or liquid form
- Not to be used as conventional food or as the sole item of a meal
- Labeled as a dietary supplement

Primary regulation of herbal supplements is under the purview of the FDA. The FDA is well known for its regulation of prescription and OTC medications, and it is equally instrumental in the regulation of herbal and other dietary supplements. The Current Good Manufacturing Practices (CGMPs) for dietary supplements is an important milestone in assuring quality, safety, and manufacturing control for supplements. CGMP requires that the FDA ensure supplements meet specific standards.

For example, in the Final Rule of the CGMP of 2007, manufacturers of dietary supplements, including herbal supplements, must:

- Have quality control procedures in the manufacturing process
- Test the listed ingredients
- Assure that the final product is free of contamination by toxins, bacteria, pesticides, glass, lead, or heavy metals
- Be packaged and labeled accurately[8]

In 2015, the New York State Attorney General began an investigation that brought several herbal supplements into question. Following DNA testing of multiple samples of the products, it was found that a number of herbal supplements being marketed contained substances that were not listed on the label. Fortunately, the extraneous substances were innocuous items such as rice, beans, pine, citrus, asparagus, and wheat. Some of the DNA testing revealed that the product contained *none* of the supplement that was on the label. This single event caused nationwide questions about the safety and quality of herbal supplements.[9]

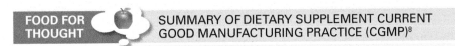

FOOD FOR THOUGHT   SUMMARY OF DIETARY SUPPLEMENT CURRENT GOOD MANUFACTURING PRACTICE (CGMP)[8]

- Manufacturers must:
  - Report adverse events related to the supplement to FDA
  - Establish quality control procedures at manufacturing plants
  - Test ingredients of the finished product and determine that the product is free of contamination
  - Assure that labeling is accurate and that the contents on the label are in the product
  - Identify the purity, strength, and composition of their products
  - Verify their products are safe

FDA regulations do not require supplements to undergo the same rigorous evaluation process that is used for prescription or OTC drugs.[9]

ADVERTISING PRACTICES AND REGULATION

Once a supplement is on the market and being used by consumers, the FDA continues its work to monitor and assure that the labeling, packaging, and insert information is correct and that claims the producer of the supplement makes are accurate. The Federal Trade Commission (FTC) also plays a role in verifying that all advertising of the product presents the product accurately.[1]

While it is best that marketing claims are based on multiple studies with large sample sizes and well-designed methods, most marketing is designed to promote sales based upon[10]:

- History of use for generations, so it must be effective (such as mother's home remedy)
- A few small, poorly designed studies that have not stood the test of replication of findings in additional studies
- Anecdotal evidence, testimonials, and hearsay, often from unqualified or inexperienced individuals

More than half of regular supplement users say they would continue using a supplement despite evidence that the supplement is ineffective. Additionally, most users have indicated that they feel supplements are safe, natural, and hold no potential harm for the users. Concerns are even further exacerbated because FDA cannot require manufacturers to use cautionary language or warnings on supplement labels.[3]

The most common sources of marketing of supplements are health food stores, pharmacies, and supermarkets, print media (newspaper and magazines), television, and Internet.[10]

- Health food store employees and owners boast of being CAM-trained herbalists; however, the credentials for complementary health practitioners vary greatly from state to state. Still, most states require significant training in health care for a practitioner to make such a claim.[11] A Canadian study indicated that consumer questions asked of health food store staff showed as much as 88% error in information provided, in that the information was unscientific and unsupported.[10] In one case study cited in research conducted in the CAM Program at the University of Iowa, a patient experiencing a recurrence of head and neck cancer sought advice from a local health food store owner who recommended numerous herbal supplements so that she could avoid radiation and chemotherapy for her cancer.[12] Although this is undoubtedly an extreme example, patients should be advised to do their own research and should know where to find the most reliable information.

- Pharmacies and supermarket pharmacies fared much better in the Canadian study in which pharmacists and staff provided accurate, well-supported information to the majority of consumer questions.[10] The National Library of Medicine has developed online resources/databases for pharmacists. The databases are an asset to pharmacists and other health care professionals who can readily access information not only on drugs but also on herbal supplements, thus adding to the truthfulness and completeness of the information they disseminate.[13]

- Print media are by far the most popular marketing tools for sellers of herbal supplements. Many of the supplements marketed are mixtures of several supplements, and almost all target a specific condition to be impacted by the supplement such as immune system, weight loss, or memory. Generally, somewhere in the small print is a disclaimer as to the effectiveness, content, and harmlessness of the product.[10]

- Television "infomercials" are relative newcomers to the marketing of herbal supplements.[10] Similar to print marketing, the products are usually combinations of herbs, vitamins, minerals, amino acids, and even hormones. And there is usually a disclaimer statement on the screen with ordering information.

- The most recent addition to sources of information about herbal supplements is the Internet. A person can search for any product and find a host of sellers and claims. Internet marketing also provides an opportunity for adding "cookies" and "spam" mail to the end user's computer so that more products can be put before the consumer. Of course, the Internet is also an excellent tool for finding valuable information about supplements. At the end of this chapter is a listing of Internet resources that provide balanced, well-informed content to help consumers decide about herbal supplements. One such resource is the **Office of Dietary Supplements** at https://ods.od.nih.gov/. The **ODS** was formed within the National Institutes of Health in the DSHEA to explore and identify the benefits of dietary supplements and to promote scientific study of supplements. Both functions are positive in regard to the consumer identifying herbal supplementation and the promotion of good health and the prevention of chronic disease.[7]

Below is a summary of sources of information about herbal supplements.[4]

- Product labels
- Television and radio
- Magazines
- Internet
- Health food stores/clerks
- Family and friends
- Physicians and CAM practitioners

HERBAL SUPPLEMENTS AND DRUG INTERACTIONS

Herbal supplements are bioactive substances[10] and are capable of participating in chemical reactions within cells and body fluids. For that reason, herbal supplements can have a number of adverse effects as well as benefits and improved health just as drugs do. In fact, many prescription and OTC drugs have their origins in herbal medicine. For example, atropine, a drug used to treat a slow heart rate, has its origins in the deadly nightshade herbal plant[14] and aspirin, an analgesic and anti-inflammatory drug, has its origins in the bark of a willow tree.

Bioactivity of a herbal supplement also varies between the brands and the combinations. In some documented cases, it even varies between the pill and capsule in the same bottle! Variations are caused by differences in soil; weather conditions during growing season, such as moisture; temperature; and harvesting time and technique. Once the product is delivered to the manufacturer, variations may occur because of contamination with metals and microbes.[15]

In a study conducted in 2012, investigators identified over 1,400 different drug interactions between 200 supplements and 500 medications.[14] Moreover, this statistic may be compounded by the underreporting of interactions by patients to their physician; it may be of even greater predominance than known.[2] Supplements are particularly popular with patients who suffer from chronic diseases and cancer.[15] This describes many of our patients, and drug interactions with herbal supplements bear serious consideration.

Indeed, a brief survey of prescription drugs reveals the side effects and drug interactions that are possible. Any substance that is taken into the body has the possibility (if not the probability) to produce an adverse event; however, the difference between drugs and herbals is that drugs are tested and the probability of an adverse event is calculated and divulged to the health care provider and the patient prior to taking the drug. In addition, the adverse effects of the drug are typically known, and the patient will know what to look for if the adverse effect occurs and can seek care immediately. In the case of herbal supplements, this is not usually the case.

Possible drug/herbal supplement interactions include hepatotoxicity (liver damage),[16] excessive bleeding, and increasing or decreasing the intended effects of the drug.[15] The pathway through which this can occur has to do with metabolism of the drug and the herbal supplement by liver enzymes. Drugs that are metabolized by liver enzymes include

- Statins (cholesterol-lowering drugs)
- Macrolide antibiotics
- Some calcium channel blockers (for various types of cardiovascular disease)
- Specific types of antidepressants
- Warfarin (a blood thinner)
- Benzodiazepines (sedatives)
- NSAIDs (ibuprofen)[2]

This is not a complete list!

If the herbal supplement is metabolized by the same liver enzyme as the drug, a competition for the enzyme can occur, and the rate of availability of the drug and rate at which it is metabolized is altered. Consequently, the effectiveness of the drug may be increased or decreased. If the drug effectiveness is increased, overdose is possible; if the drug effectiveness is decreased, the disease condition could worsen.

A sampling of serious supplement–drug interactions is given below.

Cranberry[4,6]

- Contains salicylic acid (aspirin, a mild anticoagulant) within the cranberry
- Interacts with anticoagulant medications (e.g., warfarin) to increase their effects
  - Increased bleeding risk

Echinacea[4,16]

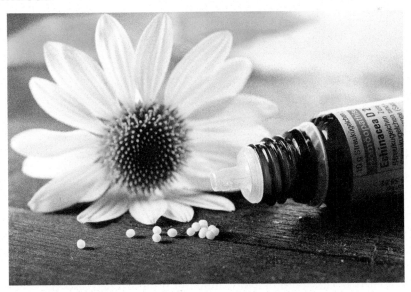

- Interacts with methotrexate, a drug used to treat psoriasis, rheumatoid arthritis, and several types of cancer (breast, lung, head and neck, lymphoma, leukemia)
  - Increases **hepatotoxicity**, resulting in liver damage

- Interacts with immunosuppression medications given to prevent transplant rejection
  - Decreases effects of the drugs and increases likelihood of rejection

Flaxseed[4]

- Functions to clear the colon
  - Decreases absorption of water and drugs from the digestive tract
  - Decreases effects of any drug that must be absorbed from the digestive tract

Garlic[2,16]

- Effects of garlic are anticoagulation.
- Interacts with warfarin, an anticoagulant medication
  - Increases bleeding risk due to additive effects
- Interacts with protease inhibitors, such as saquinavir (used to treat HIV)
  - Interacts with liver enzymes to decrease antiviral effects

Ginkgo (Ginkgo Biloba)[16]

- Interacts with warfarin due to additive effects
  - Increases bleeding risk and hemorrhage
- Interacts with omeprazole, a drug used to treat GERD and ulcers
  - Omeprazole is a proton pump inhibitor drug that decreases the production of stomach acid.
  - Decreases drug effects when combined with ginkgo and increases production of stomach acid

Ginseng[16]

- Interacts with warfarin
  - Increases clotting risk
- Interacts with prednisolone
  - Prednisolone is a corticosteroid that has anti-inflammatory effects.
  - Prednisolone is used to treat allergies, arthritis, asthma, lupus, and colitis.
  - Prednisolone has an impact on the immune system.
  - Increases effects of prednisolone due to additive effects.
- Interacts with antiglycemic medications used to treat diabetes
  - Causes additive decreases in blood sugar levels (possible hypoglycemia)
- Interacts with immunosuppression drugs
  - Decreases effect of immunosuppression and increases probability of rejection

Goldenseal[2]

- Used to treat respiratory tract infections, sore gums, and throat
- Interacts with *many* drugs to increase their effects:
  - Antiemetic drugs, used to stop vomiting
  - Antiarrhythmic drugs such as propranolol, quinidine, tocainide, and lidocaine
  - Beta-blockers used to control hypertension
  - Neuroleptic drugs (antipsychotics)
  - Tricyclic antidepressants

- ○ Statins (used to control hypercholesterolemia)
- ○ Macrolide antibiotics

Green tea[4,16,17]

- Very popular with consumers, found as part of Chinese herbal medicine regimens, and *Ayurvedic* herbal products from India
- Known to interact with anticoagulant medications to decrease their effect (increases likelihood of clotting)
- Suspected of interactions with penicillin and other antibiotics, benzodiazepines, beta-blockers, and drugs used for chemotherapy and antipsychotic and antidepressant drugs

Kava[6,16]

- Suspected of many drug interactions
- Known to cause hepatotoxicity when taken with many drugs
- Increases sedative effects of benzodiazepines

Licorice Root[16]

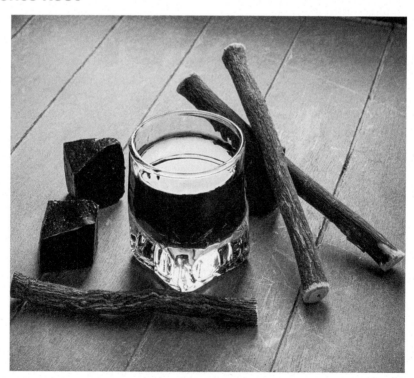

- Produces hypokalemia (low levels of potassium in the blood) when taken with prednisolone
- Decreases the effects of spironolactone, a drug used to treat heart failure, edema, liver and kidney disease, and hypertension

St. John's Wort[2,6,16]

- Many, many known drug interactions and many more suspected
- Increases the effects of
  - Warfarin
  - Methotrexate
- Decreases the effects of
  - Cyclosporine (an immunosuppression drug), thus increasing the risk of transplant rejection
  - Protease inhibitors such as saquinavir and indinavir (interacts with liver enzymes to reduce effectiveness of the inhibitors)
  - Benzodiazepines
  - Digoxin used to treat atrial fibrillation of the heart
  - Imatinib, an anticancer drug
  - Statins used to reduce cholesterol in the blood
  - Calcium channel blockers such as nifedipine and verapamil used to treat hypertension, angina, and arrhythmia
  - Tricyclic antidepressants

Be aware that this is by no means a complete list of drug interactions. It simply represents a few of the more commonly used herbal supplements. Nor does it include interactions that may occur between two or more herbal supplements.

ONGOING RESEARCH IN THE FIELD OF HERBAL SUPPLEMENTATION

The ongoing research falls into several categories. The FDA responds to research findings and reports by posting "Dietary Supplement Alerts and Safety Information" on the FDA Web site at www.fda.gov/Food/RecallsOutbreaksEmergencies?SafetyAl ertsAdvisories/default.htm. Similarly, NCCIH posts "Alerts and Advisories" on their Web site at www.nccih.nih.gov/news/. NCCIH, ODS, and the National Cancer Institute work together to support, fund, and conduct research in the area of botanicals. The particular areas of study include[1]

- Effects of herbal supplements on the human body
- Evaluation of existing research for validity
- Education of the public
- Study of the mechanisms of action and the bioactive properties of the chemical components of herbals
- Conduction of clinical trials

NCCIH also sponsors special research related to herbals[1]:

- Antioxidant therapy
- Autoimmune and inflammatory diseases and herbal remedies
- Polyphenols[18] found in herbs and their role in treatment and prevention of chronic noncommunicable and inflammatory diseases
- Treatment of pancreatic diseases
- Treatment for colorectal cancer

How exciting to know that research is progressing in this area of science and health improvement!

COMMON HERBS REPORTED ON MEDICAL AND DENTAL HISTORIES

Most of the information for this section comes from https://nccih.nih.gov/health/ herbsataglance.htm, https://www.nlm.nih.gov/medlineplus/druginfo/herb_All.html, and http://umm.edu/health/medical/altmed.

These resources are excellent sources of information to use when counseling patients about herbal supplements. The list included here is hoped to represent some of the most common herbal supplements used by patients. As research is conducted, the information will likely change and will be supported by new and stronger documented evidence. This is not intended to be a memorization exercise but a practice on finding, analyzing, and using vital information to assist patients in making good choices.

Acai

- **Functions or activity in the body**
  - Folk remedy for weight loss and "antiaging" antioxidant
  - Research in use as a contrast agent for MRI study of the GI tract
  - Lab studies indicate possible use as an anticancer and anti-inflammatory agent.
- **Cautions**
  - None when consumed as a fruit or juice in a healthy diet

Aloe Vera

- **Functions or activity in the body**
  - Treatment of skin lesions such as burns, psoriasis, and herpetic lesions
  - Powerful laxative, also causes severe abdominal cramping
  - Natural food flavoring
  - Works in a **synergistic** way to increase the effects of the following drugs in the treatment of some conditions:
    - Some antiglycemic medications to lower blood glucose level of hyperglycemia (use only under the direction of a physician)
    - Hydrocortisone to reduce swelling
- **Cautions**
  - Works synergistically with digoxin and diuretic medications to decrease potassium levels in the blood
  - May inhibit healing of deep wounds
  - May have carcinogenic effects when oral forms are used (results of animal testing)

Asian Ginseng

- **Functions or activity in the body**
  - Reduces risk of cold or flu
  - Antioxidant properties that might help lower LDL cholesterol and raise HDL (consult with physician)
  - Improves mental function. Synergistic with ginkgo biloba
- **Cautions**
  - May raise blood sugar levels in diabetics
  - Interactions with caffeine or other stimulants causing nervousness and insomnia
  - Do not use in the presence of diabetes, hypertension, HIV, or when having surgery

Bilberry

- **Functions or activity in the body**
  - Contains vitamin C
  - Antioxidant properties
  - Contains anti-inflammatory components, which reduce intestinal inflammation

- **Cautions**
  - May lower blood sugar and therefore should not be used with drugs that lower blood sugar
  - May act as a blood thinner and therefore should not be used with anticoagulant drugs

Chamomile

- **Functions or activity in the body**
  - Traditionally used for insomnia, upset stomach, and mouth ulcers
  - Treatment for mucosal ulcers resulting from chemotherapy or radiation of the head and neck
  - Ongoing research for treatment of anxiety and pain due to bowel disorders
- **Cautions**
  - Allergy

Cinnamon

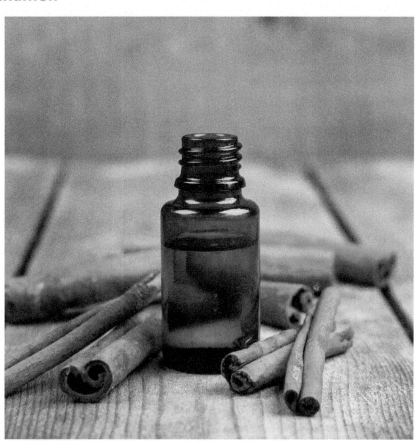

- **Functions or activity in the body**
  - ○ Used for many folk remedies; very popular supplement
  - ○ Cooking spice, great in mulled wine and coffee cake
  - ○ Contains blood-thinning compound similar to warfarin
  - ○ Insufficient scientific trials to support many of the claims
- **Cautions**
  - ○ Allergy
  - ○ Do not use with anticoagulant drugs

Clove

- **Functions or activity in the body**
  - ○ Cooking spice
  - ○ Traditionally used for toothache pain and dry socket but no longer recommended by FDA for these functions. However, clove oil does contain a compound that relieves pain in a way similar to topical anesthetic.
  - ○ Expectorant, to help in the removal of mucous from the respiratory tract
- **Cautions**
  - ○ Avoid frequent application to gingiva
  - ○ Inhaling clove smoke causes lung infections and breathing difficulties
  - ○ Slows blood clotting; do not use in presence of bleeding dyscrasia, anticoagulant, NSAIDs, or before surgery
  - ○ Interacts with other herbs that slow blood clotting: garlic, ginger, ginkgo, and turmeric

Cranberry

- **Functions or activity in the body**
  - ○ Prevention (not treatment) of urinary tract infections by preventing bacteria from adhering to the walls of the urinary tract
  - ○ Prevention of the ulcer-causing bacteria, *Helicobacter pylori*, from living in the stomach
  - ○ Ongoing studies regarding the use of cranberry in the treatment of cancer, raising HDL (good cholesterol) and fighting viral and bacterial infections
- **Cautions**
  - ○ Increased risk of kidney stones.
  - ○ Allergy to aspirin strongly predisposes person to allergy to cranberry.
  - ○ Increased risk of bleeding when taken with warfarin or aspirin.
  - ○ Do not use with medications that affect the liver; toxicity is possible.

Dandelion

- Functions or activity in the body
  - Contains vitamins A, B complex, C, and D
  - Contains minerals iron, potassium, and zinc
  - Used as flavoring in food and drinks
  - Acts as a diuretic, though no good research supports the claim
- Cautions
  - Allergy.
  - Increases occurrence of heartburn and skin irritation.
  - Because of diuretic properties, other drugs are removed from the body more rapidly, reducing their effectiveness.
  - Do not use if taking medications for diabetes, the antibiotic ciproflaxin (a derivative of dandelion), anticoagulants, or lithium for bipolar disorder.

Echinacea

- Functions or activity in the body
  - Traditional uses include treatment for scarlet fever, diphtheria, sexually transmitted disease, and colds and flu.
  - Studies indicate support of the immune system.
  - Pain relief through reduction of inflammation.
  - Antioxidant properties.
  - Antiviral properties.
- Cautions
  - Cause medications that suppress the immune system to decrease in effectiveness. Therefore, use of echinacea could cause impact on the treatment of the following diseases:
    - Autoimmune diseases
    - HIV/AIDS
    - Multiple sclerosis
    - Leukemia
    - Diabetes
    - Transplant patients
- Interactions with antifungal medications, immunosuppressants, and caffeine

Ginkgo Biloba

- Functions or activity in the body
  - May improve circulation in the legs
  - Antioxidant properties

- Many claims, little scientific evidence
  - Anxiety, schizophrenia, ADHD, autism, and depression
  - Diabetic neuropathy (nerve disease) or nephropathy (kidney disease)
  - Memory improvement, slowing the progress of Alzheimer's disease
  - Blood pressure control
  - Cancer prevention
- May be effective in treatment of macular degeneration of the retina
- **Cautions**
  - Ginkgo Evaluation of Memory study found no effectiveness for treatment of dementia, Alzheimer's, or the improvement of memory.
  - Added to nutrition bars, drinks, and fruit smoothies—beware if allergy is present.
  - Ginkgo seeds are toxic and can cause seizures and death. Most supplements do not contain seed parts.
  - Do not use prior to surgery.
  - Interactions with medications used to treat seizures and some antidepressants (SSRIs and MAOIs)
  - Interactions with medications used to treat:
    - High blood pressure and cardiac conditions (calcium channel blockers and diuretics)
    - Anxiety (alprazolam)
    - Pain and inflammation (ibuprofen)
    - Diabetes
    - Autoimmune diseases (cyclosporine)
    - Depression (trazodone)

Goldenseal

- **Functions or activity in the body**
  - Proven to kill many pathogenic microbes in test tube lab experimentation, but no human trials support findings
    - Antiseptic on minor wounds
    - Relief of sore throat caused by upper respiratory infection
- **Cautions**
  - Little scientific evidence to support any claim.
  - Touted to eliminate evidence of drug use in a drug test—no scientific support for this—not worth trying!
  - Interactions with other medications are likely.

Grape Seed Extract

- **Functions or activity in the body**
  - Antioxidant properties
  - Contains vitamin E
  - Treatment for chronic venous insufficiency (inadequate blood flow from legs back to heart)
  - Edema (inflammation) following surgery or injury
  - Prevention of growth of breast, stomach, colon, prostate, and lung cancer cells was proven in test tube laboratory research, but no documented evidence of this in humans as yet. Studies are ongoing.
- **Cautions**
  - Interactions with any medication broken down by liver enzymes
  - Interactions with anticoagulants

Kava

- **Functions or activity in the body**
  - Treatment of anxiety and insomnia
  - Tends to increase cognitive function
  - In animal studies, reduces convulsions and functions in muscle relaxation and in pain relief
- **Cautions**
  - Reported cases of liver damage, especially when combined with other herbal supplements or any drugs metabolized by the liver.
  - Avoid kava if depression, hepatitis, or Parkinson's disease is present.
  - Prolongs the effects of anesthetics.
  - Increases the effects of anticonvulsant medications, alcohol, and several anti-anxiety medications.

Lavender

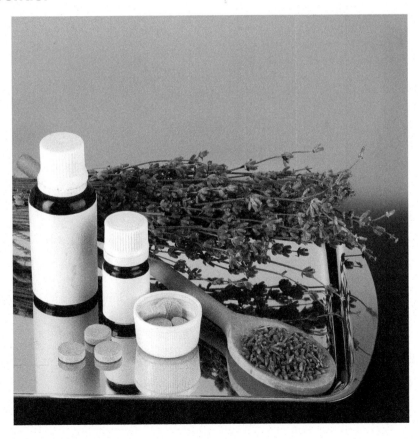

- **Functions or activity in the body**
  - Aromatherapy produces relaxing and sedative effects
  - Oil used in massage therapy
  - Ongoing studies for its antibacterial and antiviral functions
- **Cautions**
  - Oil is toxic if swallowed.
  - Allergy.
  - Interacts with narcotics, sedatives, and antianxiety medications to increase their function.

Licorice Root

- **Functions or activity in the body**
  - Many functions claimed, but poorly supported by research
    - Ulcers: peptic ulcer and aphthous ulcer
    - GERD
    - Cold and flu
    - Weight loss
- **Cautions**
  - Edema
  - Avoid licorice when following conditions are present:
    - Cardiovascular disease
    - Certain cancers
    - Diabetes
    - Kidney or liver disease
- Interacts with ACE inhibitors (for hypertension) and diuretics, corticosteroids, insulin, and oral contraceptives

Noni

- **Functions or activity in the body**
  - Popularly, the juice is used for cardiovascular disease and diabetes control.
  - Antioxidant properties
  - May have stimulating effect on immune system as indicated in laboratory tests
- **Cautions**
  - Reports of liver damage
  - High in potassium, not to be used by people with kidney disease

Passionflower

- **Functions or activity in the body**
  - Increases function of GABA in the brain causing relaxation and decreasing anxiety

- **Cautions**
  - Synergistic interaction with sedative medications
    - Anticonvulsants
    - Benzodiazepines
    - Anticoagulants

Peppermint Oil

- **Functions or activity in the body**
  - Flavoring for food
  - In the laboratory, demonstrates antibacterial, antifungal, and antiviral properties
  - Aids in digestion of fats by improving release of bile
  - Reduction in symptoms of irritable bowel syndrome (IBS)
  - Contains menthol, which is a good expectorant to relieve congestion
- **Cautions**
  - Avoid in cases of GERD.
  - Large doses are toxic.
  - Allergy.
  - Interacts with drugs that reduce stomach acid (antacids).
  - Interacts synergistically with drugs that lower blood sugar.
  - Interacts with drugs metabolized by the liver enzymes.

Pomegranate

- **Functions or activity in the body**
  - Antioxidant properties and contains polyphenol
  - Reduces infection and inflammation
  - In mouthwash, helps control plaque
  - Ongoing study on effects of pomegranate on:
    - Arthritis
    - Cancer
    - Atherosclerosis
- **Cautions**
  - Interactions with blood pressure medications, statins for cholesterol management, and warfarin

St. John's Wort

- **Functions or activity in the body**
  - Folk remedy for depression; effective for mild to moderate depression
- **Cautions**
  - Photosensitivity
  - Infertility
  - Not for use in people with major depression
  - Increases side effects of medications used to treat depression
  - Decreases effectiveness of antihistamines
  - Decreases effectiveness of immunosuppressants
  - Avoid use when taking antiviral medications for HIV

Saw Palmetto

- **Functions or activity in the body**
  - Insufficient evidence to support claim of prevention of benign prostatic hypertrophy
  - May improve urinary tract function
- **Cautions**
  - Interacts with warfarin and aspirin (anticoagulant and antiplatelet)
  - Need to assure diagnosis of benign hypertrophy over prostate cancer before considering use

Turmeric

- **Functions or activity in the body**
  - Related to ginger
  - Used in cooking, especially Indian cuisine
  - Antioxidant and anti-inflammatory properties
  - Treatment of ulcerative colitis
  - Treatment of osteoarthritis
- **Cautions**
  - Avoid when taking medications to lower blood sugar
  - Interacts with blood thinner medications
  - Increases stomach acid when used with antacids

Valerian

- **Functions or activity in the body**
  - Improves sleep by reducing time to fall asleep and improves quality of sleep
- **Cautions**
  - Research varies on the time and dosage to achieve improvements in sleep.
  - Withdrawal symptoms are possible.
  - Interacts with sedative medications and anesthetics by increasing their effects.

TRENDS IN HERBAL SUPPLEMENTS

Soy

Soy is a product used by many as a substitute for meat and dairy products. Soy comes from the soybean, which is in the pea family. It is very popular in vegetarian diets as a protein source. However, it is also a popular supplement and has been associated with providing relief from symptoms of menopause and memory loss. Today, it is used to prevent a variety of conditions from hypertension to cancer and osteoporosis.

There is a great need for additional research in the area of soy supplements for it is used very frequently and little information is available. Without doubt, soy is safe in the diet for most people. On the other hand, supplementation with soy in large amounts or over extended periods of time has been implicated in risk of endometrial hyperplasia, which could lead to cancer.

Soy contains high level of isoflavones, which are similar in chemical structure and function to female hormones and may have unexpected effects on the body.

Marijuana

Marijuana supplements come from all parts of the marijuana plant—leaves, flowers, stems, and seeds—and are called **phytocannabinoids**.[19] The active chemical in the plant is *9-tetrahydrocannabinol* or THC. In similarly, to all herbal supplements, the active ingredient, THC, varies within the supplement and the amount of variation is dependent upon the concentration THC within the plant and the plant part.[20]

THC enters the bloodstream either through the lung (if smoked) or through the intestine (if ingested) and travels to the brain and other organs. Specific receptors on neural cells of the brain interact with THC to produce the desired effects of altered sensations, altered sense of time, and altered mood. Some of the effects that are less desirable include loss of body control, impaired thought processing, and loss of memory and recall.[20]

THC, when used over extended periods of time in young people has an impact on brain development that reduces learning functions. Remember, the human brain continues development well into the twenties and the neural interactions and pathways may be altered by many chemicals during this time, which can permanently impair neural functions. Contrary to popular belief, research indicates that marijuana can be addictive, especially when used at a young age.[21]

Synthetic cannabinoids are often used for therapeutic purposes as well as the plant forms.[19] This form and natural plant forms are the subjects of numerous ongoing research projects for use as "medical marijuana."[21] As with many herbal supplements, marijuana benefits must be considered along with its negative effects. Benefits for use of marijuana include relief of chronic pain or severe pain associated with terminal illness and HIV. THC is known to improve symptoms of nausea and increase appetite in chemotherapy and radiation patients. It may also reduce inflammation. Research is also being conducted on its effects on seizures and mental illness. THC is currently undergoing trials to evaluate its effect on patients with autoimmune diseases such as HIV/AIDS, multiple sclerosis (MS), and Alzheimer's disease.[22]

For marijuana to become an accepted medical practice in all its forms, the FDA will need to complete clinical trials and approve the herb as a drug. The form of marijuana will be determined by its effectiveness in that form and for the specific medical conditions for which it is effective.

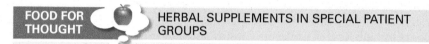

FOOD FOR THOUGHT   HERBAL SUPPLEMENTS IN SPECIAL PATIENT GROUPS

Herbal supplements in special patient groups should be used only in consultation with the physician.

- Pregnant and breast-feeding women—impact on fetal development and infant
- Children—impact on growth and development often unknown and unpredictable
- Patients with chronic diseases
- Patients taking any medication

HERBAL SUPPLEMENTS DENTAL PATIENTS USE

Much oral pain is associated with inflammation, either of the gingiva, the periapical area around the tooth, ulcerations of the mucosa, sinuses or pharyngeal area. The inflammation is typically brought about by infections, bacterial, fungal, and viral, or by trauma. Treatment of the pain of oral disease typically involves reduction of inflammation and removal of the source of the inflammation. Herbal supplements that address inflammation and are antibacterial, antifungal, or antiviral are the most effective. Patients will often resort to herbal supplementation as a temporary treatment until definitive dental treatment can be attained. Patients will also use herbal supplements as a method of preventing oral disease. Neither is a substitute for regular dental care.

A second indication for a dental patient to use herbal supplementation is bleeding. Several herbs will cause bleeding and should be avoided. Herbs that help with preventing or stopping bleeding should be used with caution, especially in patients taking cardiovascular medications or who have cardiovascular conditions. Bleeding is a significant sign of disease or disorder and professional help should be sought. This is not a matter to be neglected or treated with a home remedy or dietary supplement!

A third indication for a dental patient to use herbal supplementation is dental caries. Tooth decay is one of the most common diseases affecting the population. While there are several herbal supplements that are said to prevent decay or treat decay, the progression of the disease may be rapid in some cases. While it is true that decay may be arrested, it is a condition that, if allowed to continue, results in serious, lifelong alterations for the person. The best advice is to seek dental care.

COUNSELING DENTAL PATIENTS

Dental health care workers need to be aware of their patients' use of herbs when providing oral health care treatment. Many patients will not report taking them unless specifically asked. Many patients may not recognize their herbal supplement as one that could affect their dental condition or treatment.

The reasons for herbal use are many and varied, so it is important to ensure that herb use is reported on the medical/dental form to better serve our patients. The following are some common reasons for herb usage:

- Failure of traditional medicine to heal
- Lower cost than traditional pharmaceuticals
- Taking control of own health
- Natural and therefore good for the body

If a patient reports taking a herb for medicinal treatment or to enhance health, be sure to cross-reference the herb in a reliable reference such as the PDR's *Herbal Supplements Index* to identify herb–drug interactions. As previously discussed, there are many interactions—too many to know without looking it up!

Advice for Patients

It is strongly recommended that before taking herbs, consult is made with a physician or a professional trained in herb usage. The following is a summary of information found throughout the chapter:

- Research a herbal supplement before taking it. Seek information from reliable sources.
- Do not assume a product is safe or effective. Although touted as natural and safe, herbs act as drugs but may lack scientific study.
- Follow guidelines for dosages and length of time for which the herb can be safely taken. Often, length of usage has an effect on the body.
- Buy herbs from reliable sources. Labels should include ingredient list, precautions, manufacturer's name and address, batch or lot number, manufacture date, expiration date, and dosage information.
- Introduce herbs one at a time to monitor effectiveness and side effects. Using multiple herbal supplements puts you at a greater risk for possible adverse reactions.

- Do not give herbs to infants or young children.
- Do not take herbs if you are pregnant, nursing, or planning a pregnancy.
- Do not take herbs if you are taking any other kind of medication without discussing it with your health care provider.
- Use extreme caution with herbs purchased in other countries or through mail order. Standards for quality, purity, and content are different in every country.
- Herbs can be part of an overall health maintenance program. Before taking, investigate a product thoroughly.[4]

CHAPTER REVIEW

 PRACTICE FOR PATIENTS

Patient #1

Your patient is a 38-year-old man with a 10-year history of human immunodeficiency virus (HIV). His medical/dental history indicates use of prescription drugs and herbs. He is taking protease inhibitors (indinavir) prescribed by his physician and self-medicates with ginkgo to improve memory function and kava to aid in relief of anxiety. Upon oral examination, you note red and edematous gingival tissues that bleed freely upon probing, slow-acting salivary glands, and light retentive plaque. His third molars are partially impacted and decayed. He states that he is in pain "all over his mouth."

1. Explain to your patient the possible interactions between kava and ginkgo.
2. Discuss with your patient the impact that kava and ginkgo may have on the planned extractions of the third molars.
3. With further inquiry, you learn that your patient likes to brush his teeth with a mixture of lavender and baking soda because it helps him to relax before bed. What recommendations would you make, if any?
4. Your patient asks about a herbal supplement for his xerostomia. What recommendations would you make, if any?

Patient #2

The patient is a 16-year-old pregnant female who presents for dental hygiene treatment. The intraoral examination reveals generalized severe gingivitis with areas of sloughing tissue on the palate and attached gingiva. The patient complains of burning tongue and dry mouth. Several areas of demineralization at the cervical areas of the teeth are noted. Following the clinical assessment of the patient's oral tissues, the hygienist decides that nutritional counseling is an important feature of the treatment plan.

1. Address the possible mineral deficiencies the patient may be experiencing.
2. Associate the possible deficiencies with the specific oral conditions.
3. What additional information is the hygienist aware of about this pregnant adolescent's nutritional needs?

REFERENCES

1. Using dietary supplements wisely. (December 2012). Retrieved from https://nccih.nih.gov/health/supplements/wiseuse.htm
2. Laird J. Interactions between supplements and drugs: deciphering the evidence. *J Am Acad Phys Assist* 2011;24(12):44–49.
3. Corey RL, Rakela J. Complementary and alternative medicine: risks and special considerations in pretransplant and posttransplant patients. *Nutr Clin Pract* 2014;29(3):322–331. doi: 10.1177/0884533614528007.
4. Zelig R, Radler DR. Understanding the properties of common dietary supplements: clinical implications for healthcare practitioners. *Nutr Clin Pract* 2012;27(6):767–776. doi: 10.1177/0884533612446198.
5. Wu C, Wang C, Kennedy J. Prevalence of herb and dietary supplement use among children and adolescents in the United States: results from the 2007 National Health Interview Survey. *Complement Ther Med* 2013;21:358–363. http://.do.org/10.1016/j.ctim.2013.05.001
6. Moyad MA. Under-hyped and over-hyped drug–dietary supplement interactions and uses. *Urol Nurs* 2010;30(1):85–87.
7. Dietary supplement health and education act of 1994, public law 103-417, 103rd congress. (October 25, 1994). Retrieved from https://ods.od.nih.gov/About/DSHEA_Wording.aspx
8. Dietary supplement Current Good Manufacturing Practices (CGMPs) and interim final rule (IFR) facts. (September 19, 2014). Retrieved from http://www.fda.gov/Food/GuidanceRegulation/CGMP/ucm110858.htm
9. Herbal supplements filled with fake ingredients, investigators find. (February 3, 2015). *Rochester First.com.* Retrieved from http://www.rochesterfirst.com/news/news/herbal-supplements-filled-with-fake-ingredients-investigators-find
10. Temple NJ. Marketing of dietary supplements: a Canadian perspective. *Curr Nutr Rep* 2013;2:167–173. doi: 10.1007/s13668-013-0057-z.

11. Credentialing, licensing, and education. (October 2015). Retrieved from https://nccih.nih.gov/health/decisions/credentialing.htm
12. Nisly NL, Gryzlak BM, Zimmerman MB, et al. Dietary supplement polypharmacy: an unrecognized public health problem? *Evid Based Complement Alternat Med* 2010;7(1):107–113. doi: 10.1093/ecam/nem 150.
13. Knoben JE, Phillips SJ. New drug information resources for pharmacists at the National Library of Medicine. *J Am Pharm Assoc* 2014;54(1):49–55. doi: 10.1331/JAPhA.2014.13123.
14. Old N. Natural but not necessarily safe: nursing ethical and legal considerations when administering herbal and dietary supplements in clinical practice. *Aust Nurs Midwifery J* 2014;22(2):28–33. Retrieved from http://www.anmfvic.asn.au/
15. Schultz JD, Stegmuller M. Complementary and alternative medications consumed by patients with head and neck carcinoma: a pilot study in Germany. *Nutr Cancer* 2012;64(3):377–385. doi: 10.1080/01635581.2012.655400.
16. Bunchorntavakul C, Reddy KR. Review article: herbal and dietary supplement hepatotoxicity. Aliment Pharmacol Ther 2013;37:3–17. Print.
17. Ehrlich SD. (November 6, 2015). Green tea: overview. Retrieved from http://umm.edu/health/medical/altmed/herb/green-tea/
18. Opara EI, Chohan M. Culinary herbs and spices: their bioactive properties, the contribution of polyphenols and the challenges in deducing their true health benefits. *Int J Mol Sci* 2014;15(10):19183–19202. doi: 10.3390/ijms151019183.
19. National Institute on Drug Abuse. NIH Research on marijuana and cannabinoids. (March 2016). Retrieved from https://www.drugabuse.gov/drugs-abuse/marijuana/nih-research-marijuana-cannabinoids
20. National Institute on Drug Abuse. DrugFacts: marijuana. (March 2016). Retrieved from https://www.drugabuse.gov/publications/drugfacts/marijuana
21. Volkow ND. (May 2016). Marijuana letter from the director. Retrieved from https://www.drugabuse.gov/publications/research-reports/marijuana/letter-director
22. National Institute on Drug Abuse. DrugFacts: is marijuana medicine? (July 2015). Retrieved from https://www.drugabuse.gov/publications/drugfacts/marijuana-medicine

WEB RESOURCES

National Center for Complementary and Integrative Health www.nccih.nih.gov

Office of Dietary Supplements of National Institutes of Health https://ods.od.nih.gov/

National Center for Biotechnology Information of the National Institutes of Health www.ncbi.nlm.nih.gov/pubmed

National Center for Complementary and Integrative Health https://nccih.nih.gov/health/herbsataglance.htm

Food and Drug Administration www.fda.gov/downloads/ForConsumers/ConsumerUpdates/ucm05824.pdf

Food and Drug Administration www.fda.gov/AboutFDA/CentersOffices/OfficeofFoods/CFSAN/

United States Department of Health and Human Services www.safetyreporting.hhs.gov

National Library of Medicine, National Institutes of Health www.nlm.nih.gov/medlineplus/dietarysypplements.html

Dietary Supplement Label Database, National Institutes of Health www.dsld.nlm.nih.gov/dsld/

National Center for Complementary and Integrative Health, National Institutes of Health http://nccam.nih.gov/

American Botanical Council http://herbalgram.org

Dietitians in Integrative and Functional Medicine http://www.complementarynutrition.org

Therapeutic Research Center http://www.naturalstandard.com/

Therapeutic Research Center http://natrualdatabase.therapeuticresearch.com/home.aspx?cs=7s=ND

US Pharmacopeial Convention http://www.usp.org/

NSF International http://www.nsf.org/business/dietary_supplements/index.asp?program=DietarySups

Consumer Lab http://www.consumerlab.com/

Office of Dietary Supplements of National Institutes of Health https://ods.od.nih.gov/About/DSHEA_Wording.aspx

National Criminal Justice Reference Service https://www.ncjrs.gov/ondcppubs/publications/pdf/marijuana_myths_facts.pdf

PART III

Relationship of Nutrition to Oral Disease

Diet and Dental Caries

> I was a terrible Sugar Babies addict, so I had more cavities than the surface of the moon.
>
> *Rick Reilly—Columnist for Sports Illustrated*

Learning Objectives

- Understand the relationship between food and dental caries
- Discuss the caries process and factors that increase caries risk
- Explain how host factors can either increase or decrease caries risk
- Give examples of sugar alcohols and synthetic sweeteners and explain the difference between the two
- Suggest changes to diet that will prevent dental caries
- Recognize oral symptoms of early childhood caries
- Discuss the benefits of having ample saliva and understand concerns of xerostomia
- Name the bacteria most responsible for metabolizing carbohydrates and identify various acids created in the process
- Identify groups most at risk for dental caries
- Counsel patients on making diet changes to prevent or mitigate damage to teeth

Key Terms

Acidogenic
Aciduric
Cariogenic
Cariostatic
Critical pH
Early Childhood Caries (ECC)
Eating Event
Fermentable Carbohydrate

Lactic Acid
Lactobacillus
Salivary Gland Hypofunction
Streptococcus mutans
Sugar Alcohol
Synthetic Sweetener
Ultraprocessed Food

INTRODUCTION

Many people say, if you don't want cavities, don't eat sugar or sweets. We hear versions of this cause and effect in our practice every day. The etiology of caries and the cavitation process is more complex than this simple statement and will be explored in more depth in this chapter.[1,2] Even if there is frequent consumption of sugar, caries risk can be reduced by exposing teeth to fluoride, placing sealants, practicing better oral hygiene, and assuring ample saliva. See Table 9-1 for causative and modifying factors in the caries process.

The demineralization during acid attack and subsequent remineralization by saliva and fluoride is a dynamic process that happens multiple times throughout the day—as many times as you eat. Focusing on daily practices that remineralize enamel will offset detrimental effects of carbohydrates and acidic foods in the diet. See the two equations below: the first equation illustrates factors that promote dental caries. The second equation illustrates factors that keep teeth caries-free.

Demineralization	>	Remineralization		=	Dental Caries
Carbohydrates + Bacteria = Acid		Lack of quality saliva			Demineralized enamel
Carbohydrates		Poor oral hygiene practices			
Sugary foods		Fluoride unavailable			
Ultraprocessed foods					
Starchy foods eaten with sucrose					
Bacteria					
Streptococcus mutans					
Actinomyces					
Lactobacillus					

Demineralization	<	Remineralization		=	Caries-Free
Reduce sucrose consumption to 5%–10% of daily calorie intake		Stimulate healthy saliva by eating crunchy foods with meals and chewing sugar-free gum after a meal or snack			Intact enamel
Eat more whole fresh foods and fewer processed foods		Replace lost tooth minerals with calcium and phosphorous in saliva			
		Eat cariostatic foods with meals			
		Remove bacterial plaque every day using fluoridated dentifrice			

Table 9-1	Causative and Modifying Factors in the Dental Caries Process
At Risk	**Modifying Factors**
Frequent consumption of carbohydrates	Sucrose restriction (>5% in daily diet), inclusion of cariostatic foods, xylitol chewing gum
Presence of oral bacteria: mainly *S. mutans* and *Lactobacillus*	Reduction/elimination of bacterial plaque
Xerostomia—dry mouth	Ample quantity and quality saliva
Absence of fluoride	Use of fluoridated toothpaste and rinse, professional application
Inadequate oral hygiene	Scrupulous home care practices
Malformed dentition	Good pre-eruptive nutrition Sealants

The following facts about dental caries emerged from decades of caries research[1-3]:

- Acid *demineralizes* enamel.
- *Fermentable carbohydrates* (not just sweet foods) are used by bacteria to make acid.
- *Specific plaque bacteria* must be present to metabolize carbohydrates and produce acid.
- Demineralizing acid can also come from *extrinsic* sources, like gastric acids or acidic foods, as well as the *intrinsic* source created from bacteria metabolizing carbohydrates.
- When eaten with a simple sugar, *cooked starches* will demineralize enamel.
- The *form* of carbohydrate—liquid or solid—clears the oral cavity at different speeds and subjects teeth to varying times of acid attack.
- Although dried fruit and fruit juice are cariogenic, *fresh fruit* is not.
- Specific foods provide *protective factors* against acid attack.
- Available fluoride in food and saliva will *remineralize* enamel and protect teeth and reduce damage from acid.

FOOD FOR THOUGHT   FAMOUS VIPEHOLM STUDY

Much of what we currently know about the relationship between carbohydrates and dental caries resulted from a study conducted in 1945 to 1953, involving 436 adult residents at a mental institution in Vipeholm, Sweden.[4] Leading up to 1945, dental health in Scandinavia was very poor with 83% of 3-year-old having evidence of dental caries. The Dental Institute in Stockholm authorized the clinical trial, hypothesizing about the relationship linking sugar to dental caries—specifically if *form* of sugar and *frequency* of eating sugar had any effect on development of dental caries. Participating residents were divided into three groups. Each group received varying amounts and forms of sugar, either with their regular meals or between meals as snacks.

All groups received the basal diet (no simple sugars) plus one of the following sources of sugar:

- First group had additional 300 g of sugar in solution during meals.
- Second group ate an additional 50 g of sugary bread with their meals.
- Third group ate in-between meal snacks of toffee candy consisting of a small amount of sugar.

Results showed that the third group, eating the in-between meal sweet snacks (toffee candy), had the highest caries rate. The second highest rate was noted in the group who ate bread with a sweet spread.

Determined after 8 years of study:

1. *Frequency* of sugar consumed is the *primary* factor in caries activity.
2. *Form* and *composition* of sweets is important: solid and sticky foods that took *longer* to clear than liquids increased the rate of caries.
3. *Quantity* of sugar eaten is *not* of great importance (although studies since have proven it does make a difference): an increase from 30 to 300 g per day caused little increase in caries production.
4. Sugar exerts caries-promoting effects locally on tooth surfaces.

FACTORS OF CARIES DEVELOPMENT

You do not get a cavity after a week of binging on candy. Dental caries is a dynamic *process* that can take months or even years of destructive activity before becoming visible to the naked eye and before detection on a radiograph. Studies have shown that it can take on average 19 to 22 months for caries to progress through enamel for a person at high risk and up to 5 years if at low risk.[5] Below are some of the many factors that play a part in the development of dental caries:

1. Carbohydrates in the diet
2. Presence of specific plaque bacteria
3. Susceptible tooth structure
4. Absence of fluoride
5. Salivary gland hypofunction (SGH)
6. Poor oral hygiene

Evaluation of these factors, which vary widely from patient to patient, determine a patient's risk for dental caries. The demineralization/mineralization process can begin as soon as the first primary tooth erupts into the oral cavity as evident in early childhood caries (ECC) and continues throughout the life cycle manifesting as recurrent and root caries in older adults with gingival recession.

Demineralization

When carbohydrates enter the mouth, plaque bacteria begin metabolizing sugar and produce acid. Every **eating event**, meal or snack, is an opportunity for bacteria to produce acid. Landmark research conducted by Stephan and Miller in 1943 demonstrated that oral pH begins to drop within 3 minutes of rinsing with sucrose and remains low for up to 40 minutes. Acid is continually produced until the carbohydrate is cleared from the mouth.[1,3] The longer the carbohydrate remains in the mouth, the more acid produced, and the lower oral pH drops. When pH drops enough to reach the **critical pH** of **5.5**, demineralization (net mineral loss) of enamel occurs.[1,3] Movement of acid through enamel tubules increases solubility of calcium hydroxyapatite, and demineralization occurs as calcium leaches from the tooth surface.

Once the food clears the mouth, oral pH gradually returns to normal, which is around 6.8 to 7.0. The goal in preventing demineralization is to keep the pH as close to neutral as possible for as long as possible. Eating certain foods with the meal or snack can inhibit bacteria from producing acid, and swishing with water (7 pH) after eating can neutralize acids.

See the Stephan curve below (named after Dr. Robert Stephan, an officer in the US Public Health Service), which demonstrates how eating and drinking alter the pH of the mouth (Figure 9-1).

For a close-up view of porous enamel, watch the YouTube video on The Structure of a Tooth: https://www.youtube.com/watch?v=f_Gdl0C4CnY

Figure 9-1 Stephan curve.

If there has not been enough remineralization activity, whether due to absence of time between eating events, unavailable fluoride or low-quality saliva, net mineral loss exceeds remineralization and you will see a rough parchment-white spot. It is typical for first sight of demineralization to be at the gingival 1/3, where bacterial plaque accumulates.[6-8] The white spot indicates dissolution of hard tooth structure. When demineralization activity is more frequent or severe than remineralization, cavitation occurs. After a good percentage of the hard structure is demineralized, the lesion appears as a radiolucent area on a radiograph.

Remineralization

The importance of saliva is often taken for granted. It mixes with chewed food to make swallowing easier, contains enzymes to start digestion, and flushes food from the oral cavity. It feels like water in the mouth but in fact, it contains important minerals that are needed to minimize acid's destruction of teeth. Even though acid may erode enamel, there is opportunity between eating events for the area to be remineralized, as long as there is ample saliva and daily use of fluoridated dentifrice.[9,10] During the times between eating events, saliva bathes teeth with calcium, phosphates, and fluoride, replacing lost minerals to rejuvenate enamel. The minerals take the same pathway as the acid, deep into enamel matrix.[3] This action reverses or halts the carious process before the lesion reaches a stage where restoration is required.[3]

ROLE OF FOOD IN FORMATION OF DENTAL CARIES

Most people are aware that sugar contributes to dental caries. According to the USDA, global sugar *consumption* now outpaces sugar *production*. Over the last two decades, sucrose consumption in the United States has increased steadily, whereas the incidence of dental *caries has decreased*. This is because although there is a scientifically established cause-and-effect relationship between sugar and dental caries, other host factors can mitigate the damages. Because of a robust body of dental caries research, more is known about how to manipulate host factors to preserve the tooth.

All *sugars* are not the same; some carbohydrates have a more deleterious effect on teeth than others. Even though a potato chip does not in any way resemble a piece of sweet candy, it can actually be more detrimental to tooth enamel than a teaspoon of sugar. A potato chip is a *cooked starch*, which is a form of carbohydrate that gets stuck in teeth giving longer opportunity for acid production. Salivary amylase breaks down the starch to a disaccharide, which is metabolized by plaque bacteria. This results in acid production for as long as the potato chip remains in the mouth.[1,11] Starchy foods like bread, rice, and crackers can become packed between teeth and remain in the oral cavity longer than a piece of hard candy. Imagine a piece of bread topped with jelly surrounding teeth. That combination of a starch with sucrose is perhaps the most detrimental of all food choices for teeth. So yes, sugar does cause dental caries, but so do other forms of carbohydrates.

In regard to dental caries, food in the modern diet can be labeled one of three ways:

- Cariogenic—contributes to the caries process
- Cariostatic—does not contribute to the caries process
- Acidic—contains acid and erodes hard structures

Cariogenic Foods

Cariogenic foods are rich in fermentable carbohydrates. This would include any food considered a monosaccharide or disaccharide, plus sweeteners used in manufacturing: fruit juices, honey, high-fructose corn syrup, glucose, and refined starch. All forms of these sugars are used by bacteria to create acid.

According to the USDA, the average American consumes about ¼ lb of sugar each day. This is equivalent to about four cans of soda. Even if you are not a soda drinker, sugar in the diet can add up fast. Whole or unprocessed foods typically have zero sucrose; processed food may contain up to 2% sucrose; ultraprocessed foods may contain over 20% sucrose. Ultraprocessed foods account for 90% of all *added sugars* in the diet. By definition, ultraprocessed foods are cheap, ready to consume, high in fat and sugar, and low in fiber.[12] Any food product that has industrial additives not used when preparing whole food in your kitchen is ultraprocessed: flavor enhancers, sucrose additives, colorants, trans fats, and emulsifier. In the United States, ultraprocessed foods account for on average 57% of daily energy intake, which means that added sucrose is readily consumed in food products.[13] Examples of ultraprocessed foods besides soft drinks are sweet or spicy boxed/packaged baked goods and snacks, frozen convenience meals, chicken nuggets, instant noodles and soups, cereals, crackers, boxed or packaged potatoes and rice, and reconstituted meat.[14] Figure 9-2 provides examples of manufactured food. Multiple research studies found that those who consume in excess of 10% daily calories from sugar have increased caries and reducing that amount, especially in childhood, reduced incidence throughout the life cycle.[15-17] Awareness must be developed of the many sources of sugar in the diet in order to keep sugar to a minimum.

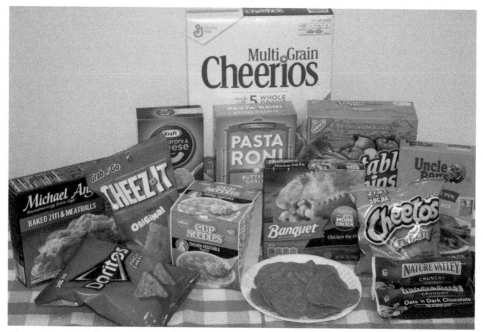

Figure 9-2 Ultraprocessed food. (Photo courtesy of Kevin Brown, Zolfo Springs, FL.)

FOOD FOR THOUGHT UBIQUITOUS HIGH-FRUCTOSE CORN SYRUP

On your next trip to the grocery store, examine food product labels. You might be surprised at the volume of products containing one of the following sugars: high-fructose corn syrup, HFCS-90, fructose syrup, corn sugar, maize syrup, glucose syrup, crystalline fructose, and corn syrup solids. High-fructose corn syrup received FDA approval for inclusion in our food supply in 1983. Since then, it has made its way into many food products including some you would not even think need sweetener.

According to the Corn Refiners Association Web site (www.corn.org), corn syrup is chemically close to sucrose and is formulated at a level of sweetness so that consumers will not notice the substitution in a food product. It has the same number of calories per gram and is used as a preservative, to retain moisture and give baked goods a crunchy surface. It is the ingredient that gives bread its golden-brown crust and breakfast bars a chewy consistency. Food manufacturers appreciate the fact that corn syrup remains stable when freezing, melting, and boiling. Costwise HFCS is less expensive than either cane or beet sugar.

In a study conducted by researchers at the Shanghai Jiao Tong University's Laboratory of Stomatology in Shanghai, China, high-fructose corn syrup displayed the same level of cariogenicity as sucrose. This is vital information as high fructose appears on labels of food in which you would not expect to see it. When counseling patients with current dental caries, be sure to educate them on identifying all sources of sugar in their diet. See Figure 9-3 for examples of foods containing high-fructose corn syrup.

From Sun M, et al. Effect of high-fructose corn syrup on Streptococcus mutans virulence gene expression and on tooth demineralization. Eur J Oral Sci 2014;122(3):216–222.

Acidic Foods

All foods and beverages considered carbohydrates have the potential to cause dental caries. *Equally as bad* are naturally *acidic foods* that *erode* enamel.[18] Either acid by-products from metabolized carbohydrates *or* acidic foods can cause

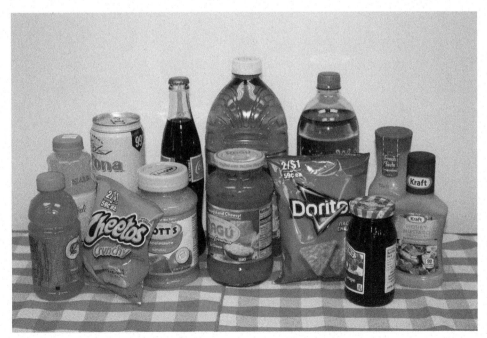

Figure 9-3   Foods containing HFCS. (Photo courtesy of Kevin Brown, Zolfo Springs, FL.)

destruction to enamel. Erosion begins by softening the enamel surface. As each newly exposed "surface" dissolves, enamel volume is lost.[19] As enamel continues to disappear and the surface rests closer on dentin, the area will appear darker than areas covered by healthy enamel. Citric, phosphoric, malic, tartaric, lactic, ascorbic, and carbonic acids are ingredients found on labels of many foods. Examples of highly acidic food and beverages that erode enamel are soda (phosphoric acid); citric fruits lemons, limes, grapefruit, and oranges (citric acid); yogurt (lactic acid); and grapes and wine (tartaric acid). Preliminary results from in vitro studies of cow's milk fortified with fluoride indicate effectiveness in reducing erosion.[20]

See Figure 9-4 for examples of foods that contain acid. See Table 9-2 for pH of other common foods and beverages that are acidic pH.

Cariostatic Foods

Cariostatic foods are those that do not contribute to initiation of enamel demineralization or continue the caries process. Cariostatic foods may have properties that actually help *prevent* dental caries. Foods that fall under this category can

Figure 9-4 Acidic foods. (Photo courtesy of Kevin Brown, Zolfo Springs, FL.)

Table 9-2	pH of Common Foods and Beverages (Approximate)
Nondiet soda	2.5–4.0
Diet soda	3.0
Bottled iced tea	3.2–4.0
V8	4.3
Grapefruit/orange juice	3.7
Cranberry juice	3.0
Gatorade	2.9
Ice cream	6.5–7.0
Bottled water	5.5–6.4
Beer	4.3
Wine	3.1–3.6
Mouthwash	3.2–5.0
Apple (including juice and applesauce)	3.1–3.5
Avocado	6.4
Banana	4.5
Beans	5.6–6.0
Blueberries	3.1
Broccoli	6.4
Cabbage	5.2
Carrots	5.8
Cherries	4.1
Corn	5.8
Cucumber (including dill pickle)	3.2–5.1
Grapes	2.8
Lemons/limes	2.0
Mushroom	6.0
Nectarine/peach	3.3–3.9
Onion	5.3
Pears	3.5
Peas	5.8
Green pepper	5.2
Plum	2.8
Spinach	5.5
Squash	5.1–5.7
Strawberry	3.0
Sweet potato	5.3
Tomato	3.7
Vinegar	2.4
Watermelon	5.1
Zucchini	5.7

mitigate or prevent acid production when consumed with carbohydrate-rich meal or snack. They can moderate the pH by maintaining a more basic environment, put a protective coating on enamel, provide fluoride, and interfere with or reduce acid-producing bacteria.

Researchers have been studying the effects of food components on the growth and virulence of *S. mutans*. They have found that polyphenols, which are plant molecules, inhibit production of acids.[21] Cranberries, cocoa, coffee, black tea, and red wine are examples of foods that contain polyphenols. Both in vivo and in vitro tests show compounds in these foods, as well as apples, red grape seeds, nutmeg, caraway, and garlic show potential of either reducing the colonization or interfering with *S. mutans* acid production.[22]

Low-acid nutrients like protein, fats, phosphorous, and calcium moderate oral pH when eaten with carbohydrates. Meat, milk, cheese, and nuts in the meal will maintain the oral pH closer to 7.0.[23] Eating cheese after a sugary food can prevent the steep decline in oral pH by stimulating saliva flow, which counteracts acid production. Several studies have demonstrated plaque pH remains neutral after drinking cow's milk that is rich in calcium, phosphorous, and casein.[24]

See Figure 9-5 for examples of healthy snacks and beverages.

Figure 9-5   Cariostatic foods. (Photo courtesy of Kevin Brown, Zolfo Springs FL.)

Starchy Foods

Foods considered starches are *reduced* to glucose, maltose, and maltotriose by salivary amylase and are then utilized by bacteria to create acid. A **cooked starch**—rice, potatoes, bread—are by themselves low on the cariogenicity list as they have half the caries causing potential of sucrose-containing foods. But combining a cooked starch with sucrose has more potential of causing dental caries than either of the two alone as the starch typically is sticky and clings to teeth, keeping sugar (or acid) close to the tooth. A good example of this is bread with jelly.[1,11] See Figure 9-6 through 9-8 showing

Plaque retention in area
slightly out of alignment

Figure 9-6 Disclosed plaque. (Reprinted from Bob Sconyers, with permission.)

Bread with jelly stuck between #26 and #27.
Area of retention traps food and bacteria
have longer acid production time.

Figure 9-7 Retained bread and jelly. (Reprinted from Bob Sconyers, with permission.)

Cheese puffs stuck between
teeth #26 and #27

Figure 9-8 Retained Cheetos. (Photo courtesy of Bob
Sconyers, Wauchula FL.)

disclosed plaque with bread and jelly (sucrose rich) and Cheetos (contains lactic acid)
accumulating in the same area.

Detrimental Effects of Soda

Sodas are double trouble as they destroy enamel both ways—chemical erosion from
acid and cariogenic potential from sugar. This means that even though *diet soda* does
not have sugar, it still has erosive potential.

Sip All Day, Get Decay. This abbreviated version of American Dental Association's
publication called Sip and Snack All Day? Risk Decay! Sends the message that sipping
on soda has devastating oral effects. Enamel can be softened by acids within 1 hour
of exposure to sodas.[25] But exposure to calcium-rich foods like milk and cheese while
drinking soda in a meal or immediately afterward may moderate the drop in pH.[26,27]

See Figure 9-9 through 9-11 for an example of caries from soda sipping throughout the day.

Regular and diet sodas have citric and **phosphoric acid** with a pH of 2.3 to 2.6
added as flavor enhancers, which dissolves enamel without the help of bacteria producing acid.

Additionally, one 12-oz can of regular soda contains 10 teaspoons of sugar, give
or takes a few depending on the brand. Noncola drinks and canned iced teas are actually more harmful to enamel than Coke, Dr. Pepper, and Pepsi because flavor additives like malic and tartaric and other acids aggressively demineralize enamel. Sprite,
Mountain Dew, Ginger Ale, and Arizona Iced Tea are the *most* harmful, and root
beer, brewed black tea, black coffee, and water are *least* harmful to enamel. It is recommended to wait 30 minutes after drinking erosive beverages before toothbrushing
to protect softened dentin.[28]

Placement of these three photos showing damage from soda sipping belong after Detrimental Effects of Soda

Figure 9-9 Damage from soda sipping—right side. (Reprinted from Dr. Rick Foster, with permission.)

Figure 9-10 Damage from soda sipping—anterior. (Reprinted from Dr. Rick Foster, with permission.)

Figure 9-11 Damage from soda sipping—left side. (Reprinted from Dr. Rick Foster, with permission.)

Suggestions for reducing the caries potential of soda in the diet[29-33]:

- Drink the whole can or bottle of soda with a meal and rinse the mouth with water to reduce amount of sugar available for bacteria to make acid.
- Restrict consumption of soda by drinking 100% fruit juice, unsweet tea, and water instead.
- Drink through a straw to bypass teeth.
- Once the bottle or can is opened, drink fast.
- Wait 30 minutes after finishing the soda before brushing to allow opportunity for remineralization.

ANALYZING THE FACTS

Food factors that determine cariogenicity of the diet are as follows:

1. *Frequency* of eating events—meals or snack. A snack is a small amount of carbohydrate food or beverage consumed 20 minutes on either side of a meal. Snacks are separate opportunities for bacteria to feed and produce acid.[34,35] Sipping and grazing are two extremely devastating behaviors for teeth. Constant acid production leaves little time for remineralization. Below is a typical example of seven eating events in a day.

8 AM Breakfast	11:30 AM Snack	12 PM Lunch	2:30 PM Snack	4 PM Snack	6 PM Dinner	9 PM Snack
Coffee with Cremora and sugar Scrambled eggs with cheese Toast Orange juice	Breakfast bar	Lettuce Grilled chicken Walnuts Dried cranberries Soda Raspberry vinaigrette dressing	Apple Creamy peanut butter Soda	Chips Sports drink	Stouffer's frozen 3-cheese lasagna Garlic bread 3-bean salad with vinegar and oil Water	Chocolate chip cookies
	60		30	60		60 = 210

2. *Physical form* of food—liquids clear the oral cavity twice as fast as solid foods and sticky cooked starches are retained in the oral cavity the longest.[36] Sticky simple carbohydrates like caramels, jellybeans, and gumdrops (any chewy candy) are perceived as being the most cariogenic food. In fact, cookies, crackers, and potato chips are more cariogenic because they are

retained longer in the mouth, which means longer exposure to acid as bacteria metabolize the carbohydrate.[37] Oral clearance times for food items in the example are given below. (Some foods fall into multiple categories.) *Snacks* alone provide 210 minutes of acid attack to hard tooth structures (numbers are on the bottom of snack columns in the example). Including meals, it is almost 400 minutes:

Form		Approximate Clearance Time
Liquid	Soda, sports drink	20–30 minutes
Solid	Breakfast bar, chocolate chip cookies	45–60 minutes
Starch	Bread, lasagna noodles, chips	60 minutes
Acidic	Orange juice, soda, sports drink, green beans with vinegar, raspberry vinaigrette salad dressing	20–30 minutes

3. *Sequence* in which foods are eaten can minimize effects of acid attack. Alternating bites of cariogenic and cariostatic foods minimizes effects of local acid.[1,35–37] Fats and proteins consumed with a meal generate a fatty coating on teeth, protecting them from sugars that are eaten later. Consuming dairy products keeps the saliva rich in calcium and phosphorus, offering the benefit of remineralization.[37] Cheese eaten after a carbohydrate encourages salivation and prevents the pH from dropping below 5.5.[38] Below are cariostatic foods in the example:

   Eggs with cheese, coffee
   Chicken, walnuts
   Apple
   Cheese in lasagna, oil

4. *Quantity* of sugar consumed in the diet has an impact on dental caries. The more fermentable carbohydrates eaten in a day, regardless of available fluoride for remineralization, the greater incidence of caries.[39,40] According to the 2015 WHO dietary guidelines, the goal for amount of total sugar intake per day should be less than 10% of total calorie intake. A goal of less than 5% would add extra benefits. Below are foods containing sugar in the example: they add up fast:

Breakfast	(Coffee) with Cremora and Sugar, Orange Juice, Toast
Snack	Breakfast bar
Lunch	Soda, dried cranberries, raspberry vinaigrette dressing
Snack	Soda, creamy peanut butter
Snack	Chips, sports drink
Dinner	Lasagna, bread
Snack	Chocolate chip cookies

Advice for making meals/snacks in the example less cariogenic:

- Include a crunchy food with each meal to stimulate saliva: add crunchy fresh vegetables.
- Eat cariostatic foods with each meal to interfere with acid production: cheese and other dairy products, nuts, meats.
- Eat cariostatic foods as snacks: fresh fruits and vegetables, nuts, cheese.
- Reduce amount of sugar in the diet to less than 10% of total calories.
- Choose water or unsweet tea as beverage of choice.
- Use sugar substitute in coffee.
- Drink milk with cookies to offer protective factors of calcium and phosphorous.

See Figure 9-12 for an example of the dynamic demineralization/remineralization of teeth through the day in the previous example.

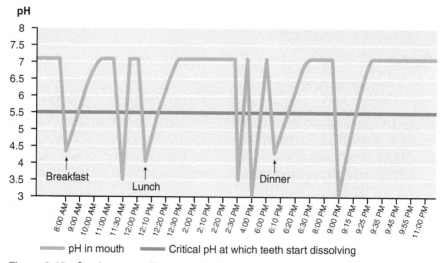

Figure 9-12 Stephan curve illustration for the 7 eating event in the example. Notice all the accumulated time when the oral cavity is below 5.5 critical pH.

FOOD FOR THOUGHT ARE ALL SWEETENERS EQUALLY AS CARIOGENIC?

- Natural sugars like honey, molasses, and raw sugar (turbinado) are just as cariogenic as refined sugars. (Honey may be more cariogenic because of its thick and sticky properties.)
- Corn syrup added to food is just as cariogenic as refined sugars.
- Powdered sugar is more cariogenic than granulated sugar because it is concentrated and fine.
- Fruits, vegetables, and their juices are not as cariogenic as sucrose because of water dilution.
- Food that is 80% sucrose may not be any more harmful than one that is 40% sucrose.
- A starch combined with sucrose is more retentive (bread and jelly).

BACTERIA ASSOCIATED WITH DENTAL CARIES

Human oral environment nurtures hundreds of known bacterial species. Those that play a role in developing dental caries must be either **acidenogenic**, which means ability to produce acid, and/or **aciduric**, which means able to tolerate and thrive in an acidic environment.[41] All acidenogenic bacteria have the ability to dissolve enamel but depend on carbohydrates to provide sugar.[3,11,42] Following are predominant acids resulting from bacteria metabolizing carbohydrates[43]:

1. Lactic acid—most abundant
2. Formic
3. Proprionic
4. Acetic

The following are popular hypotheses regarding acid-producing bacteria:

- *Specific plaque* hypothesis proposes that only a few identified species of bacteria in plaque are involved in the caries process.
- *Nonspecific* plaque hypothesis proposes that activity from *all* oral bacteria plays a role in the disease process.
- *Ecological plaque* hypothesis proposes that a shift in balance of resident oral bacteria, caused by a change in local environment, causes initiation and continuance of dental caries process.

This last hypothesis, ecological plaque hypothesis, is the most popular among researchers as it allows that acid can be produced by *many species* of bacteria, not just a few select one or two, and there can be a *proliferation* of certain species at any one point in time. Oral flora differs from one person to the next, and many types of acidogenic bacteria can

Figure 9-13   Incipient dental caries between the lateral and central incisors. Notice the white halo (etched enamel) around the darker spot. (Reprinted from Dr. Rick Foster, with permission.)

proliferate and dominate the environment. In health, acidogenic bacteria accounts for less than 1% of total oral flora; in a mouth with dental caries, the balance shifts to a much higher percentage with several species of bacteria capable of producing acid. *S. mutans*, *Actinomyces*, *Veillonella*, *Lactobacillus*, *Bifidobacterium*, and *Propionibacterium* (and more) have all been cultivated at the site of caries development.[11,44] Most caries studies indicate that **Streptococcus mutans**, **Streptococcus sobrinus** (*anaerobic* gram-positive coccus), **Actinomyces**, and *Lactobacillus* (anaerobic gram-positive rods) are the *main* microbial species that initiate dental caries with *Lactobacillus* even more predominate at the site of dentinal and root caries[3,44–47] (see Figures 9-13 and 9-14).

Figure 9-14   Caries in dentin on the lateral incisor and canine. (Reprinted from Dr. Rick Foster, with permission.)

Figure 9-15 Rampant caries in mixed dentition. (Reprinted from Dr. Rick Foster, with permission.)

Visit https://www.youtube.com/watch?v=anyjIcL_PUc and http://youtu.be/rOW80FKs2HQ for a microscopic view of oral bacteria.

Oral flora can differ between primary dentition and permanent dentition. *Candida albicans* is commonly found at the site of smooth surface caries in ECC. When both *S. mutans* and *C. albicans* are present in the mouth at the same time, they create a more virulent environment indicating a synergistic effect. The two together are more destructive than either one by itself.[48] There is strong evidence that a mother (or caregiver) can transmit *S. mutans* to a child thereby increasing incidence of ECC[49–52] (see Figure 9-15).

IMPACT OF TOOTH STRUCTURE AND TOOTH ALIGNMENT ON DENTAL CARIES

Generally, a good gene pool and good maternal nutrition can make the difference between carious and caries-free teeth. Ample consumption of vitamin D and calcium during fetus development, well functioning will result in generation of well-calcified teeth for the child.[53] Adequate protein intake during pregnancy will also improve lifetime caries resistance by helping to form well-aligned dentition.[54,55] Straight teeth offer fewer places for plaque to accumulate and are easier to clean during daily oral care. Inclusion of vitamin A–rich foods during gestation will assure well-formed salivary glands which is important for remineralization throughout the lifecycle. Characteristics of teeth that reduce caries risk are as follows:

- Teeth with shallow pits and fissures
- Well-calcified teeth free of enamel defects
- Perfectly aligned teeth

Posterior molars with shallow grooves are less susceptible to dental caries because they do not retain plaque and food as do molars with very deep grooves. Teeth with deeper grooves retain plaque and food because toothbrush bristles cannot reach to the depth during daily cleaning. See Figure 9-16 for an example of toothbrush bristles unable to reach depth of occlusal groove. Dental sealants should be placed prophylactically to prevent bacteria from reaching the depth of a deep groove.

Teeth that are rotated or crowded offer protected areas for bacterial plaque to accumulate and are not cleansed by chewing action or quick toothbrushing. See Figure 9-17 for an example of teeth out of alignment being more difficult to keep clean.

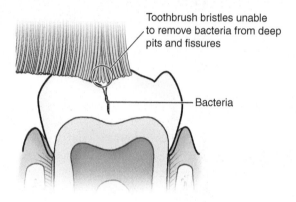

Toothbrush bristles unable to remove bacteria from deep pits and fissures

Bacteria

Figure 9-16   Toothbrush bristles unable to reach depth of occlusal groove.

Figure 9-17   Teeth out of alignment. Notice plaque and stain teeth in facial and lingual version and in crossbite.

The action of chewing has a cleansing effect on teeth that are all in alignment and with shallow grooves; however, there are no such detergent foods that replace good oral hygiene practices.

IMPACT OF FLUORIDE'S REMINERALIZING EFFECT ON DENTAL CARIES

Fluoride in plaque fluid and saliva will inhibit detrimental effects of acid.[56–59] It alters rate of demineralization when incorporated into enamel matrix by binding to crystalline surfaces that have been partially dissolved. Fluoride converts hydroxyapatite into fluorapatite, which reinforces the matrix, fortifying the structure against future acid attacks.[32]

Presence of fluoride in the oral cavity *throughout* the day is very important as there is an ebb and flow of minerals traveling back and forth through enamel tubules. Acid produced during an eating event causes dismantling of enamel, and fluoride is needed to infiltrate as part of the remineralizing process.

When fluoride enters the mouth, whether from food, water, toothbrushing, rinsing, or professional application, it passes through the oral cavity within minutes with each swallow. But enough residual fluoride remains in the oral cavity where it gets absorbed by mucosal tissues, infiltrates plaque, and adds to minerals in saliva. This becomes the "reservoir" of available fluoride each day for use during the remineralization process.[32]

Fluoridated dentifrices have been available for over 40 years, and their effect on caries is well established.[60,61] Although fluoridated toothpaste is the most common source of daily applied fluoride, certain foods will contribute small amounts: black tea, iceberg lettuce, citrus fruits, potatoes, and shellfish.[62]

Other sources of fluoride will occasionally boost the daily supply. Fluoridated rinses provide even more available fluoride to oral reservoirs than fluoridated toothpaste as it has a better absorption rate. Patients with high caries risk should be encouraged to use a fluoridated mouthrinse as part of daily oral care routine.[63,64]

Professionally applied fluoride preparations like sodium fluoride varnish and fluoride gels arrest enamel caries.[65,66] Patients can receive these added benefits during oral hygiene therapy visits.

Early results from fluoride studies that mix fluoride with other agents like silver diamine, arginine, and gallium show promise, but further research is needed before products are available for the public.

For information about the effects of systemic water fluoridation on dental caries, visit the American Dental Association, www.ada.org, and search for: Fluoridation Facts, published in 2005. Other opinions have been published in a

Review Article: Water Fluoridation: A Critical Review of the Physiological Effects of Ingested Fluoride as a Public Health Intervention by Stephen Peckham and Niyi Awofeso, Scientific World Journal Volume 2014, Article 293019.

IMPACT OF QUALITY SALIVA ON DENTAL CARIES

As with fluoride, adequate saliva is a great protector of teeth.[67,68] The watery nature of saliva is deceptive; although it is 99% water, the remaining 1% contains a plethora of organic and inorganic elements. Protein, urea, and lipids make up most of the organic nutrients, and calcium, bicarbonate, phosphate, and fluoride make up most of the inorganic nutrients. Also in saliva are enzymes, mucins, antimicrobials, and pain-killing substances (see Figure 9-18 for components and functions of saliva).

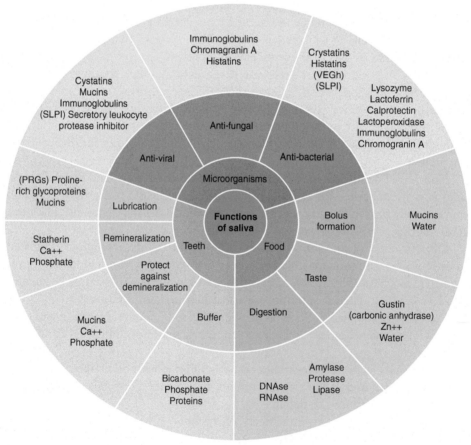

Figure 9-18 Functions of saliva.

The following are important anticaries factors of saliva:

- Saliva flushes food and beverages from the mouth thereby reducing the amount of time bacteria can feed on carbohydrates and manufacture acid. Fluid saliva is more efficient at this function than viscous (thicker) saliva. Watery saliva can be swished more vigorously around the mouth and forced between teeth to dislodge retained food so it can be swallowed. If there is no carbohydrate present in the mouth, bacteria will not manufacture acid.
- Saliva keeps the oral cavity in basic pH range. During noneating times, pH of the mouth hovers around 6.8 to 7.0. A basic pH level indicates absence of acid production and is conducive for remineralization activity. Elements in saliva that keep it basic are bicarbonate phosphate and proteins.
- Minerals in saliva contribute to the oral reservoir for remineralizing enamel.[69] Calcium, phosphates, and fluoride are used to strengthen enamel. Studies have shown that salivary calcium and phosphate levels are higher in those who are caries-free than those who have active caries.[70]

Trying to maintain adequate levels of saliva can be a challenge for some individuals. Saliva production diminishes when we sleep, as we age, take certain medications, or with specific disease processes. Eating crunchy or chewy foods will increase salivation, bringing all of its great benefits to the oral cavity. Chewing gum will do the same.

It is recommended to include at least one chewy or crunchy food with each meal.

FOOD FOR THOUGHT   SALIVARY GLAND HUPOFUNCTION

Decreased volume of saliva is called salivary gland hypofunction (SGH). Underproduction of saliva causes xerostomia and is evident during an oral exam when mucosa appears dull and gloves stick to oral tissue.

The elderly are at high risk for SGH and are at higher risk for dental caries because aging process reduces the sense of thirst, and many are prescribed medications that have xerostomia as a side effect. A mouth without the benefit of saliva needs *aggressive intervention* to head off rampant caries.[71] Without the remineralizing benefit of saliva, the net loss of minerals exceeds replacement, and cavitation is inevitable. When xerostomia is combined with gingival recession, there is a very high risk for dentinal root cavities. See Figure 9-19 for an example of dry mouth with root caries.

Figure 9-19 Dry mouth with root caries. (Reprinted from Dr. Rick Foster, with permission.)

IMPACT OF GOOD ORAL HYGIENE ON DENTAL CARIES

The motivation and ability to remove bacterial plaque play a modifying role in keeping teeth caries free. If the caries equation includes both bacterial plaque and carbohydrates, eliminating one half of the formula will improve the outcome. Scrupulous removal of bacterial plaque on a daily basis reduces colonies of *S. mutans*, *Actinomyces*, and *Lactobacillus*. Both brushing and interdental cleaning should be demonstrated and taught to patients to assure all tooth surfaces are cleared of plaque to the best of their ability on a daily basis. Research indicates the incorporation of tongue brushing into the daily oral care routine greatly reduces the number of *S. mutans* colonies.[72]

EARLY CHILDHOOD CARIES

Worldwide, ECC is the most chronic *infectious disease* in childhood.[73] The scope of worldwide research expands each year as scientists continue to identify etiology and modifying factors like cultural practices, parental knowledge, feeding habits, paths of bacterial transmission, and preventive treatments. ECC is diagnosed by the presence of one or more missing, decayed, or filled primary teeth (even if just one tooth surface), within the first 3 years of life.[74] As soon as teeth erupt into the oral cavity, they become vulnerable to decay. The American Dental Association states in their position paper on ECC that "unrestricted consumption of liquids, beverages and foods containing fermentable carbohydrates can contribute to dental caries after *eruption of first tooth*." Smooth surface of maxillary incisors are usually the first sites involved, whereas they are usually the last sites involved in adult caries. It is not unusual for

Figure 9-20 Early childhood caries. (Photo courtesy of Dr. Rick Foster.)

all teeth to be involved, and sadly, it often goes untreated. See Figure 9-20 for an example of ECC.

Etiology of ECC is the same as that for adult caries: it is a combination of oral bacteria, carbohydrate-rich diet, and poor oral hygiene. *Streptococcus, Porphyromonas,* and *Actinomyces* are the bacteria associated with the disease.[74] *Candida albicans* is often detected along with *S. mutans,* and the two together make for a very virulent, aggressive form of ECC.[48] Initially, infants can acquire oral bacteria as they descend down the birth canal or from skin contact with the mother if born by C-section.[75] Research has shown mothers and other caregivers in close contact can transmit *S. mutans* to the infant.[76,77] Treating a mother with active caries will reduce the amount of bacteria transmitted to the child and result in less incidence of caries later in life.[78]

Prior to 1994, ECC was called "bottle-mouth caries," and parents were strongly encouraged to wean the child off the bottle by 9 months of age. Infants quit sucking when they fall asleep, allowing whatever is in the bottle (formula, milk, juice, breast milk) to pool around teeth, thus beginning the demineralization process. It is suggested that if a bottle is needed at bedtime, let the child empty the bottle before putting them to bed or fill the bottle with water.

As the child grows and starts choosing their own food, parents need to be vigilant in offering less sugary foods and assisting with good oral hygiene.

Recent research concludes there is lower ECC incidence with breast-feeding vs. bottle-feeding in children younger than 12 months, yet there is no consensus in research conducted with children still being breast-fed over the age of 12 months.[79,80] Breast-feeding does not routinely require use of a bottle, and sugars are not added to breast milk. Because of this and its many benefits, the World Health Organization encourages breast-feeding for infants/children up to 2 years old.

Whether or not an infant/child is bottle-fed or breast-fed, the equation remains the same; the combination of bacteria plus carbohydrates produces acid that is detrimental to early calcified teeth. The clinician should instruct parents on healthy feeding practices and daily plaque removal.

FOOD FOR THOUGHT — **SUGAR CONTENT IN COMMONLY USED ADULT AND PEDIATRIC MEDICATIONS**

Ninety-five percent of pediatricians prescribe liquid medications for their young patients. Doctors will prescribe liquid medications for adult patients who either do not like or are physically unable to swallow a pill. Due to a potentially bitter taste, pharmaceutical manufacturers will add sugar to the liquid formula to make it more agreeable to the palate, thereby increasing compliance. It is estimated that there are over 50 such prescribed syrupy medications. Some more recognized medications with the highest content of sucrose are codeine, azithromycin, cephalexin, erythromycin, and acetaminophen. Over-the-counter medications and preparations can be equally as cariogenic, like NyQuil, Robitussin, cough drops, lozenges, and vitamins. Oral medications may need to be taken two or three times a day, and each occurrence is an opportunity for bacteria to metabolize sugar into acid.

From Donaldson, M, Goodchild J, Epstein J. Sugar content, cariogenicity, and dental concerns with commonly used medications. JADA 2015;146(2):129–133.

SUGAR SUBSTITUTES

A sugar substitute is sweetener used in place of regular table sugar. There are two main classifications of sugar substitutes: synthetic sweeteners and sugar alcohols. Both synthetic sweeteners and sugar alcohols are **noncariogenic**, but only the synthetic sweeteners are *noncaloric*.[81]

Synthetic Sweeteners

Synthetic sweeteners, also called intense sweeteners, are popular sugar substitutes. Pink, yellow, and blue packets of the powders are offered aside packets of cane sugar in restaurant condiment containers and on grocery store shelves. Examples of the most common synthetic sweeteners are aspartame, saccharine, acesulfame K, and sucralose. Synthetic sweeteners are not metabolized by oral microorganisms to form acid so do not cause dental caries.[82] Artificial sweeteners are used in diet soft drinks, candy, pudding, jams and jellies, dairy products, and baked goods. They are helpful for weight control and a good sugar alternative for those with diabetes since they are not true carbohydrates. Many people report incompatibility with most of the sugar substitutes, the major complaints being headaches, bloating, and diarrhea. This is important to know when recommending suggestions for making better food and beverage choices.

- Aspartame (Equal and NutraSweet) is 200 times sweeter than sucrose and is used by more than 100 million people globally. Aspartame is made of aspartic acid and the amino acid phenylalanine. Those with phenylketonuria (PKU) should be made aware that aspartame is toxic to them. Aspartame has been around since the mid-seventies and is a popular choice to sweeten beverages. Even though it has a bitter aftertaste, it is less so than other sweeteners. It is not heat tolerant so is not used often when cooking and baking.
- Saccharin (Sweet 'N Low, Sugar Twin) is 300 to 400 times sweeter than sucrose. Discovered over 100 years ago, it is used to sweeten food and beverages. It has a bitter metallic aftertaste so is usually combined with other artificial sweeteners in products.
- Acesulfame K (Sunett, Sweet One) is 200 times sweeter than sucrose. It is very stable when frozen or heated so is a common sweetener in frozen foods. It has a bitter taste requiring addition of other sweeteners in the food product. You will find acesulfame K on food labels for soda, Kool-Aid, Jell-O, cocoa mix, ice cream, yogurt, syrup, and even alcoholic drinks.
- Sucralose (Splenda) is the only sugar substitute made from sugar. It is produced by chemically changing the structure of sugar molecules by substituting three chlorine atoms for three hydroxyl groups. With this chemical change, the body is unable to burn sucralose for energy. Sucralose remains stable at high temperatures, making it an ideal substitute for sugar in recipes. Consumers report no bitter aftertaste as with saccharin and aspartame.

Sugar Alcohols

Sugar alcohols, also called polyols, are neither sugar nor alcohol so the name is a bit misleading. Their chemical structure is similar to sugar and alcohol but they do not contain any *ethanol*. Sugar alcohols are naturally occurring in some fruits and vegetables but are also manufactured from sucrose, glucose, and starch. Placed next to regular table sugar, polyols look the same, but they are different in that they do not raise blood glucose levels like sucrose. Calorie content for sugar alcohol ranges from 1 to 3 calories/g versus 4 calories/g for sucrose. When sugar alcohol enters the intestines, it can cause cramping, bloating, and diarrhea. Sugar alcohols are prolific in chewing gum, which stimulates saliva and is great for enamel remineralization.

Examples of sugar alcohols:

- **Xylitol** is the alcohol form of xylose and is made by extracting the carbohydrate from corn cobs or birch wood. Xylitol is about 60% as sweet as sucrose but does not raise blood sugar. It has the ability to *reduce bacteria* in saliva, so is one of the most desirable sugar substitutes. Not only does it reduce bacterial count, but oral bacteria are unable to metabolize xylitol to create acid. The ability of xylitol chewing gum and candy to reduce *S. mutans* in plaque continues to be studied and shows promise in control of dental caries.[83–85]
- Sorbitol, also called glucitol, is made by adding hydrogen to glucose. Most sorbitol is made from corn syrup but can be found naturally in prunes, apples, peaches, and pears. Sorbitol draws water into the large intestines for a laxative effect. It has some unusual uses such as humectant in cosmetics and cigarettes and is a component in rocket fuel. Chewing gum with sorbitol has shown anticaries properties.[82]
- Erythritol is made by fermenting glucose with a yeast (*Moniliella pollinis*). It is 60% to 70% as sweet as sugar but has close to zero calories. Ninety percent of erythritol is absorbed before it enters the large intestines, eliminating laxative effects that other polyols have. Found naturally in soy sauce, grapes/wine, watermelon, and pears, it is also regularly used to sweeten chewing gum.
- Maltitol is the alcohol form of mannose and naturally occurs in pineapples, olives, asparagus, sweet potatoes, and carrots. It is 80% to 90% as sweet as sucrose and has a pleasant taste. It is a known ingredient in sugar-free hard candy and gum, chocolates, ice cream, and baked goods. Since maltitol is slowly absorbed, the rise in blood glucose is reduced and is a good sugar substitution for diabetics. With just 2 calories/g, it is also a good choice for those counting calories for weight reduction.

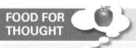

FOOD FOR THOUGHT THE FAMOUS TURKU STUDY

The Turku Study conducted in Finland in 1970s sought to discover if type of sugar made a difference in incidence of dental caries. Subjects (125) were divided into three groups, and each group sweetened food for 25 months with only one sweetener, depending on the group in which they were placed: sucrose, fructose, xylitol. 85% caries reduction in dental caries was noted in the xylitol group. The ability of xylitol chewing gum to reduce *S. mutans* in plaque continues to be studied and shows promise in control of dental caries.[83,85]

The American Diabetes Association (ADA) does not suggest complete elimination of sugar for people with diabetes although many may choose to avoid it and use artificial sweeteners.

The ADA's position on the use of sugar by people with diabetes is: "Sucrose foods may be substituted for other carbohydrate if it is part of the meal plan and covered by insulin or medication. It is advised to avoid excess energy intake from sweet foods."

If your patient has diabetes and is not amenable to using sugar substitutes, the following can be suggested as possible alternatives:

- Stevia (Truvia, SweetLeaf) is considered a natural sweetener as it is a plant derivative from South America. Like artificial sweeteners, stevia is not metabolized by the human body like sugar.

Other natural sweeteners that can be used in place of sucrose in recipes are agave nectar, date sugar, fruit juice concentrate, honey, maple syrup, and molasses. Sucanat, another natural sweetener, is whole cane sugar with water removed.

GROUPS AT RISK FOR DENTAL CARIES

Patients of all ages and socioeconomic status can develop dental caries, but those considered most at risk are children and elderly.[86,87] The following are other patient groups that can be at risk for dental caries:

- Patients who report carbohydrate-rich diets: frequent snacks consisting of added sugar (nibblers, grazers, or sippers of sodas and sugared coffee and tea)
- Patients with past experience with dental caries: visible caries, restorations placed within the last 3 years
- Patients with xerostomia; elderly and patients on antihypertensive, antidepressant, antihistamine, diuretic, analgesic, and other drugs that decrease saliva; those with diseases that contribute to dry mouth such as cancer, diabetes, anemia, salivary gland dystrophy, stroke, Alzheimer's, Sjögren's syndrome, autoimmune diseases, Parkinson's, and palsy
- Patients with low exposure to systemic fluoride
- Patients with poor oral hygiene habits or physical limitations preventing thorough oral care
- Patients reporting use of herbal supplements like Ma huang and ephedra, which cause dry mouth

- Patients prescribed soft diets, eliminating hard crunchy foods that stimulate saliva
- Young patients whose parents or caregivers have current caries

RELATE TO PATIENTS

Not all patients are in need of diet counseling for dental caries, so it is imperative to identify those groups at high risk. An evaluation for **caries risk** should be completed on every new and returning patient of any age to formulate the best plan for preventive treatment. There are many existing caries assessment forms available for use at chairside. Patient assessment findings and answers to additional questions are weighed, giving a numeric value. For example, previous experience with caries, source and amount of fluoride, meal/snacking habits, socioeconomic status, amount of bacterial plaque, nature of saliva, and frequency of dental visits. Scores fall in categories that indicate levels of risk from low to high. Depending on where the patient falls on the risk matrix, diet counseling may be needed.

The following is an example of Caries Risk Matrix:

CAMBRA = Caries Management by Risk Assessment

- ☐ Irregular dental care/poor family oral health
- ☐ Poor oral hygiene (reasons include reduced physical/mental ability or homelessness)
- ☐ Tooth morphology and defects (deep grooves, crowding, malformed arch, enamel defects)
- ☐ Current orthodontic appliances
- ☐ Exposed root surfaces
- ☐ Current restorations, overhangs, open margins
- ☐ Xerostomia-reduced salivary flow or poor quality of saliva (including polypharmacy, chemotherapy, or radiation therapy)
- ☐ Substance abuse (includes tobacco, alcohol, or drugs)
- ☐ Prolonged nursing (bottle or breast)
- ☐ Cariogenic diet (see 24-hour diet survey)

_____

- ☐ TOTAL

1–2 checked boxes = *Low* Risk
3–6 checked boxes = *Moderate* Risk
7–10 checked boxes = *High* Risk

Disease Indicators (WREC)	Risk Factors (BADD)	Protective Factors (SAFER)
White spot	Bad bacteria	Saliva and sealants
Restorations <3 years	Absence of saliva	Antibacterials
Enamel lesions	Dietary habits are poor	Fluoride
Cavities in dentin	Destructive lifestyle habits	Effective diet and lifestyle habits
		Risk-based reassessment

Adapted from "The Caries Imbalance" by John Featherstone, MSc, PhD.

1–2: Low Risk: No incipient or new lesions within the last 3 years

- ☐ Provide oral hygiene instructions emphasizing complete plaque removal and routine dental visits.
- ☐ Use fluoride toothpaste on a daily basis (pea sized for young children).
- ☐ Determine need for sealants.
- ☐ In-office fluoride if indicated.

3–6: Moderate Risk: No incipient or new lesions within the last 3 years and one or two risk factors that may increase caries risk

- ☐ Provide oral hygiene instructions emphasizing complete plaque removal and routine dental visits.
- ☐ Use fluoride toothpaste on a daily basis (pea sized for young children).
- ☐ Determine need for sealants.
- ☐ Complete a 24-hour food recall—stress frequency, sequence of eating carbohydrates, and give examples of cariostatic foods.
- ☐ In-office fluoride if indicated.
- ☐ Prescribe fluoride supplements if under 6 years old, and OTC fluoridated mouthwash if able to rinse and spit or supply with tray for gel fluoride.

7–10: High Risk

- ☐ Provide oral hygiene instructions emphasizing complete plaque removal and more frequent dental visits (3 months).
- ☐ Use fluoride toothpaste on a daily basis (pea sized for young children).
- ☐ Determine need for sealants.
- ☐ Complete a 24-hour food recall or 3-Day Diet Diary—stress frequency, sequence of eating carbohydrates, and give examples of cariostatic foods.
- ☐ Frequent in-office fluoride if indicated.
- ☐ Prescribe fluoride supplements if under 6 years old, and OTC fluoridated mouthwash if able to rinse and spit or supply with tray for gel fluoride.
- ☐ Antimicrobial mouth rinse if over 6 years old.

It is important to explain the relationship of food to disease in the oral cavity and discuss factors that can lessen the impact of sugar in the diet. It is impractical to think that your patients will eliminate all carbohydrates from their diet and unwise to suggest eliminating any favorite food or drink. Work at raising the oral pH by including the following cariostatic foods in the diet:

- Cheese: Aged cheddar, Swill, Blue, Monterey Jack, Mozzarella, Brie, Gouda
- Peanuts
- Artificial sweeteners
- Crunchy foods
- Sugar-free chewing gum[88,89]

It is important to teach patients how to calculate approximate amount of acid attack on teeth per day. Keeping the time to a minimum, no more than 60 minutes each day, will moderate caries incidence.[3] Snacks eaten 20 minutes before a meal or 20 minutes after a meal count as a separate eating event and contribute to calculations for total acid production. For example, if it takes 30 minutes for liquids to clear the oral cavity, then limit sweet beverage consumption to twice a day. If sipping on soda throughout the day, each sipping interval counts as 20 minutes of acid attack. Since cookies take about 60 minutes to clear the oral cavity, then you would only want to eat them as a snack once a day.

Eating patterns to reduce amount of acid attack can be manipulated for healthier teeth. The best advice would be to rearrange the sequence of foods and beverages within meals and throughout the day. For example:

If an acidic food or fermentable carbohydrate is eaten with a meal, they will clear with the rest of the food in the meal. Certain foods included with the meal may help neutralize acids, and the act of chewing will bring saliva into the mouth.

Rinsing with water or chewing on an antacid tablet after eating has some neutralizing effect.[90]

After sugared gum has lost its flavor, the chewing action can do the same thing as the sugar-free gum.

Other good suggestions are as follows:

- If at all possible, greatly reduce *frequency* of consuming sugary and acidic foods.[91-95]
- Eliminate carbohydrate snacks before bedtime.
- Combine foods—eat sweets after proteins and fats or follow sugared foods with cheese.
- Combine raw, crunchy foods (that stimulate saliva) with cooked foods.
- Citrus fruits (citric acid) stimulate saliva production.
- Limit sweetened beverages to meals.
- Eat cookies with milk for benefits of calcium and phosphate.

- Drink iced tea instead of soda—tea will still work as a stimulant but also contains fluoride.[96]
- Drink orange juice with calcium—calcium helps remineralize.
- Do not rush to brush after acidic beverages—let the oral cavity remineralize enamel on its own for about **30** minutes. (Brushing may remove demineralized structure before it has a chance to remineralize.)
- Chewing sugar-free gum stimulates salivary flow that may be effective in neutralizing interproximal plaque acid through mechanical action.
- Use a fluoridated toothpaste.

Develop a "script" on what to teach your patient about dental caries. Watch the YouTube video on Tooth Decay—how to Avoid It: http://youtube/Z3rheJVWNt4.

CHAPTER
REVIEW

PRACTICE FOR PATIENTS

Patient #1

Your doctor has referred a patient to you for advice on limiting amount of dietary sugar. The patient is a 28-year-old marathon runner who reports carbohydrate loading and drinking on average 10 sports drinks throughout the week as he trains for the next marathon. As a result, his oral exam revealed three new carious lesions and two broken amalgams with recurrent decay. Watch the Truth about Sugar—Part 1—Nutrition by Natalie on www.Psychetruth.net and formulate an educational program to help the patient manage the amount of sugar consumed in his diet.

Patient #2

Your client is a 23-year-old female graduate student who presents at your dental practice after a 5-year absence from professional dental care. She reports good health with use of antihistamines as needed for seasonal allergies. Radiographic and clinical examinations reveal five new posterior interproximal carious lesions and recurrent caries around two existing anterior restorations. A quick inquiry into her diet indicates high intake of carbohydrates, preference for soft foods, and frequent use of sugared breath mints. Home care consists of daily brushing for about 45 seconds and flossing two or three times per week.

1. List all factors in the above scenario that could contribute to dental caries formation, explaining in detail their relationship to each other.
2. Write the advice you would give this client to help reduce future caries development.

RELATE TO YOU

Assignment #1

Purchase online or borrow litmus paper from your Chemistry Department. Litmus paper will determine acidity or alkalinity of a substance. A good brand is Hydrion as it offers a full-range color chart. Another good source is A.T.Still University: ASDOHtext2floss@atsu.edu or www.Text2Floss.com

Use the litmus paper to test the pH of your oral cavity and record in the following chart:

Oral pH	Time Interval
	Immediately before drinking a soda
	5 minutes after you start drinking
	Immediately after finishing the soda
	10 minutes after drinking
	20 minutes after drinking
	30 minutes after drinking

How quickly did the oral pH drop when drinking the soda?
How many minutes did it take to reach a pH of 5.5?
How long did it take for the pH to start returning to normal?

Assignment #2

Conduct variances of change to pH by following pH change when eating a jelly bean, piece of bread with jelly, and potato chip.
Which example cleared the fastest?
Does rinsing with water right after chewing speed oral clearance time?

REFERENCES

1. Moynihan P, Petersen PE. Diet, nutrition and the prevention of dental disease. *Public Health Nutr.* 2004;1(1A):201–226. (WHO Collaborating Centre for Nutrition and Oral Health)
2. Sheiham A, James WP. Diet and dental caries: the pivotal role of free sugars reemphasized. *J Dent Res* 2015;94(10):1341–1347.
3. Featherstone JD. The continuum of dental caries—evidence for a dynamic disease process. *J Dent Res* 2004;83(Spec Iss C):39–42.
4. Gustaffson BE, Quensel CE, Lanke LS, et al. The Vipeholm dental caries study: the effect of different levels of carbohydrate intake on caries activity in 436 individuals observed for five years. *Acta Odontol Scand* 1954;11(3–4):232–264.
5. Lagerweij MD, vanLoveren C. Declining caries trends: are we satisfied? *Curr Oral Health Rep* 2015;2(4):212–217.
6. Bowen WH. Dental caries-not just holes in teeth! A perspective *Mol Oral Microbiol* 2015;31(3):228–233.
7. Linke HA, Moss SJ, Arav L, et al. Intra-oral lactic acid production during clearance of different foods containing various carbohydrates. *Z Ermahrungswiss* 1997;36(2): 191–197.
8. Kalesinskas P, et al. Reducing dental plaque formation and caries development. A review of current methods and implications for novel pharmaceuticals. *Stomatologia* 2014;16(2):44–52.
9. Islam B, Khan SN, Khan AU. Dental caries: from infection to prevention. *Med Sci Monit* 2007;13(11):RA196–RA203.
10. Sharma G, Puranik MP, KR S. Approaches to arresting dental caries: an update. *J Clin Diagn Res* 2015;9(5):ZE08–ZE11.
11. Bradshaw DJ, Lynch RJ. Diet and the microbial etiology of dental caries: new paradigms. *Int Dent J* 2013;63(suppl 2):64–72.
12. Monteiro CA, et al. Ultra-processed products are becoming dominant in the global food system. *Obes Rev* 2013;14(S2):21–28.
13. Martinez-Steele E, et al. Ultra-processed foods and added sugars in the US diet: evidence from a nationally representative cross-sectional study. *BMJ Open* 2016;6(3):e009892.
14. Yeung CA, Goodfellow A, Flanagan L. The truth about sugar. *Dent Update* 2015;42(6):507–510.
15. Meyer BS, Lee JY. The confluence of sugar, dental caries, and health policy. *J Dent Res* 2015;94(10):1338–1340.
16. Moynihan PJ, Kelly SA. Effect on caries of restricting sugars intake. Systematic review of WHO guidelines. *J Dent Res* 2014;93(1):8–18.
17. Peres MA, et al. Sugar consumption and changes in dental caries from childhood to adolescence. *J Dent Res* 2016;95(4):388–394.
18. Barbour ME, Lussi A. Erosion in relation to nutrition and the environment. *Monogr Oral Sci* 2014;25:143–154.
19. Kanzow P, et al. Etiology and pathogenesis of dental erosion. *Quintessence Int* 2016;47(4):275–278.
20. Cassiano LP, et al. Protective effect of whole and fat-free fluoridated milk, applied before or after acid challenge, against dental erosion. *Caries Res* 2016;50(2):111–116.

21. Ferrazano GF, et al. Plant polyphenols and their anti-cariogenic properties: a review. *Molecules* 2011;16:1486–1507.
22. Gazzani G, Daglia M, Papetti A. Food components with anticaries activity. *Curr Opin Biotechnol* 2012;23(2):153–159.
23. Lussi A, et al. Dental erosion-an overview with emphasis on chemical histopathological aspects. *Caries Res* 2011;45(suppl 1):2–12.
24. Aimutis WR. Bioactive properties of milk proteins with particular focus on anticariogenesis. *J Nutr* 2004;134(4):989S–995S.
25. Ehlen LA, et al. Acidic beverages increase the risk of in vitro tooth erosion. *Nutr Res* 2008;28(5):299–303.
26. Setarehnejad A, et al. The protective effect of caseinomacropeptide against dental erosion using hydroxyapatite as a model system. *Int Dairy J* 2010;20(9):652–656.
27. Naval S, et al. The effects of beverages on plaque acidogenicity after a sugary challenge. *J Am Dent Assoc* 2013;144(7):815–822.
28. Attin T, et al. Brushing abrasion of softened and remineralized dentin: an in-situ study. *Caries Res* 2004;38(1):62–66.
29. Kumar S, et al. Dental caries experience in high risk soft drinks factory workers of South India: a comparative study. *Indian J Dent Res* 2014;25(2):174–177.
30. Skinner J, et al. Sugary drink consumption and dental caries in New South Wales teenagers. *Aust Dent J* 2015;60(2):169–175.
31. Bemabe E, et al. Sugar-sweetened beverages and dental caries in adults: a 4 year prospective study. *J Dent* 2014;42(8):952–958.
32. Jain P, Gary JJ. Which is a stronger indicator of dental caries: oral hygiene, food, or beverage? A clinical study. *Gen Dent* 2014;62(3):63–68.
33. Marshall TA. Preventing dental caries associated with sugar-sweetened beverages. *J Am Dent Assoc* 2013;144(10):1148–1152.
34. Punitha VC, et al. Role of dietary habits and diet in caries occurrence and severity among urban adolescent school children. *J Pharm Bioall Sci* 2015;7(suppl 1):S296–S300.
35. Geddes DA. Diet patterns and caries. *Adv Dent Res* 1994;8(2):221–224.
36. Touger-Decker R, van Loveren C. Sugars and dental caries. *Am J Clin Nutr* 2003;78(4):881S–892S.
37. Tanaguchi H, et al. Correspondence between food consistency and suprahyoid muscle activity, tongue pressure, and bolus transit times during the oropharyngeal phase of swallowing. *J Appl Physiol (1985)*. 2008;105(3):791–799.
38. Herod EL. The effect of cheese on dental caries: a review of the literature. *Aust Dent J* 1992;36:120–125.
39. Sheiham A, James WP. A new understanding of the relationship between sugars, dental caries and fluoride use: implications for limits on sugar consumption. *Public Health Nutr* 2014;17(10):2176–2184.
40. ten Cate JM. Contemporary perspective on the use of fluoride products in caries prevention. *Br Dent J* 2013;214:161–167.
41. Belda-Ferre P, et al. The human metaproteome reveals potential biomarkers for caries disease. *Proteomics* 2015;15(20):3497–3507.
42. Aas JA, Griffin AL, et al. Bacteria of dental caries in primary and permanent teeth in children and young adults. *J Clin Microbiol* 2008;46(4):1407–1417.
43. Struzycka, I. The oral microbiome in dental caries. *Pol J Microbiol* 2014;63(2):127–135.

44. Bizhang M, et al. Detection of nine microorganisms from the initial carious root lesions using a TaqMan-based real-time PCR. *Oral Dis* 2011;17(7):642–652.

45. Chen L, et al. Extensive description and comparison of human supra-gingival microbiome in root caries and health. *PLoS One* 2015;10(2):e0117064.

46. Do T, et al. Transcriptomic analysis of three *Veillonella* spp. Present in carious dentin and in the saliva of caries-free individuals. *Front Cell Infect Microbiol* 2015;5:25.

47. Badet C, Thebaud NB. Ecology of lactobacilli in the oral cavity: a review of the literature. *Open Microbiol J* 2008;2:38–48.

48. Falsetta ML, et al. Symbiotic relationship between *Streptococcus mutans* and *Candida albicans* synergizes virulence of plaque biofilms in vivo. *Infect Immun* 2014;82(5): 1968–1981.

49. deSouzaa PM, et al. Association between early childhood caries and maternal caries status: a cross-section study in Sao Luis, Maranhao, Brazil. *Eur J Dent* 2015;9(1): 122–126.

50. Yates C, Duane B. Maternal xylitol and mutans streptococci transmission. *Evid Based Dent* 2015;16(2):41–42.

51. Milgrom P, et al. Counseling on early childhood caries transmission by dentists. *J Public Health Dent* 2013;73(2):151–157.

52. Mitchell SC, et al. Maternal transmission of mutans streptococci in severe-early childhood caries. *Pediatr Dent* 2009;31(3):193–201.

53. Schroth RJ, et al. Prenatal vitamin D and dental caries in infants. *Pediatrics* 2014;113(5):e1277–e1284.

54. Martin AE, et al. Facial development disorders due to inhibition to endochondral ossification of mandibular condyle process caused by malnutrition. *Angle Orthod* 2014;84(3):473–478.

55. Garat JA, et al. Orthodontic implications of protein undernutrition in mandibular growth. A cephalometric study in growing rats. *Acta Odontol Latinoam* 2007;20(2): 73–78.

56. TenCate JM, Featherstone JD. Mechanistic aspects of the interactions between fluoride and dental enamel. *Crit Rev Oral Biol Med* 1991;2(3):283–296.

57. Armfield JM, et al. Water fluoridation and the association of sugar-sweetened beverage consumption and dental caries in Australian children. *Am J Public Health* 2013;103(3):494–500.

58. Rosen-Grget K, Peros K, Sutej I, et al. The cariostatic mechanisms of fluoride. *Acta Med Acad* 2013;42(2):179–188.

59. Yeung CA. Fluoride prevents caries among adults of all ages. *Evid Based Dent* 2007;8(3):72–73;50(suppl 1):22–37.

60. Lynch RJ, Navada R, Walla R. Low-levels of fluoride in plaque and saliva and their effects on the demineralisation and remineralisation of enamel; role of fluoride toothpastes. *Int Dent J* 2004;54(suppl 1):304–309.

61. Mielczarek A, Gedrange T, Michalik J. An in vitro evaluation of the effect of fluoride products on white spot lesion remineralization. *Am J Dent* 2015;28(1):51–56.

62. Waldbott G. Fluoride in food. *Am J Clin Nutr* 1963;12(6):455–462.

63. Duckworth RM, et al. Effects of flossing and rinsing with a fluoridated mouthwash after brushing with a fluoridated toothpaste on salivary fluoride clearance. *Caries Res* 2008;43:387–390.

64. Hellwig E, Lennon AM. Systemic versus topical fluoride. *Caries Res* 2004;38:258–262.

65. Gao SS, et al. Caries remineralization and arresting effect in children by professionally applied fluoride treatment—a systematic review. *BMC Oral Health* 2016 Feb;16:12.
66. ADA Center for Evidence-Based Dentistry Position Paper. Topical fluoride for caries prevention. BioMed Central The open Access Publisher: 2016.
67. Buzalaf MA, Hannas AR, Kato MT. Saliva and dental erosion. *J Appl Oral Sci* 2012;20(5):493–502.
68. Lagerlof F, Oliveby A. Caries-protective factors in saliva. *Adv Dent Res* 1994;8(2):229–238.
69. Lenander-Lumikari M, Loimaranta V. Saliva and dental caries. *Adv Dent Res* 2000;14:40–47.
70. Rajesh KS, et al. Assessment of salivary calcium, phosphate, magnesium, pH, and flow rate in healthy subjects, periodontitis and dental caries. *Contemp Clin Dent* 2015;6(4):461–465.
71. Su M, et al. Caries prevention for patients with dry mouth. *J Can Dent Assoc* 2011;77:b85.
72. Manju M, et al. Evaluation of the effect of three supplementary oral hygiene measures on salivary mutans streptococci levels in children: a randomized comparative clinical trial. *Eur J Dent* 2015;9(4):462–469.
73. Colak H, et al. Early childhood caries update: a review of causes, diagnoses and treatments. *J Nat Biol Med* 2013;4(1):29–38.
74. Kononen E. Development of oral bacteria flora in young children. *Ann Med* 2000;32:107–112.
75. Gilbert S. A holobiont birth narrative: the epigenetic transmission of the human microbiome. *Front Genet* 2014;5:282–330.
76. Tanner AC, et al. Similarity of the oral microbiota of pre-school children with that of their caregivers in a population-based study. *Oral Microbiol Immunol* 2002;17:379–387.
77. Ma C, Chen F, Zhang Y, et al. Comparison of oral microbial profiles between children with severe early childhood caries and caries-free children using the human oral microbe identification microarray. *PLoS One* 2015;10(3):e0122075.
78. Boggess KA, Edelstein BL. Oral health in women during preconception and pregnancy: implications for birth outcomes and infant oral health. *Matern Child Health J* 2006;10(suppl 1):169–174.
79. Tham R, et al. Breast feeding and the risk of dental caries: a systematic review and meta-analysis. *Acta Paediatr* 2015;104:62–84.
80. Walesca AM, et al. Breast and bottle feeding as risk factors for dental caries: a systematic review and meta-analysis. *PLoS One* 2015;10(11):e0142922.
81. Kinghorn D, et al. Noncariogenic intense natural sweeteners. *Med Res Rev* 1998;18(5):347–360.
82. Gupta P, et al. Role of sugar and sugar substitutes in dental caries: a review. *ISRN Dent* 2013;2013:519421.
83. Soderling E, et al. The effect of xylitol on the composition of the oral flora: a pilot study. *Eur J Dent* 2011;5(1):24–31.
84. Ribelles LM, et al. Effects of xylitol chewing gum on salivary flow rate, pH, buffering capacity and presence of *Streptococcus mutans* in saliva. *Eur J Paediatr Dent* 2010;11(1):9–14.
85. Parizi MK, et al. Sugar alcohols efficacy on dental caries incidence: a review article. *Res J Pharm Biol Chem Sci* 2015;6(3):1871–1874.

86. Llena C, et al. Association between the number of early carious lesions and diet in children with a high prevalence of caries. *Eur J Paediatr Dent* 2015;16(1):7–12.
87. Gati D, Vieira A. Elderly at greater risk for root caries: a look at the multifactorial risks with emphasis on genetics susceptibility. *Int J Dent* 2011;2011:Article ID 647168. 6 pages.
88. Emamieh S, et al. The effect of two types chewing gum containing casein phosphopeptide–amorphous calcium phosphate and xylitol on salivary *Streptococcus mutans*. *J Conserv Dent* 2015;18(3):102–105.
89. Thabuis C, et al. Effects of maltitol and xylitol chewing-gums on parameters involved in dental caries development. *Eur J Paediatr Dent* 2013;14(4):303–308.
90. RLindquist B, Lingstrom P, Fandriks L, et al. Influence of five neutralizing products on intra-oral pH after rinsing with simulated gastric acid. *Eur J Oral Sci* 2011;119(4): 301–304.
91. Freeman R. Moderate evidence support a relationship between sugar intake and dental caries. *Evid Based Dent* 2014;15(4):98–99.
92. No Authors. Sugar consumption reduction needed to prevent caries, study says. *J Am Dent Assoc* 2014;145(11):1110.
93. Kmietowicz Z. Reduce sugar intake to 3% to protect against tooth decay, say researchers. *BMJ* 2014;15:349.
94. Moynihan PJ, Kelly SA. Effect on caries of restricting sugar intake: systematic review to inform WHO guidelines. *J Dent Res* 2014;93(1):8–18.
95. Marshall TA. Nomenclature, characteristics, and dietary intakes of sugars. *J Am Dent Assoc* 2015;146(1):61–64.
96. Peng CY, et al. Analysis of naturally occurring fluoride in commercial teas and estimation of its daily intake through tea consumption. *J Food Sci* 2016;81(1):H235–H239.

10

Nutrition and Periodontal Disease

Learning Objectives

- Describe the proposed roles of micronutrients and macronutrients in periodontal disease
- Discuss the link between obesity and periodontal disease
- List some oral symptoms associated with ascorbic acid deficiency gingivitis
- Explain the role of dental health care providers in addressing nutrition in the management of periodontal disease
- Suggest healthy food choices for patients with periodontal disease

> A diet low in important nutrients can compromise the body's immune system and make it harder for the body to fight off infection. Because periodontal disease begins as an infection, poor nutrition can worsen the condition of your gums.
>
> *American Academy of Periodontology (perio.org)*

Key Terms

Antioxidants
Ascorbic Acid Deficiency Gingivitis
Body Mass Index (BMI)
Coenzyme Q10
Dietary fiber
Gingivitis
Hyperlipidemia
Macronutrients
Micronutrients
Modifying Role

National Health and Nutrition Examination Survey (NHANES)
Obesity
Periodontal Diseases
Periodontitis
Periodontium
Primary Role
Probiotic Supplements
Susceptible Host

INTRODUCTION

Traditionally, the impact of nutrition on oral health has focused on the effects of diet on caries risk. It is well known that the caries process can be modified through changes in eating habits and food selection. Diet is a major factor in the development of dental caries; however, its role in the development and progression of periodontal diseases is less well understood. While diet plays a **primary role** in the development of dental caries, diet primarily plays a **modifying role** in the progression of periodontal disease.

The **periodontium** consists of the hard and soft tissues that surround the teeth including the gingiva, gingival connective tissue, periodontal ligament, alveolar bone, and cementum. **Periodontal diseases** are bacterial/inflammatory diseases that lead to the destruction of the supporting tissues of the teeth. Gingivitis and periodontitis are the two basic categories of periodontal disease. **Gingivitis** is a bacterial infection that is confined to the gingiva (Figure 10-1). **Periodontitis** is a bacterial infection of all parts of the periodontium including the gingiva, periodontal ligament, bone, and cementum (Figure 10-2).

While bacteria are the primary etiologic factors for periodontal disease, a **susceptible host** is also necessary for disease initiation. Nutrition may be a modifying factor that impacts the host's immune response and the integrity of the tissues of the periodontium.[1-3]

Figure 10-1 Gingivitis. Note the *red* gingiva and bulbous interdental papilla in this patient with gingivitis. (From Gehrig J, Willmann D. *Foundations of Periodontics for the Dental Hygienist.* 4th ed. Baltimore, MD: Lippincott Williams & Wilkins; 2016, with permission.)

Figure 10-2 Periodontitis. An example of periodontitis with loss of soft tissue and bone support around the teeth. (From Gehrig J, Willmann D. *Foundations of Periodontics for the Dental Hygienist.* 4th ed. Baltimore, MD: Lippincott Williams & Wilkins; 2016, with permission.)

This chapter reviews possible links between nutrition and periodontal disease. Nutrients may be categorized as major or minor based on the amounts consumed in our diets. **Macronutrients** are the class of nutrients, which humans consume in the largest quantities—gram quantities—and which provide humans with the bulk of energy.[4] There are five primary macronutrients: carbohydrate, protein, fat, fiber, and alcohol. **Micronutrients** are nutrients that are required only in minuscule amounts—milligram to microgram quantities—and include vitamins and minerals. Micronutrients enable the body to produce enzymes, hormones, and other substances essential for proper growth and development.[5] In addition to nutrients, other molecules provided by diet, such as antioxidants, might play a role in the health of the periodontium.

WHAT'S GOOD FOR THE BODY IS GOOD FOR THE PERIODONTIUM

The body needs both macronutrients and micronutrients to *maintain* health in the various tissues of the body. Likewise, the tissues that support the teeth—the periodontium—require the presence of nutrients to develop and remain healthy. The health of the periodontium depends on the intake of sufficient protein, folic acid, and various micronutrients.[2,3] If a patient is undernourished or malnourished, his or her periodontium will suffer a diminished resistance to disease (as will the rest of the body).

It is reasonable to consume a nutritionally adequate diet to help maintain the integrity of the periodontal tissues (Table 10-1). Examples of nutrients that are important for a healthy periodontium are as follows:

- Omega-3 fatty acids
- Fiber
- Protein
- Vitamin C
- Vitamin A
- Vitamin B complex
- Vitamin D
- Calcium
- Magnesium
- CoQ 10

Table 10-1	Periodontal Benefit of Vitamins and Minerals		
Nutrient	**Function**	**Mineral**	**Function**
Vitamin A	Builds and maintains healthy epithelium Aids immune system	Calcium	Builds and maintains strong alveolar process
Vitamin B complex	Forms new cells	Iron	Forms collagen
	Keeps immune system healthy		Aids with wound healing Regulates inflammatory response
Vitamin D	Aids with calcium, magnesium, and phosphorus absorption	Zinc	Forms collagen Aids with wound healing Regulates inflammatory response
Vitamin C	Aids with wound healing	Copper	Aids with wound healing
	Helps the body resist infection	Selenium	Prevents harm to cells
Protein	Promotes growth, maintenance, and repair all body tissues	Magnesium	Works with vitamin D and calcium to build and maintain strong alveolar bone

MACRONUTRIENTS AND THE PERIODONTIUM

Lipids

Lipids help provide energy and insulation for the body and are needed to for the body to *absorb* the lipid-soluble vitamins A, D, E, and K. Omega-3 fatty acids are a class of essential fatty acids found in fish oils, especially from salmon and other cold-water fish. EPA (eicosapentaenoic acid) and DHA (docosahexaenoic acid) are the two principal omega-3 fatty acids. The body has a limited ability to manufacture EPA and DHA by converting the essential fatty acid, alpha-linolenic acid, which is found in flaxseed oil, canola oil, or walnuts.

Omega-3 fatty acids have *anti-inflammatory* properties, and their presence in the diet may help to reduce the inflammation associated with periodontal disease. In an in vivo study, rats on an omega-3 fatty acid diet showed a reduced alveolar bone loss associated with an infection by *Porphyromonas gingivalis*.[6,7] A study by Naqvi et al. looked at the data from the **National Health and Nutrition Examination Survey (NHANES)**—a population-based survey conducted by the National Center for Health Statistics designed to assess the health and nutritional status of Americans—of 9,182 adults aged 20 years and older who participated in the survey between 1999 and 2004. In this nationally representative sample, higher dietary intakes of DHA and to a lesser degree EPA were associated with lower prevalence of periodontitis.[8] In another study, Iwasaki et al. found that low DHA intake was significantly associated with more periodontal disease in older individuals.[9] These studies suggest that diets enriched for omega-3 fatty acids may modulate the host response to periodontal disease.

Hyperlipidemia is the condition that occurs when a body has too many lipids or fats in the blood. In proper quantities, lipids—which include cholesterol and triglycerides—are an important part of a body's overall health. Having higher levels of lipids may lead or contribute to blocked arteries and an increased chance of heart disease or stroke.

Obesity occurs when body weight is so high that it puts an individual's health in danger. Obesity is defined as a medical condition of excess body fat that has accumulated overtime. According to the **body mass index (BMI)**, a BMI between 25 and 29.9 is considered overweight, while a BMI of over 30 is generally an indication of obesity. Some very fit athletes will have a BMI over 30, but that is an exception. The most recent national data on obesity prevalence indicate that more than one third of adults and 17% of youth in the United States are obese.[10]

Obesity is a *risk factor* for periodontal disease.[11,12] Recent studies suggest that periodontal disease affects glucose metabolism both in individuals with and without diabetes.[12] Figure 10-3 illustrates a proposed relationship between obesity and periodontitis. Adipose tissues release inflammatory agents, including enlarged adipocytes, which contribute to the body's inflammatory response. They also predispose the

Figure 10-3   Obesity as a risk factor for periodontal disease. Relationships between obesity and periodontal disease. The *black arrows* indicate established relationships; *blue arrows* indicate proposed associations.

body to insulin resistance. A poorly nourished host will have a poorly functioning immune system, which fails to fight off inflammation. The relationship between obesity and periodontal disease was examined in the Third National Health and Nutrition Examination Survey (NHANES III) for a population of 12,367 individuals without diabetes. These data show that body mass index is positively related to the severity of periodontal attachment loss.[12–15]

Dietary Fiber

Carbohydrates nondigestible by humans are considered **dietary fiber**. Examples of foods that are a good source of dietary fiber include bananas, apples, pears, oranges, prunes, peas, and beans.[16] Interest in dietary fiber and periodontal health stems from fiber's effect on body weight. Fiber controls serum glucose levels and lowers lipids, body mass index, and *inflammatory* agents excreted by adipose tissue, which are associated with periodontal disease.

There is some evidence to support the beneficial role of dietary fiber, although the reason behind this is not entirely clear. Dietary habits including low intakes of fiber have been noted in edentulous women compared with women with 25 to 32 teeth.[17] In two cross-sectional studies, a low dietary fiber intake *increased* periodontal *inflammation*[18] in middle-aged women and gingivitis risk[17] in adolescent females. A study by Schwartz et al. shows that each serving of good to excellent sources of total fiber is associated with lower risk of alveolar bone loss progression, but only in men aged 65 or older.[16]

Years ago, it was thought that chewing fibrous foods could remove plaque biofilm at the gingival margin, but that theory has been proved incorrect. There is no such thing as "detergent" foods," and the act of chewing fibrous foods will not increase gingival keratinization.

Proteins

The effect of protein-energy malnutrition (PEM) on periodontal disease risk was extensively reviewed by Enwonwu, who observed that aggressive periodontal disease is more prevalent and severe in undernourished individuals than in well-nourished ones.[19-21] Enwonwu found marked *changes in the oral microbial ecology* resulting in an increase in pathogenic anaerobic organisms in individuals with protein deficiencies.[21] Despite these findings, epidemiological studies of protein deficiencies are complicated. Protein deficiencies in malnourished individuals are accompanied by deficiencies in other nutrients. In addition, there are many other risk factors present in malnourished individuals such as inadequate plaque biofilm control.[22]

MICRONUTRIENTS AND THE PERIODONTIUM

Vitamin C

Vitamin C—also known as ascorbic acid—is named for its ability to cure scurvy. Humans are unable to synthesize ascorbic acid and depend on dietary sources to meet vitamin C needs. Vitamin C is found in fresh fruits and vegetables such as oranges, berries, tomatoes, leafy greens, and kiwifruit. Consumption of fruits and vegetables or fortifying the diet with vitamin C supplements is essential to avoid ascorbic acid deficiency. **Ascorbic acid deficiency gingivitis** is an inflammatory response of the gingiva caused by plaque biofilm that is aggravated by chronically low vitamin C levels. Ascorbic acid deficiency gingivitis manifests clinically as bright red, swollen, ulcerated gingival tissue that bleeds with the slightest provocation.[23,24] An example of ascorbic acid deficiency gingivitis is shown in Figure 10-4.

Nishida et al. evaluated the role of dietary vitamin C as a contributing risk factor for periodontal disease utilizing the NHANES III.[25] Dietary intake of vitamin C showed a weak, but statistically significant, relationship with periodontal disease in current and former smokers as measured by clinical attachment. Cross-sectional studies show that low serum levels of vitamin C led to a higher relative risk for periodontal disease and to the number of teeth with periodontal disease progression.[26-28]

Vitamin A

Vitamin A—a fat-soluble vitamin—is needed for the maturation of epithelial tissues. Preformed vitamin A is found primarily in animal fats and fish oils as retinoids, which can be toxic when taken in high doses. Carotenoids—precursors of vitamin A—are present mainly in vegetables and fruits. The main carotenoid found in foods, beta carotene, is nontoxic in high doses and functions as an antioxidant.

Figure 10-4 Ascorbic acid deficiency gingivitis. A photograph of a patient with scurvy. Note the *bright red*, swollen, and ulcerated gingival tissue. (From Gehrig J, Willmann D. *Foundations of Periodontics for the Dental Hygienist.* 4th ed. Baltimore, MD: Lippincott Williams & Wilkins; 2016, with permission.)

Two cross-sectional studies found that levels of vitamin A are significantly lower in men with periodontitis.[29,30] *Excess* vitamin A can lead to periodontal *inflammation*. In a case report, a 20-year-old woman exhibited gingival ulcerations, bleeding, swelling, and xerostomia. Headache and hair loss were also noted. The woman reported taking 2,000,000 IU of vitamin A daily for 6 months. When the vitamin supplementation was stopped, improvement in the gingival tissues was noted within 1 week. At 2 months, the appearance of the oral tissue was normal.[31]

Vitamin B Complex

Thiamin, niacin, riboflavin, pantothenic acid, pyridoxine, folic acid, cyanocobalamin, and biotin together form the water-soluble vitamin B complex. (See Chapter 5 for more information.) The B-complex vitamins are a group of related substances involved in energy production, red blood cell formation, and protein and amino acid metabolism. Folic acid and vitamin B_{12} are two closely related B complex vitamins that are necessary for bone marrow to produce red blood cells. The vitamin B complex may be important to periodontal wound healing. Biotin—important for collagen synthesis—is necessary for growth and muscle function. Cross-sectional studies found that low serum folate level was independently associated with periodontal disease.[32] Yu et al. studied 844 dentate elderly subjects aged 60 and older (mean age 70.6) who completed a periodontal examination and laboratory test for serum folate levels. Data analysis showed a statistically significant association between low folate level and periodontal disease. Thus, a low serum folate level was independently associated with periodontal disease in older adults.[32] The results suggest that serum folate levels, important indicators of periodontal disease in older adults, may provide an important clinical target for intervention to promote oral health.

Vitamin D

Vitamin D may be obtained from the diet and can be synthesized in the body as a result of adequate exposure to sunlight. In northern latitudes, sunlight is often inadequate, especially during the winter months, necessitating the intake of vitamin D in the diet. The active vitamin D hormone, 1,25-dihydroxyvitamin D, plays a significant role in the regulation of bone metabolism.[33] Vitamin D deficiency has been linked to many immune-deficient diseases as well as periodontal disease.[34] Low serum levels of vitamin D are linked with increased gingival inflammation and a loss of periodontal attachment.[35] Data from NHANES III were analyzed in more than 11,000 subjects for serum vitamin D levels and attachment loss.[36] In individuals under 50 years of age, there was no significant association between vitamin D levels and attachment loss. In individuals over 50 years of age or older, *low* serum vitamin D levels were associated with *attachment loss* for both men and women.

MINERALS

Calcium

Calcium is needed for normal bone metabolism and therefore has a role in the formation and maintenance of alveolar bone. A study by Nishida et al. suggests that a low dietary intake of calcium results in more severe periodontal disease.[37] In this study, an analysis of data from the NHANES III found that periodontal disease in young men and women, and in older men, was associated with low levels of dietary calcium. Calcium provided by dairy products—such as milk, cheese, and yogurt—seems to be important in relation to periodontitis. Dairy product intake, particularly from milk and fermented foods, such as yogurt, appears to have a beneficial effect on inhibiting the development of periodontal disease.[38-41]

Magnesium

Magnesium is present in all tissues. The average person contains about 25 g of magnesium, with the majority stored in bone and about 25% present in the soft tissues.[3] A matched-pair study by Meisel et al. compared 60 subjects using oral magnesium-containing drugs with 120 subjects not taking oral magnesium-containing drugs.[42] In subjects aged 40 years and older, increased serum calcium/magnesium was significantly associated with reduced probing depth, less attachment loss, and a higher number of remaining teeth. Subjects taking magnesium drugs showed less attachment loss and more remaining teeth than did their matched counterparts. These results suggest that nutritional magnesium supplementation may improve periodontal health in individuals aged 40 years and older.

NUTRITIONAL SUPPLEMENTS

In adequately nourished individuals, current evidence is insufficient to support recommendations of vitamin and mineral supplementation in the treatment of periodontal disease. A PubMed and Cochrane database literature search reveals only a possible relationship between vitamins and minerals and periodontal disease.[43] However, the efficacy of prophylactic nutrient supplementation for the prevention of the onset and progression of periodontal disease, or for the enhancement of periodontal wound healing, remains to be determined.[3,43-46] More randomized controlled trials are needed to explore this association.

It may be reasonable to suggest vitamin and mineral supplementation for patients with periodontal disease whose nutrition might be inadequate.[3,44,47,48]

Probiotic Supplementation

Probiotic supplements are usually a dairy food or dietary supplement containing potentially beneficial live bacterial cultures that replace or add to the beneficial bacteria normally present in the gastrointestinal tract. These bacteria are believed to strengthen the body's immune system and inhibit the ability of harmful microorganisms to colonize. Kassee et al. conducted a randomized, placebo-controlled, double-blind study with 59 patients with moderate to severe gingivitis.[49] The patients were given one of two different *Lactobacillus reuteri* formulations or a placebo. After 14 days, the groups receiving *Lactobacillus reuteri* showed a significant change in plaque index and reduction in gingivitis from baseline compared with the placebo group. The researchers concluded that *Lactobacillus reuteri* is efficacious in reducing both gingivitis and plaque biofilm in patients with moderate to severe gingivitis. More research is needed before recommending probiotics as a component of periodontal therapy.

Coenzyme Q10

Coenzyme Q10 is found in every cell in the body, where it helps to bring oxygen into the cells and is used in the production of energy. Coenzyme Q10 is thought to improve the function of mitochondria, the "powerhouses" that produce energy in cells. Coenzyme Q10 is also an antioxidant, a substance that protects cells from highly reactive chemicals called free radicals that can damage cells and their DNA. Coenzyme Q10 has been proposed as a modulator of periodontal disease. Reports in the literature suggest that periodontally diseased tissues had lower levels of coenzyme Q10 than healthy gingival tissues and that treatment with this coenzyme might improve a patient's periodontal disease status.[50–55] With the limited number of studies in the literature, it is premature to recommend treatment of periodontal disease with coenzyme Q10.

Antioxidant Supplementation

Antioxidants are substances—such as vitamins—that prevent or repair damage that has been done to the body by oxidation. Oxidation is a chemical reaction that can produce free radicals, leading to chain reactions that may damage cells. Oxidation stress occurs with the production of harmful molecules called free radicals. Free radicals containing oxygen, known as reactive oxygen species, are the most biologically significant free radicals.

Well-known antioxidants include enzymes and other substances, such as vitamin C, vitamin E, and beta carotene, which are capable of counteracting the damaging effects of oxidation. Antioxidants are widely used in dietary supplements and have been investigated for the prevention of diseases such as cancer or coronary heart disease. The hypothesis that antioxidant supplements might promote health has not been confirmed experimentally. In fact, some authors argue that the hypothesis that antioxidants could prevent chronic diseases has now been disproved and that the idea was misguided from the beginning.[56–58]

Oxidative stress is involved in the initiation and progression of periodontal disease.[59] In response to plaque biofilm, polymorphonuclear leukocytes produce reactive oxygen species during phagocytosis as part of the host response to infection. Thus antioxidant effects on periodontal disease are a notable topic in periodontal research. Several studies have demonstrated a correlation between reactive oxygen species and periodontal disease activity.[60,61]

Many studies have been conducted on the effects of antioxidants on periodontal disease. However, there have been few randomized controlled studies on the effects in humans, and these studies have yielded contradictory results.[44,62,63] The use of antioxidant supplementation thus requires further investigation. In it's publication,

"Antioxidants: Beyond the Hype", the Harvard School of Public Health Newsletter states that eating *foods* rich in antioxidants like whole fruits, vegetables, and whole grains will provide protection from oxidative damage. Results published from both the Carotene and Retinol Efficacy Trial (CARET) and also the Alpha-Tocopherol, Beta-Carotene Cancer Prevention Study (ATBC) support the idea of absorbing antioxidants from food vs. supplements.[64]

THE ROLE OF THE DENTAL TEAM IN PROMOTING GOOD NUTRITION FOR THE HEALTH OF THE PERIODONTIUM

Making appropriate connections among the general health of a patient and diet, nutrients, and periodontal disease can allow clinicians to make specific suggestions to improve a patient's diet. As individuals live longer due to advances in medical treatment, members of the dental team will see more patients with chronic diseases that place them at risk for inadequate nutrition. Clinicians should consider dietary intake when managing patients with periodontal disease. The recommendations of the 2011 European workshop on Periodontology suggest that the dental team should consider including advice to patients on *increasing* levels of:

- fish oils
- fiber
- fruit and vegetables
- and to *decrease* levels of *refined* sugars.[44]

"Disease, oral medications, or unhealthy lifestyle choices may increase a person's risk for periodontal disease. A patient can't change the fact that he has a chronic disease or takes prescribed medications, however he does have the choice to improve his eating habits. In general, nutritional recommendations for periodontal health are the same as those suggested for overall health (Table 10-2). After assessing the patient's current diet, the hygienist may provide suggestions for improving the patient's eating habits, such as:

- Follow the plan on www.choosemyplate.gov.
- Include foods rich in calcium, B complex, vitamins, protein, complex carbohydrates, antioxidants, and stay hydrated.
- Follow the new Dietary Guidelines for Healthy Americans.

Table 10-2	Food Sources of Nutrients
Nutrient	**Foods Source**
Vitamin A	Carrots, sweet potatoes, pumpkin, spinach, collards, kale, green beans, red peppers
B Complex	Fortified cereals, pork, liver, brewer's yeast, soybeans, peas, nuts, fortified whole grains, dairy products
Vitamin C	Guava, red and green peppers, kiwi, citrus fruit, cantaloupe, strawberries, broccoli, cabbage, Brussel sprouts
Protein	Beef, pork, eggs, milk, fish, poultry, legumes, tofu, and soy products
Complex carbohydrate	Whole grain bread, rice, pasta, oat meal, all-bran cereal, corn, yams, peas, lentils
Calcium	Milk, cheese, yogurt, fortified orange juice, tofu, tahini, sardines, turnip greens, okra, kale
Vitamin D	Milk, soy beverage, trout, salmon, sardines, tuna
Omega-3	Fish, salmon, tuna, sardines, eggs
CoQ 10	Organ meats, beef, sardines, spinach, broccoli, cauliflower
Fiber	Bran cereal, almonds, lima beans, black beans, lentils, raspberries, quinoa

CHAPTER REVIEW

PRACTICE FOR PATIENTS

Your patient is a 29-year-old single male with a history of infrequent dental visits. Results of initial assessment:

Medical/Dental

- Weight 185 lb, height 5 ft 10 in.
- Blood pressure 140/90 mm Hg
- No significant disease factors

Intra-/Extraoral Examination

- Multiple facial piercings—bilateral ear lobe, left nares of nose, corner of right eyebrow, and tongue
- Clicking of temporomandibular joint (TMJ) upon opening
- Bilateral swollen submandibular lymph nodes
- Coated tongue
- Bilateral linea alba

Periodontal/Gingival Examination

- Generalized marginal and papillary redness
- Heavy marginal plaque biofilm and light subgingival calculus
- Localized blunted papilla in mandibular anterior/facial and lingual
- Moderate generalized bleeding upon probing
- Pocket depth range of 3 to 6 mm
- No significant recession of the gingival margin or furcation involvement

Dental Charting

- Class I amalgam restorations in first molars
- Porcelain crown maxillary left incisor
- Suspicious area occlusal mandibular right second molar
- Impacted third molars

Nutritional Survey Assessment

- Irregular eating habits
- Patient is a musician and is primarily nocturnal
- Meals consist of fast food and convenient microwavable meals
- Lactose intolerant

1. Outline the source of his nutrient deficiency based on the information given regarding his eating habits.
2. List some ideal foods with specific nutrients and state why the food/nutrient is needed in his diet.

RELATE TO YOU

A healthy immune system that works to reduce inflammation helps to support the health of the periodontium. Choose two nutrients that are considered anti-inflammatory and list foods that supply them. Complete a 24-hour diet diary on yourself to determine whether your diet provides the two nutrients.

REFERENCES

1. Boyd LD, Lampi KJ. Importance of nutrition for optimum health of the periodontium. *J Contemp Dent Pract* 2001;2(2):36–45.
2. Schifferle RE. Nutrition and periodontal disease. *Dent Clin North Am* 2005;49(3): 595–610, vii. doi: 10.1016/j.cden.2005.03.008.
3. Schifferle RE. Periodontal disease and nutrition: separating the evidence from current fads. *Periodontol 2000* 2009;50:78–89. doi: 10.1111/j.1600-0757.2008.00297.x.
4. Prentice AM. Macronutrients as sources of food energy. *Public Health Nutr* 2005;8(7A):932–939.
5. Proceedings of a workshop on micronutrients and infectious diseases: cellular and molecular immunomodulatory mechanisms. Bethesda, Maryland, USA. 16–17 September 1999. *J Infect Dis* 2000;182(suppl 1):S1–S143. doi: 10.1086/512573.
6. Kesavalu L, Bakthavatchalu V, Rahman MM, et al. Omega-3 fatty acid regulates inflammatory cytokine/mediator messenger RNA expression in Porphyromonas gingivalis-induced experimental periodontal disease. *Oral Microbiol Immunol* 2007;22(4):232–239. doi: 10.1111/j.1399-302X.2007.00346.x.
7. Kesavalu L, Vasudevan B, Raghu B, et al. Omega-3 fatty acid effect on alveolar bone loss in rats. *J Dent Res* 2006;85(7):648–652.
8. Naqvi AZ, Buettner C, Phillips RS, et al. n-3 fatty acids and periodontitis in US adults. *J Am Diet Assoc* 2010;110(11):1669–1675. doi: 10.1016/j.jada.2010.08.009.
9. Iwasaki M, Yoshihara A, Moynihan P, et al. Longitudinal relationship between dietary omega-3 fatty acids and periodontal disease. *Nutrition* 2010;26(11–12):1105–1109. doi: 10.1016/j.nut.2009.09.010.
10. Ogden CL, Carroll MD, Fryar CD, et al. Prevalence of obesity among adults and youth: United States, 2011–2014. *NCHS Data Brief* 2015(219):1–8.
11. Jenzsch A, Eick S, Rassoul F, et al. Nutritional intervention in patients with periodontal disease: clinical, immunological and microbiological variables during 12 months. *Br J Nutr* 2009;101(6):879–885. doi: 10.1017/S0007114508047776.
12. Saito T, Shimazaki Y. Metabolic disorders related to obesity and periodontal disease. *Periodontol 2000* 2007;43:254–266. doi: 10.1111/j.1600-0757.2006.00186.x.
13. Al-Zahrani MS, Bissada NF, Borawskit EA. Obesity and periodontal disease in young, middle-aged, and older adults. *J Periodontol* 2003;74(5):610–615.

14. Genco RJ, Grossi SG, Ho A, et al. A proposed model linking inflammation to obesity, diabetes, and periodontal infections. *J Periodontol* 2005;76(11 suppl):2075–2084. doi: 10.1902/jop.2005.76.11-S.2075.

15. Wood N, Johnson RB, Streckfus CF. Comparison of body composition and periodontal disease using nutritional assessment techniques: Third National Health and Nutrition Examination Survey (NHANES III). *J Clin Periodontol* 2003;30(4):321–327.

16. Schwartz N, Kaye EK, Nunn ME, et al. High-fiber foods reduce periodontal disease progression in men aged 65 and older: the Veterans Affairs normative aging study/Dental Longitudinal Study. *J Am Geriatr Soc* 2012;60(4):676–683. doi: 10.1111/j.1532-5415.2011.03866.x.

17. Petti S, Cairella G, Tarsitani G. Nutritional variables related to gingival health in adolescent girls. *Community Dent Oral Epidemiol* 2000;28(6):407–413.

18. Yamori M, Njelekela M, Mtabaji J, et al. Hypertension, periodontal disease, and potassium intake in nonsmoking, nondrinker African women on no medication. *Int J Hypertens* 2011;2011:695719. doi: 10.4061/2011/695719.

19. Enwonwu CO. Cellular and molecular effects of malnutrition and their relevance to periodontal diseases. *J Clin Periodontol* 1994;21(10):643–657.

20. Enwonwu CO. Interface of malnutrition and periodontal diseases. *Am J Clin Nutr* 1995;61(2):430S–436S.

21. Enwonwu CO, Phillips RS, Falkler WA Jr. Nutrition and oral infectious diseases: state of the science. *Compend Contin Educ Dent* 2002;23(5):431–434; 436, 438 passim; quiz 48.

22. Enwonwu CO, Phillips RS, Ibrahim CD, et al. Nutrition and oral health in Africa. *Int Dent J* 2004;54(6 suppl 1):344–351.

23. Moran JR, Greene HL. The B vitamins and vitamin C in human nutrition. II. 'Conditional' B vitamins and vitamin C. *Am J Dis Child* 1979;133(3):308–314.

24. Riepe FG, Eichmann D, Oppermann HC, et al. Special feature: picture of the month. Infantile scurvy. *Arch Pediatr Adolesc Med* 2001;155(5):607–608.

25. Nishida M, Grossi SG, Dunford RG, et al. Dietary vitamin C and the risk for periodontal disease. *J Periodontol* 2000;71(8):1215–1223.

26. Iwasaki M, Manz MC, Taylor GW, et al. Relations of serum ascorbic acid and alpha-tocopherol to periodontal disease. *J Dent Res* 2012;91(2):167–172. doi: 10.1177/0022034511431702.

27. Eklund SA, Burt BA. Risk factors for total tooth loss in the United States; longitudinal analysis of national data. *J Public Health Dent* 1994;54(1):5–14.

28. Iwasaki M, Moynihan P, Manz MC, et al. Dietary antioxidants and periodontal disease in community-based older Japanese: a 2-year follow-up study. *Public Health Nutr* 2013;16(2):330–338. doi: 10.1017/S1368980012002637.

29. Freeland JH, Cousins RJ, Schwartz R. Relationship of mineral status and intake to periodontal disease. *Am J Clin Nutr* 1976;29(7):745–749.

30. Linden GJ, McClean KM, Woodside JV, et al. Antioxidants and periodontitis in 60-70-year-old men. *J Clin Periodontol* 2009;36(10):843–849. doi: 10.1111/j.1600-051X.2009.01468.x.

31. de Menezes AC, Costa IM, El-Guindy MM. Clinical manifestations of hypervitaminosis A in human gingiva. A case report. *J Periodontol* 1984;55(8):474–476. doi: 10.1902/jop.1984.55.8.474.

32. Yu YH, Kuo HK, Lai YL. The association between serum folate levels and periodontal disease in older adults: data from the National Health and Nutrition Examination Survey 2001/02. *J Am Geriatr Soc* 2007;55(1):108–113. doi: 10.1111/j.1532-5415.2006.01020.x.
33. Liu K, Meng H, Tang X, et al. Elevated plasma calcifediol is associated with aggressive periodontitis. *J Periodontol* 2009;80(7):1114–1120. doi: 10.1902/jop.2009.080675.
34. Lucas RM, Gorman S, Geldenhuys S, et al. Vitamin D and immunity. *F1000Prime Rep* 2014;6:118.
35. Stein SH, Livada R, Tipton DA. Re-evaluating the role of vitamin D in the periodontium. *J Periodontol Res* 2014;49(5):545–553.
36. Dietrich T, Nunn M, Dawson-Hughes B, et al. Association between serum concentrations of 25-hydroxyvitamin D and gingival inflammation. *Am J Clin Nutr* 2005;82(3):575–580.
37. Nishida M, Grossi SG, Dunford RG, et al. Calcium and the risk for periodontal disease. *J Periodontol* 2000;71(7):1057–1066.
38. Adegboye AR, Christensen LB, Holm-Pedersen P, et al. Intake of dairy products in relation to periodontitis in older Danish adults. *Nutrients* 2012;4(9):1219–1229. doi: 10.3390/nu4091219.
39. Adegboye AR, Christensen LB, Holm-Pedersen P, et al. Intakes of calcium, vitamin D, and dairy servings and dental plaque in older Danish adults. *Nutr J* 2013;12:61. doi: 10.1186/1475-2891-12-61.
40. Al-Zahrani MS. Increased intake of dairy products is related to lower periodontitis prevalence. *J Periodontol* 2006;77(2):289–294. doi: 10.1902/jop.2006.050082.
41. Shimazaki Y, Shirota T, Uchida K, et al. Intake of dairy products and periodontal disease: the Hisayama study. *J Periodontol* 2008;79(1):131–137.
42. Meisel P, Schwahn C, Luedemann J, et al. Magnesium deficiency is associated with periodontal disease. *J Dent Res* 2005;84(10):937–941.
43. Kulkarni V, Bhatavadekar NB, Uttamani JR. The effect of nutrition on periodontal disease: a systematic review. *J Calif Dent Assoc* 2014;42(5):302–311.
44. Chapple IL, Milward MR, Ling-Mountford N, et al. Adjunctive daily supplementation with encapsulated fruit, vegetable and berry juice powder concentrates and clinical periodontal outcomes: a double-blind RCT. *J Clin Periodontol* 2012;39(1):62–72. doi: 10.1111/j.1600-051X.2011.01793.x.
45. Neiva RF, Steigenga J, Al-Shammari KF, et al. Effects of specific nutrients on periodontal disease onset, progression and treatment. *J Clin Periodontol* 2003;30(7):579–589.
46. Van der Velden U, Kuzmanova D, Chapple IL. Micronutritional approaches to periodontal therapy. *J Clin Periodontol* 2011;38(suppl 11):142–158. doi: 10.1111/j.1600-051X.2010.01663.x.
47. Elkhouli AM. The efficacy of host response modulation therapy (omega-3 plus low-dose aspirin) as an adjunctive treatment of chronic periodontitis (clinical and biochemical study). *J Periodontal Res* 2011;46(2):261–268. doi: 10.1111/j.1600-0765.2010.01336.x.
48. Sculley DV. Periodontal disease: modulation of the inflammatory cascade by dietary n-3 polyunsaturated fatty acids. *J Periodontal Res* 2014;49(3):277–281. doi: 10.1111/jre.12116.
49. Krasse P, Carlsson B, Dahl C, et al. Decreased gum bleeding and reduced gingivitis by the probiotic *Lactobacillus reuteri*. *Swed Dent J* 2006;30(2):55–60.

50. Hansen IL, Iwamoto Y, Kishi T, et al. Bioenergetics in clinical medicine. IX. Gingival and leucocytic deficiencies of coenzyme Q10 in patients with periodontal disease. *Res Commun Chem Pathol Pharmacol* 1976;14(4):729–738.

51. Iwamoto Y, Nakamura R, Folkers K, et al. Study of periodontal disease and coenzyme Q. *Res Commun Chem Pathol Pharmacol* 1975;11(2):265–271.

52. Littarru GP, Nakamura R, Ho L, et al. Deficiency of coenzyme Q 10 in gingival tissue from patients with periodontal disease. *Proc Natl Acad Sci U S A* 1971;68(10): 2332–2335.

53. Nakamura R, Littarru GP, Folkers K, et al. Deficiency of coenzyme Q in gingiva of patients with periodontal disease. *Int J Vitam Nutr Res* 1973;43(1):84–92.

54. Nakamura R, Littarru GP, Folkers K, et al. Study of CoQ10-enzymes in gingiva from patients with periodontal disease and evidence for a deficiency of coenzyme Q10. *Proc Natl Acad Sci U S A* 1974;71(4):1456–1460.

55. Wilkinson EG, Arnold RM, Folkers K. Bioenergetics in clinical medicine. VI. adjunctive treatment of periodontal disease with coenzyme Q10. *Res Commun Chem Pathol Pharmacol* 1976;14(4):715–719.

56. American Institute for Cancer Research, World Cancer Research Fund. *Food, Nutrition, Physical Activity and the Prevention of Cancer: A Global Perspective: A Project of World Cancer Research Fund International.* Washington, DC: American Institute for Cancer Research; 2007; xxv, p. 517.

57. Hail N Jr, Cortes M, Drake EN, et al. Cancer chemoprevention: a radical perspective. *Free Radic Biol Med* 2008;45(2):97–110. doi: 10.1016/j.freeradbiomed.2008.04.004.

58. Stanner SA, Hughes J, Kelly CN, et al. A review of the epidemiological evidence for the 'antioxidant hypothesis'. *Public Health Nutr* 2004;7(3):407–422.

59. Ekuni D, Firth JD, Nayer T, et al. Lipopolysaccharide-induced epithelial monoamine oxidase mediates alveolar bone loss in a rat chronic wound model. *Am J Pathol* 2009;175(4):1398–1409. doi: 10.2353/ajpath.2009.090108.

60. Cao CF, Smith QT. Crevicular fluid myeloperoxidase at healthy, gingivitis and periodontitis sites. *J Clin Periodontol* 1989;16(1):17–20.

61. Marton IJ, Balla G, Hegedus C, et al. The role of reactive oxygen intermediates in the pathogenesis of chronic apical periodontitis. *Oral Microbiol Immunol* 1993;8(4): 254–257.

62. Abou Sulaiman AE, Shehadeh RM. Assessment of total antioxidant capacity and the use of vitamin C in the treatment of non-smokers with chronic periodontitis. *J Periodontol* 2010;81(11):1547–1554. doi: 10.1902/jop.2010.100173.

63. Chandra RV, Sandhya YP, Nagarajan S, et al. Efficacy of lycopene as a locally delivered gel in the treatment of chronic periodontitis: smokers vs nonsmokers. *Quintessence Int* 2012;43(5):401–411. PubMed PMID: 22536592.

64. Ilkay J. Debate on antioxidants—some studies suggest efficacy while others question safety. *Today's Dietician* 2010;12(4):14.

WEB RESOURCES

American Academy of Periodontology www.perio.org

Food Guidelines

11

Choosing Foods for Health and Fitness

> To keep the body in good health is a duty....otherwise we shall not be able to keep our mind strong and clear.
>
> *Buddha*

Learning Objectives

- Explain why the typical American diet is called S.A.D.
- Make healthy food choices to prevent disease
- Locate dietary guidelines for other cultures and eating styles
- Explain the U.S. Department of Agriculture's (USDA) MyPlate graphic and discuss key points in using it as a resource for healthy eating
- Identify four types of vegetarians and their food eliminations
- Counsel patients on how to locate guidelines for making healthy food selections and using MyPlate
- Demonstrate four steps in keeping food safe
- Discuss common kitchen dangers

Key Terms

Cruciferous
Dietary Guidelines
Energy Balance
Food-Borne Illnesses
Fruitarian
Lacto-Ovo-Vegetarian

Mindful Eating
MyPlate
Pescatarian
S.A.D. Diet
Unified Dietary Guidelines
Vegan

WE ARE SAD

Twenty-first century nutrition textbooks are not worth their salt if they fail to emphasize what a *sad* state of affairs our eating habits have become; amount of sugar, saturated fat, and salt in our diet has increased exponentially.[1] The Western Pattern Diet, also called S.A.D. (Standard America Diet), is aptly titled, as instead of providing life-sustaining qualities, it increases morbidity. How *sad* that this gradual shift in eating patterns, now recognized worldwide, has contributed to soaring disease rates.[2-4] Like everything else, S.A.D. has its ups and downs, and neither direction is good. Scientists have tracked the *rise* in obesity, diabetes, heart disease, and cancer to our modern way of eating. Others suggest *declining* athletic performance and mental cognition for the same reasons.[5-8] Rate of obesity has more than doubled in the last 30 years with 39% of adults over the age of 18 being overweight.[1] We are all well aware of this cause and effect; none of this is news. So why then, do we continue our bad habits and maintain this sorry state?

TARGET MARKETING

It is hard to cultivate good eating habits when so much of our waking moments are inundated with different-minded messages. Our senses are constantly transferring information from our environment to our brains. According to the Nielsen Trust in Advertising Report (www.nielsen.com/us/en/insights/news/2013/under-the-influence), consumers are more trusting of advertisements now than in the past regardless of the format—TV, newspaper online, or mobile devices. Half of those surveyed said they trusted ads in search engine results and on social networks. For a nonbeliever, the numbers are astounding!

Be on high-alert advertising is all about making money, not about offering what is good for you: So get it straight....*nobody* is looking out for your best interest, *but you*. Read the facts below and then play the YouTube Video: 25 Facts that Might Convince You to Eat Healthier—By List 25 (2015).

> **Without your conscious consent, your brain absorbs advertising messages.**

- We are bombarded with over three to five TV food advertisements in a 2-hour viewing period, encouraging us to eat fast food (Yale Rudd Center: fastfood-marketing.org).
- Fast-food marketing has invaded social media with viewers able to "like" ads.
- Six billion fast-food ads appeared on Facebook: Starbucks, Subway, and McDonalds are at the top with 23 million *likes*.
- Taco Bell YouTube videos were viewed nearly 14 million times last year.
- SmartPhone APPS now allow us to call in our fast-food order right from our phones improving the *fast* in fast food.

- Children 2 to 7 years old are exposed to about 4,400 food ads a year; 8 to 12 years old 7,600; 13 to 17 years old 6,000. Of these food ads, 34% are for candy and snacks, 28% for cereal, and 10% for fast food. None are for fruits and vegetables (kaiserfamilyfoundation.files.wordpress.com).
- Upward trends in fast-food advertising and consumption parallel increase in obesity rates among children.[9-15]
- Words of promotion and accompanying music (jingles) to advertisement are deliberately created to induce chanting and enjoyable repetition. A 2010 article in Forbes Magazine state that Coke's 1971 "I'd Like to Buy the World a Coke" is still the most successful advertising jingle to date. Consumption of Coke doubled in the 1970s.

PORTION DISTORTION

Portion distortion is rampant in the restaurant industry; restaurants promote *bigger* and *more* for your buck. If you don't believe me, watch the video Super Size Me: "A Film of Epic Portions" that details what fast-food marketing has done to our health. To keep customers frequenting their businesses, fast-food restaurants offer monstrous portions to make consumers feel good about getting more for less. Feeling like our dollar was stretched makes us feel good. Brain imaging has shown that losing money can cause you to experience the same brain pattern of activity as stubbing a toe or hitting your funny bone. But stop for a moment and think about this psychological ploy... feeling mentally great about getting more for less is actually worse for our physical health. Opting for smaller portions, even though cost is not proportional, is better in the long run.[16]

 FOOD FOR THOUGHT   ARE WE DOOMED TO WANT HIGH-CALORIE FOOD?

Jonah Lehrer wrote in an article called "The Neuroscience of McGriddles" (The Frontal Cortex) that as our craniums grew, the digestive tract shrank. The result is that humans developed a taste for more energy-dense foods that are high in calories and easier to digest. The most satisfying emotion about eating fast food is the amount of calories we can eat in a short while.

For a peek into how fast-food restaurants load us up with fat, sugar, and salt, go to YouTube archives and watch these two videos:

Celebrity chef, Jamie Oliver's Food Revolution and Pink Slime Videos. (2013)
Proof That Fast Food Salads are Anything but Healthful—a HuffPost Video (2013)

DEVELOP IMPULSE CONTROL TO GET YOUR MIND BACK

Humans have poor impulse control. Dopamine in the brain's reward center disrupts our brain's decision-making ability by interfering with the prefrontal cortex—the brain's impulse control region. When we want sugar or immediate relief from hunger, we want it right now.

The brain is wired to spend as little time thinking as possible, so when given a choice, it takes the easiest way out.[17] S.A.D. is all about convenient routine and it is way too comfortable for the brain to give it up. Frozen meals and fast food are laden with salt, sugar, and artery-clogging fat, all of which contribute to disease. They can't be good, and we know it, but they are addicting and convenient.

- Fixing breakfast before leaving the house takes more time and thought than picking up a sandwich at a fast-food drive-through.
- Preparing the evening meal at home requires premeditation: grocery shopping for food on hand, thawing, or precooking.
- Searching for recipes that create healthy food dishes can take hours.

CHANGING BAD HABITS

DNA programs the brain to acknowledge that change can be dangerous. Shifts in wind patterns, obnoxious smells, unexpected movement, or bitter tasting food alert the mind that something is up.

Making a change in eating habits—food preparation and food choices—is hard and requires more than just information. You need motivation and *deliberate intent* for at least 3 or 4 weeks to make a change stick. Brains need to be reprogrammed anytime a routine flexes. Twenty-one days is the average time needed to reprogram the brain to incorporate any change in routine: driving a new route to work, writing the new year's date on documents, changing daily routine for a new baby in the house, learning a new job, or choosing different foods and ways to prepare them. Deciding to make a change is just the start. Figure out what you need to do to improve food choices and then make a deliberate intent to stay on course for 21 days. Soon you will be making good choices without much effort.

EATING REAL FOOD IS COMPLICATED

Deciding to rewire the brain to make healthier food choices is a good thing. But figuring out what to choose is another matter. When you are feeling well, you wish for many things: bigger houses, nicer car, new fashionable clothes—the list goes on and on. But when you are ill, the only thing you wish for is restored health. Because there is a scientific link between good nutrition and good health, changing bad food habits is a must to maintain health. With backward advertising, how do you go about choosing foods wisely to maintain good health and keep you disease-free? The amount of nutrition information is daunting; some of it is credible and some absolutely untrue. Learn to decipher opinion from science. Filtering through nutritional information to choose what is best for your family is a skill that takes conscious practice. Following guidelines developed by credible sources with proven track records is a good place to start. Most countries have developed plans for good nutrition that include guidelines and pictorial representations of culturally preferred foods as suggestions to help maintain health. Following established dietary guidelines, making your food selections according to a healthy food graphics, and utilizing good food-handling and safety measures will ensure a course for better health and possibly a longer life.

FOOD FOR THOUGHT   **MEAL KIT SERVICES—ARE THEY WORTH IT?**

Instead of the convenience of fast food, try a meal kit service for healthier, fresher option. Although meals are not as immediate, the shopping, deciding on what to cook, and finding recipes are all done for you. Meal ingredients are fresh, locally grown, and often chemical free, and there is very little waste. Chilled boxes containing everything you need to prepare three meals for two or more arrive on your doorstep each week. Three of the most successful and kitchen tested are as follows:

1. Blue Apron—www.blueapron.com
2. HelloFresh—www.hellofresh.com
3. Plated—www.plated.com

   Here is the convenience you can expect:

- You don't have to go to the grocery store.
- All you need on hand are oil, salt, and pepper.
- You can opt out of any week if vacationing.
- Easy to follow recipe cards included.
- All spices and incidentals included.
- Affordable—about 10 to 13 per restaurant quality meals per kit.

DIETARY GUIDELINES

Dietary guidelines are typically government documents carefully crafted by nutritional experts that, if followed, will serve as a foundation for making good food choices for healthy eating habits to prevent certain chronic diseases.[18,19] Dietary Guidelines for Americans made its debut in 1980 and is updated by law every 5 years (www.health.gov/DietaryGuidelines). The format has changed dramatically over the years from simple bulleted statements to a lengthy document that includes food selection for age-groups, necessity for physical activity and weight management, and food sources of specific nutrients. The US guidelines were developed by nutritional experts from the USDA and Department of Health and Human Services (HHS). Its purpose is to guide Americans, over the age of 2, to choose a healthy, well-balanced diet and to set standards for federal nutrition programs such as school lunch programs.

Other countries have established their own guidelines, taking into account cultural preferences and seasonal availability of foods. Because we live in a globally connected world, many of our patients may be following their home country's nutritional guidelines, and for better compliance while counseling, it is wise to make suggestions that align with what they use. Reading other countries' nutritional guidelines emphasizes the fact that the intended use for all is to keep people healthy. Visit www.fnic.nal.usda.gov—Dietary Guidelines from Around the World—to see other country's food guides.

UNIFIED DIETARY GUIDELINES

Before 1999, major health organizations for cancer, heart disease, diabetes, and hypertension each had their own set of dietary guidelines for people to follow to reduce their risk of the specific disease. It is not unusual for a person to have more than one disease, such as the combination of diabetes and heart disease or having hypertension and high cholesterol. Having several guidelines to follow is confusing, and oftentimes, they fall by the wayside. To help with compliance, the organizations united their suggestions and developed one set of guidelines for healthy eating—the Unified Dietary Guidelines. The Unified Dietary Guidelines have been approved by the American Cancer Society, American Heart Association, American Dietetic Association, American Academy of Pediatrics, and National Institute of Health and, if followed, will reduce the risk for many chronic diseases. The following is a list of their suggestions:

- Eat various foods; choose most of what you eat from plant sources.
- Eat six or more servings of breads, cereals, pasta, and grains each day.
- Choose five or more servings of vegetables per day.
- Eat high-fat foods sparingly, especially those from animal sources. Choose fats and oils with 2 g or less saturated fat per tablespoon, such as liquid and tub margarines, canola oil, and olive oil.

- Keep your intake of simple sugars to a minimum.
- Balance the number of calories you eat with the number you use each day.
- Eat less than 6 g of salt (sodium chloride) per day (2,400 mg of sodium).
- Have no more than one alcoholic drink per day if you are a woman and no more than two if you are a man.

5-A-DAY PROGRAM

Even with the major health organizations recommending the **5-A-Day** program for fruits and vegetables, Americans consume less than three servings a day. Unless fruit and vegetable dishes are dripping in butter or sugar, they are considered an excellent low-fat source of vitamins, minerals, and fiber. Avocados, coconut, and olives are the exception because they are high in fat, but remember, not all fat is bad. The National Cancer Institute (branch of the National Institutes of Health) refers to fruit and vegetables as the *original fast food*. Grapes, cherry tomatoes, and bananas can be eaten on the spot without any preparation. Visit www.fns.usda.gov/5-day for more information. **Cruciferous vegetables**, plants with leaf structure that resembles as cross, are important to include in the diet for their nutrient dense properties: Vitamin A, carotenoids, Vitamin C, folic acid and fiber.

Cruciferous Vegetables

- Bok choy
- Broccoli
- Brussels sprouts
- Cabbage
- Cauliflower

Good Sources of Fiber

- Apples
- Bananas
- Blackberries/blueberries/raspberries/strawberries
- Brussels sprouts
- Carrots
- Cherries
- Cooked beans and peas
- Dates/figs
- Grapefruits/oranges
- Kiwi
- Pears
- Prunes
- Spinach
- Sweet potatoes

Table 11-1 indicates source of vitamins A and C in fruits and vegetables.

Table 11-1	Good Source of Vitamins A and C	
	A	C
Acorn squash	×	
Apricots	×	×
Bell peppers		×
Broccoli		×
Brussels sprouts		×
Cabbage		×
Cantaloupe	×	×
Carrots	×	
Cauliflower		×
Chili peppers		×
Collards	×	×
Grapefruit		×
Honeydew melon		×
Kale	×	
Kiwi		×
Leaf lettuce	×	
Mangoes	×	×
Mustard greens	×	×
Oranges		×
Pineapple		×
Plums		×
Potato with skin		×
Pumpkin	×	
Romaine lettuce	×	
Spinach	×	×
Strawberries		×
Sweet potatoes	×	
Tangerines		×
Tomatoes		×
Watermelon		×
Winter squash	×	

Keeping Vegetables Safe (*Adapted from Johns Hopkins Health Alert*)

- Do not buy vegetables that are bruised or damaged
- Avoid pre-cut vegetables or packaged salads that are not refrigerated
- Wash your hands for 20 seconds before and after handling vegetables
- Using soap and water, clean all surfaces and utensils used before and after preparing vegetables
- Rinse all vegetables under cold running water for 2 minutes before cutting since bacteria can be transported to the flesh
- Scrub the skin of root vegetables such as potatoes and carrots with a brush under cold running water
- Wash bagged salads and pre-cut vegetables even if the package says "ready to eat"
- Cook sprouts before using them in recipes, as bacteria grows inside sprouts
- Keep vegetables away from raw meat, seafood, and poultry even when in the shopping cart, refrigerator, and on the counter
- Refrigerate all cut, peeled, and cooked vegetables within 2 hours

WHICH IS BEST: FRESH, FROZEN, OR CANNED?

Fresh, frozen, canned, or dried fruits and vegetables all provide vitamins, minerals, and fiber; fruit and vegetable juice also provide vitamins and minerals. A wise shopper, however, knows it makes a difference as to what form of fruit or vegetable is bought:

1. Fresh is best. Food is freshest if picked ripe off the vine and eaten immediately. If picked unripe, it may not have had enough time to accumulate all its nutrients. Many fruits and vegetables are harvested too early and then sprayed to retard spoilage as they travel to the grocery store and sit on the produce shelf waiting for purchase.
2. Frozen is the next best choice after fresh with nutrient levels being high. When choosing produce from the frozen food section, shake the bag to make sure the contents move around. If the contents do not move around and the bag is one big block of ice, this indicates that the contents have been allowed to thaw, which causes the nutrients to leach out of the food and into the water. When refrozen, the nutrients are in the block of ice instead of in the vegetables themselves.
3. Canned is the least desirable, as the canning process requires intense heat, which can destroy many of the B vitamins.

FOOD PYRAMIDS AND GRAPHICS

In addition to regional food guides, illustrated food selection graphics are another dynamic way to visually give patients ideas for making better food choices for overall health.[20]

The graphics are geometric and, depending on the country, can be triangular, circular, square, or three-dimensional (3D) pyramids with sections that represent various food groups. The idea is that the larger the section, the more foods in that group should be eaten. A picture is worth a thousand words and having examples of foods in each group can trigger ideas for similar foods that may not be pictured, allowing for greater food choices.

The US food graphic, formerly Food Guide Pyramid, is called **MyPlate** and was updated by the USDA and HHS. Figure 11-1 illustrates MyPlate. Medical and nutrition organizations/groups are able to take the concept of MyPlate and adapt it to make their own recommendations, taking main staples and cultural preferences into considerations. Just as an example, Mayo Clinic Web site has several color-ful pictorial food graphics based on MyPlate that depict food selections for Asians, Mediterraneans, Latinos, vegetarians as well as their own design for healthy eating (http://www.mayoclinic.com/health/healthy-diet/NU00190).

Points to consider when interpreting food pyramids are as follows:

- A healthy diet should be combined with exercise and weight control.
- Eat whole grains versus refined at most meals for satiety and more stable blood glucose levels.
- Include good sources of unsaturated fats in your daily diet, such as olive, canola, and other vegetable oils and fatty fish such as salmon, to lower choles-terol and offer protective factors for the heart.
- Eat various fresh fruits and vegetables throughout the week.

Figure 11-1 MyPlate.

- Choose fish, poultry, eggs, nuts, and legumes as a source of protein over fatty meats such as beef and pork.
- Choose low-fat dairy products or take a calcium supplement daily.
- Eat red meat, pork, and butter sparingly.
- Eat refined and simple carbohydrates such as white rice, white bread, pasta, potatoes, and sweets sparingly.
- Take a multivitamin/mineral supplement as a backup.
- Drink alcohol in moderation: one to two drinks per day for males and less than one drink per day for females.

Because MyPlate is based on a **2,000**-calorie diet for Americans, different age-groups and those with differing activity levels should alter the recommendations to fit their needs. Children have different food preferences and require fewer calories. See Figure 11-2 for the USDA Children's MyPlate. Those with a sedentary lifestyle require fewer calories than those who are in a state of growth or are very active. The serving size suggestions for each food group are given in a range, so inactive or small people should use the lower end and the very active should use the upper range.

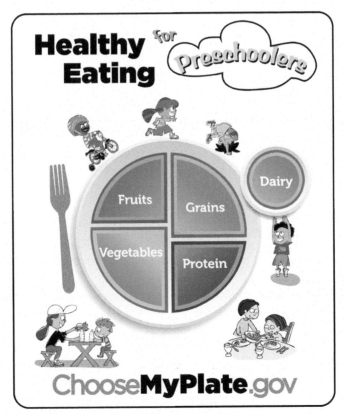

Figure 11-2 MyPlate for young children.

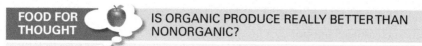

IS ORGANIC PRODUCE REALLY BETTER THAN NONORGANIC?

You no longer have to seek out a health food store to purchase organic produce. Local grocery stores stock not only organic but also locally grown organic. The term organic indicates the grower did not use harmful pesticides or fertilizers and used a farming method that reduced pollution and encouraged soil and water conservation. To earn the right of using the label organic, producers must complete a rigorous U.S. Department of Agriculture certification program. There are some noticeable differences between organic and nonorganic fruits and vegetables:

Organic	Nonorganic
Small in size	Plump and large
Physically imperfect	Perfect consistent shape
Irregular color	Bright consistent color

Reasons for choosing organic:

- No pesticide residue
- No artificial coloring or flavoring
- Unadulterated fresh food tastes better
- Benefits the environment by reducing pollution
- Conserves water and soil

Foods that carry high levels of pesticide residues:

- Spinach
- Scallions
- Green peas
- Green beans
- Apples, grapes, peaches, and pears
- Berries—strawberries, raspberries, and blackberries

OK—so bottom line…is organic produce healthier than nonorganic? Not exactly…..

Choosing to eat organic foods may reduce exposure to antibiotic-resistant bacteria and pesticides, but there is no evidence that it makes you healthier. Smith-Spangler C, et al. Are organic foods safer or healthier than conventional alternatives? A systematic review. *Ann Intern Med.* 2012;157(5):348–366.

For sane advice on how to choose wisely at your local supermarket, read the handy reference book, **Eat This Not That** *Supermarket Survival Guide* by David Zinczenko. Inside, he provides tips on making healthy choices to keep you fit and lean.

BALANCING DIET AND PHYSICAL ACTIVITY

In 1994, the National Weight Control Registry was created to keep track of and identify the habits of individuals who were successful in losing and maintaining weight. (Visit www.nwcr.ws to join the study.) More than 5,000 individuals are now in the database, making it one of the largest studies of its kind. Years of research reveal why these individuals were successful in losing an average of 60 lb and maintaining the loss for at least 5 years: they were highly motivated and had increased their daily physical activity level. Weight loss was not necessarily a result of the foods they chose or excluded from their diets. Physical activity and a sensible diet work together for better health.

Energy balance is when calories consumed are adequate for maintenance or growth. When there is an excess of calories consumed—more than needed for maintenance—weight increases. A decrease in calories results in weight loss. Weight gain or loss is referred to as "energy imbalance." We need to eat each day to provide our bodies with energy to keep our hearts beating, lungs expanding, liver and kidneys filtering waste, and sodium pumps maintaining water balance. Energy (calories) is delivered to all parts of our bodies from metabolism of carbohydrates, protein, fat, and alcohol. The energy our body needs just to stay alive accounts for two thirds of all energy spent throughout the day, leaving one third for our physical activity. For some, there are more calories left to spend than are spent, and if physical activity is minimal, weight gain is inevitable.

Obesity is now considered to be of epidemic proportions not just in the United States, but all over the world, for all age groups, and is the second major cause of death. Decreased activity levels as well as increased portion sizes have swelled our waists and given us heart disease, hypertension, stroke, diabetes[21], certain kinds of cancer (colon, postmenopausal breast cancer, and endometrial as well as others still being studied). What we eat and whether we exercise are both important choices to make. Hours spent sitting at a desk (or chairside), surfing the Internet, watching television, and playing video games create overweight, sedentary people. Being aware of activity levels and rethinking ways to incorporate physical activity into daily routines prevent the downward spiral into obesity and its accompanying diseases. It takes a conscious effort to keep a healthy weight, keeping track of calories in and calories out.[22] If the number of calories consumed consistently exceeds the number spent, weight increases. If you expend 3,500 more calories each week than you take in, you will lose a pound. Over time, that adds up. See Figure 11-3.

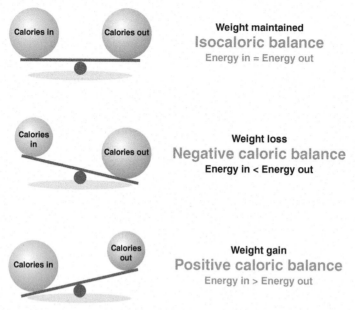

Figure 11-3   Calorie balance.

TIPS FOR EATING TO MAINTAIN PROPORTIONAL WEIGHT

The best way to assure weight maintenance is to practice portion control. Eat everything you normally eat, but make a conscious effort to eat a little less. If you have a craving, give in to it by eating a few bites of the food you desire. Avoid eating when you are stressed or feel rushed and chew slowly; enjoy your food. Sip water throughout the day and munch on raw vegetables. Try dividing your daily ratio of food into six small meals versus three large meals. It keeps your metabolism working at top efficiency and you would not feel as hungry between meals. Choose snacks that require some work, like cracking nuts and peeling fruit. The effort in preparation will reduce amount eaten. Select low-fat dairy products and choose whole grain versus refined grain foods. The bulk will give you a sense of fullness quicker. Avoid using a lot of sauces and gravies. Eat for better health, not to lose weight, and the pounds will gradually roll off.

Here are some other tips that help in weight loss efforts:

- Make a point to eliminate as much sugar from your diet as possible.
- Sniff peppermint when you feel hungry—it is an appetite suppressant.
- Stare at the color blue—yes, this really works so use blue tablecloth, blue plate, you get the idea.
- Shut down your kitchen after dinner and don't open until it is time for breakfast.
- Serve food portions on a plate, not platter.
- Make a point to leave three or four bites of food on your plate—taking the top hamburger bun off will do it.

- Use chopsticks for a week—they slow down eating.
- Put your fork down between each bite—this also slows you down.
- Avoid white foods—refined wheat and sugar.
- Drink regular coffee instead of the sweet coffees served at coffee shops.
- Use Cajun seasoning—you can only eat so much of that hot stuff.
- Eat most of the day's food for breakfast and lunch.
- Make dinner your smallest meal—you have already expended the lion's share of energy needed.
- Practice mindful eating.
- Aim for slow weight loss versus rapid weight loss.
- Stay away from diets that promise rapid results.
- Reducing your *weekly* diet by 3,500 calories will result in a 1-lb weight loss.
- Reduce your daily caloric intake by 200 calories. This amounts to leaving the last few bites of food from each meal on your plate.

FOOD FOR THOUGHT MINDFUL EATING

In the book *Mindless Eating: Why We Eat More Than We Think,* Food Psychologist Brian Wansink states that every day, the average person makes well over 200 decisions about food. If you are unable to explain why you eat what you do, then you are in a mindless eating mode. It is possible that not paying attention to what and how you are eating can cause you to be overweight or not lose those last remaining pounds. Thinking about and being aware of your food as you prepare and then eat it play a role in improving food choices and eating patterns. You have probably been told at one time in your life to chew each bite of food 25 times before swallowing and there is good reason for that wisdom. Besides contributing to more efficient digestion, counting your chews and saying grace are the simplest habits to create more mindful eating.

Steps to more mindful eating:

- Turn off the TV and other outside distractors. Eat in silence or turn on pleasant background music.
- Begin by doing a self-check to determine your conscious need to eat. Ask yourself if you are hungry, stressed, or eating because everyone else is.
- Contemplate your food (similar to saying grace).
  - Your meal is a gift, created with loving hands.
  - Eat with gratitude.
  - Remind yourself to eat with moderation.

- Take a full deep breath before you begin.
- Cut your solid food into small pieces. Smaller food particles passing to the stomach and then small intestine reduce bacterial overgrowth that leads to indigestion, bloating, and constipation.
- Sense when the saliva enters the mouth and chew until your food liquefies. Chewing triggers hydrochloric acid production, which speeds up the digestive process and relaxes the lower stomach.
- Concentrate on the flavors and texture of each bite of food. Breathe slowly through the nose and take the first bite with your eyes closed.
- Take an occasional long deep breath to calm the mind and body. Be present in the moment.
- Feed yourself with your non-dominant hand. This slows you down by about 30%.
- Consciously determine when your stomach is full. Eat what you need NOT what you can possibly eat. If you say to yourself that you can't possibly take one more bite, you have gone too far. Overfilling the stomach puts stress on it and affects the digestive process.

All types of physical activity are beneficial. The recommended 30 minutes of physical activity per day does not have to be accomplished all at once. Short bursts of activity throughout the day are also acceptable, although sustained activity levels are best for weight loss. If exercise has not been part of your daily routine, remember to start out slow and gradually increase intensity. Starting out fast and furious can only lead to pain and injury.

Aerobic exercise speeds up your heart rate and breathing, keeping the circulatory system strong. Strength training, such as lifting weights, helps maintain bone strength and prevent osteoporosis. Stretching while dancing or doing yoga can increase flexibility, making other activities more enjoyable. The following are examples of moderate exercise that can burn 100 extra calories per day:

- Washing and waxing a car for 45 minutes
- Gardening for 45 minutes
- Mowing the lawn 20 minutes
- Raking leaves for 30 minutes
- Shooting baskets for 30 minutes
- Riding a bike for 30 minutes
- Swimming laps for 20 minutes
- Walking stairs for 6 minutes
- Practicing yoga for 20 minutes

- Zumba for 11 minutes
- Elliptical machine for 8 minutes
- Bowling 30 minutes
- Dancing in the living room 20 minutes
- Carrying an infant 24 minutes
- Pushing a stroller 35 minutes
- Shopping for 38 minutes
- Walking the dog for 26 minutes
- Ice skating 18 minutes
- Treading water 23 minutes

Suggestions to incorporate more physical activity into your day without even trying:

- Limit time spent in front of the TV or computer and spend the time moving your body.
- Always opt for the stairs versus elevators or escalators.
- Ride the exercise bike as you watch TV.
- Dance to your favorite music while you are waiting for the pot to boil.
- Organize play outside with your children instead of sitting in front of the TV or computer.
- Trade a sit-down lawn mower for push mower.
- Park as far away from work, mall, or arena entrances as possible, and while doing so, think about how fortunate you are to be healthy enough to walk the distance.
- If safe, ride your bike when possible; ride with your children to school or sports practice.
- Form a walking group in your neighborhood and establish a specific meeting time and place.
- Conduct a walking meeting instead of sitting around a conference table.
- Walk with coworkers to restaurants for lunch.
- Spend 15 minutes longer walking the dog or play fetch.
- Wash your car yourself.
- Window shop.
- Walk over to a coworkers desk or office instead of calling or emailing.

EATING TO DECREASE RISK OF CANCER

A nutrition text would not be complete without including suggestions on what we should and should not eat to decrease the risk of cancer. If approximately one-third of all cancer in the world can be prevented with proper diet and physical activity, it is worth learning to choose which foods are best, and those we should avoid.[23-26]

Decide to make one small dietary change and practice it for 3 weeks and then choose another. Before long, you will be incorporating more grains, fruits, and vegetables into meals that will change body fat ratio in just a few months. Just say "no" to high-fat and sugared foods (but maybe not to chocolate).

Incorporating daily activity is suggested to decrease cancer risk. The human body was designed to move, and we should move it until the day of our last sunset. Park farther from the entrance, place frequently used objects so you have to stretch (reach) to get them, or exaggerate movements when doing simple chores like folding clothes. Small changes can lead to big improvements if practiced over time. The American Institute for Cancer Research publication titled Food, Nutrition, Physical Activity and the Prevention of Cancer: A Global Perspective suggests the following:

- Be as lean as possible within your normal body weight range.
- Be physically active as part of everyday life.
- Limit consumption of calorie-dense food (those high in fat and sugar) and avoid sugary drinks.
- Eat mostly foods of plant origin—fruits, vegetables, and whole grains.
- Limit intake of red meat (beef, pork, and lamb) and avoid processed meats, such as bacon, sausage, and lunchmeat—bologna, ham, and salami.
- Limit your intake of alcoholic beverages.
- Limit your salt intake.
- Aim to meet your nutritional needs through diet alone.
- Mothers should breastfeed their babies as it is good for both mother and child; it lowers the risk of breast cancer and the child is less likely to become obese.
- Cancer survivors should be encouraged to follow the report on recommendations for cancer prevention and, of course, seek and take the advice of a trained nutrition professional.

For more information, visit www.aicr.org/foods-that-fight-cancer/the American Institute for Cancer Research's Web site for Foods that Fight Cancer.

POPULAR WEIGHT LOSS DIETS

Anyone who eats food is on a diet because the literal meaning of the word **diet** is food and drink regularly consumed. But a more common meaning of **diet** is restriction of food and drink, and that is what most people think of when you say you are on a diet. With obesity being of global concern, many of your patients presenting with oral disease—dental caries or periodontal concerns—will be on a specific diet that must be considered when counseling to prevent/reduce oral disease. Demonstrating respect for a patient's wish to follow a particular diet enforces your concern for their overall health and earns respect for the suggestions you make for better oral health.

There are many diet or weight reduction organizations that are very specific with food choices and eating suggestions, even to the point of providing exclusive pre-packaged food products. Keep in mind that companies selling products guaranteeing weight loss are in business to make money. They may or may not work. *Hungry for Change*, a 2012 documentary exposes the diet industry's strategies to keep people from losing weight and keeping the pounds at bay. There are as many weight loss strategies as the mind can comprehend; so although you may be a proponent of one weight loss regime, it may not work for someone else. A 2010 video, *Fat, Sick, and Nearly Dead*, follows Australian entrepreneur, Joe Cross, on a quest to regain his health by consuming nothing more than juice. You can imagine the motivation needed to permanently eliminate solid food from the diet. Below is a list of some of the more common diets that patients may be following and that should be researched before offering suggestions to assure better compliance with their dental nutritional counseling.

Zone Diet

The Zone Diet was developed by Dr. Barry Sears and published in his best-selling book aptly titled The Zone in 1995. Dr. Sears, a well-known research scientist who has spent more than 30 years studying and writing about lipids and hormones and their effect on heart disease, uses the premise that if we treat food as a drug, we can keep ourselves healthy and disease-free (http://www.zonediet.com/). The five simple components to follow with this diet are as follows:

1. Balance every meal and snack with carbohydrate, protein, and fat. Meal composition should be 40-30-30, respectively.
2. Include anti-inflammatory omega-3 fats.
3. Include polyphenols (phytochemicals) that are found abundantly in fruits and vegetables for anti-inflammatory and antioxidant benefits.
4. Moderately exercise for 30 minutes 6 days a week.
5. Take daily supplements.

Meals prepared for individuals on this diet are fairly balanced, but if counseling a patient subscribing to this diet, it would be important to suggest foods high in omega-3 and fruits and vegetables high in antioxidants.

Atkins Diet

The Atkins Diet is the most marketed and well-known low-carbohydrate nutritional program. Dr. Robert Atkins found himself in need of a way to lose weight in the 1960s and adapted a diet published in the Journal of American Medical Association to serve his needs. In 1998, after many years of successful weight loss and maintenance, he published the diet in his best-selling book titled Dr. Atkins Diet Revolution. The success of the diet depends on the individual's ability to know how much carbohydrate there is in each food choice. Most eating choices are from the protein food group. Visit this link for an example of a low-carbohydrate food pyramid: http://lowcarbdiets.about.com/OD/whattoeat/IG/Low-Carb-FOOD-Pyramid/lowcarb-pyramid1-IG.htm. Counseling patients on this diet can be tricky as proportion of food choices are not according to what is usually suggested in MyPyramid. If counseling a patient on this diet, it would be important to suggest food choices illustrated on the low-carbohydrate food pyramid. Be aware that very-low-carbohydrate diets can cause your body to use ketones for fuel in the absence of carbohydrates.[27]

South Beach Diet

The South Beach Diet was developed in 1990s by Miami cardiologist Dr. Arthur Agatston and emphasizes eating good carbohydrates and good fats. Foods with a high glycemic index and saturated or trans fats are eliminated. Success of this diet depends on knowing which foods are acceptable versus those that are prohibited. The first phase of the diet lasts 2 weeks and allows only specific foods, called "authorized foods," to eliminate food cravings for sugar and refined starches. If counseling a patient on this diet, it would be important to know which phase of the diet your patient is in and to have a list of foods you can and cannot suggest (http://www.southbeachdiet.com/sbd/publicsite/index.aspx).

Weight Watchers

Weight Watchers organization is one of the oldest nutritional programs, dating back to the early 1960s. It is a weight reduction plan that teaches participants how to make better food choices and use portion control. There are no forbidden foods or restrictions but plenty of suggestions for creating a healthy eating environment and balancing food intake with exercise. A four-pillar scientific foundation was created using 45 years of trial and error and includes food, behavior, support, and exercise that can be incorporated into any lifestyle. If counseling a patient on this diet, it would be important to consider following suggestions for portion control and have a list of foods and point value for each (http://www.weightwatchers.com/plan/index.aspx).

Spectrum Diet

The Spectrum Diet was developed by Dr. Dean Ornish and works well for those wanting to lose weight and especially for those at risk for heart disease. Dr. Ornish is known for reversing the damage of heart disease. Suggestions and techniques are backed by science and lauded as one of the few ways to stay off statins. As its title indicates, there is a spectrum of foods from which to choose all the way from the most healthy of choices to favorite indulgent foods. Diets can be customized to individual preferences. Predominant is the focus on limiting intake of high-fat proteins from animals and increasing complex carbohydrates. Additionally, followers are encouraged to include moderate exercise and some form of stress reduction technique like yoga, meditation, and joining support groups. Visit www.ornishspectrum.com for more information on this diet.

HEALTHY LIVING DIET ALTERNATIVES

Vegetarianism

Vegetarianism is the practice of excluding animal foods from the diet, including dairy items, eggs, honey, and purchasing/wearing clothes from animal products, like wool, silk, or leather (The Vegetarian Resource Group—www.vrg.org). Reasons for choosing this lifestyle and eating pattern are varied and include health, religion, ethics, weight, fashion, and environment.

Many famous and productive people were practicing vegetarians: Socrates, Leonardo da Vinci, Benjamin Franklin, Mahatma Gandhi, Albert Einstein, and Clara Barton, just to name a few. Paul and Linda McCartney even started their own line of convenience vegetarian meals (not available in the United States or Canada) called Linda McCartney Foods. Vegetarianism is practiced worldwide, and the numbers increase each year. Percent of various countries population who identify as vegetarian are as follows:

31% India
13% Taiwan
10% England
10% Italy
9% Germany
9% Austria
5% Australia, United States, Israel, and Switzerland
4% Canada and Russia

The Vegetarian Resource Group Web site offers information on how to choose a meatless diet but still consume all the needed nutrients. Diets rich in vegetables, fruits, leafy greens, whole grains, nuts and seeds, and legumes can meet the protein needs of people from all age groups and all walks of life.[28] Research has proven that there is a health benefit to those who actively practice vegetarianism compared to those with non-vegetarian diets.[29-31] The 2011 documentary *Forks Over Knives* presents information on how eating a plant-based diet will eliminate diseases like cancer and diabetes.

When meat is excluded from a diet, it leaves room for more carbohydrates, and oftentimes, plant sources of protein are forgotten. The type of carbohydrates substituted matters, because eating more simple sugars opens the door for increased incidence of caries and diseases.[32,33] Vegetarians should choose foods wisely and include complex carbohydrates to ensure that there is enough protein in the diet. Vegan diets are typically lower in protein than the standard diet; however, the recommendations are very generous and diets high in protein do not appear to have any health advantages. (Protein is needed in very small quantities, approximately 1 out of every 10 calories.) There are several levels of vegetarianism, depending on what is *included* in the diets:

- **Vegan**—eliminates all foods of animal origin
- **Lactovegetarian**—includes dairy products
- **Ovovegetarian**—includes egg products
- **Lacto-ovo-vegetarian**—includes dairy and egg products
- **Pollotarian**—includes poultry (no red meat or fish)
- **Pescatarian**—includes fish
- **Fruitarian**—eats only fruits

In addition to the above list, there are two other categories related to vegetarianism:

A flexitarian is semivegetarian who eats meat every once in a while.

- **Raw vegan**—unprocessed vegetables that are not heated above 115 degrees so nutritional value is not destroyed by heating
- **Macrobiotic**—unprocessed vegan foods, with emphasis on Asian vegetables, and avoiding sugar and oil as well

Vegetarians include specific foods with their meals to serve as good protein sources. Some examples are as follows:

- Beans
- Nuts
- Seeds
- Tofu
- Soy foods
- Vegetarian meat substitutes
- Eggs
- Dairy products

Completely eliminating animal protein from the diet can create a deficiency in *vitamin B₁₂*, which is found only in animal foods.[34] The deficiency develops over time, affecting the central nervous system, and is not manifested until after the body's stores are depleted, usually 4 years' worth. Once the deficiency manifests, its symptoms are irreversible. Lacto-ovo-vegetarians need not worry, because B_{12} is supplied in cow's milk.[35] A true vegan, however, must supplement his or her diet with fortified soy milk or meat replacement. Vitamin B_{12} deficiency symptoms are as follows:

- Anemia
- Fatigue
- Constipation
- Anorexia
- Numbness and tingling of hands and feet
- Depression
- Confusion
- Poor memory
- Sores in mouth and on tongue

Concerns of Vegetarianism

Lack of animal foods can cause deficiencies in certain nutrients, but if you are aware of the possibility, corrective action can be taken. See Table 11-2 Vegetarian Nutrient Deficiencies.

Ecological concerns have been raised concerning grazing cattle versus growing plant crops. It takes *17 acres* of grazing land to produce 1 million calories of animal protein, but *one* well-developed *acre* of plants can raise 1 million calories of plant-based protein. Another complaint or accusation is that emissions from animal agriculture surpass transportation emissions, which contribute greatly to global warming.[36] There are many articles and Web sites arguing for change in the animal farming industry, and those concerns are being addressed. There is a growing shift toward *regenerative agriculture* that actually heals the land as it is used for food production. Visit www.upliftconnect.com for more information on farming that heals the earth.

Table 11-2	Vegetarian Nutrient Deficiencies
Nutrient Deficiency	**Corrective Action**
Vitamin B_{12}	Take a daily supplement
Vitamin D	Take a supplement or expose skin to 20 minutes of sun each day
Iron	Cook with cast iron or take a daily supplement
Calcium and riboflavin	Include soy products or calcium-fortified foods like orange juice

Benefits of Vegetarianism

Research has established that there are many benefits to eating vegetarian diets. Aside from curtailing obesity and controlling hypertension and diabetes,[37] the following are advantages of vegetarian diets:

- Usually maintains desired weight for height
- Lower blood cholesterol
- Lower rates of some forms of cancer
- Better digestive function
- Benefits the earth
- Higher in fiber than animal protein
- Rich in vitamins A and C
- Lower in fat than animal protein

Paleo

The Paleo diet consists mainly of foods that were eaten by our ancient hunter-gatherer relatives. Sometimes called the Caveman Diet, followers choose foods heavy in protein and light in carbohydrates. There is a lack of evidence to determine if cavemen suffered from diet-induced diseases, but we are sure of the cause and effect of the modern S.A.D. diet and many chronic life-altering, life-limiting, diseases. Going back to the earliest way of eating might not be such a bad idea.

Just imagine a caveman, armed with spears and rocks, hunting for food as his stomach growls. Traveling in groups, they foraged for nuts and berries and went on hunts for free-range animals. Today, we can find everything we want at the local grocery store. Making choices as to what to put in the cart is all that stands between eating the heavily marketed fat-, sugar-, and salt-laden processed foods and healthier choices that resonate with our genes.

It is thought that adopting this eating pattern works with human genetics to keep our bodies lean and strong. Recommended foods are all whole fruits and vegetables, lean meats (including venison and buffalo), seafood, nuts and seeds, and monounsaturated and omega-3 fats. Alcohol, dairy, grain, and processed food heavy in sugar and starch should be avoided. So, nix the soda if you are going to follow this eating pattern.

Followers of this diet will find there are many *benefits*:

- Plant nutrients, nuts, and healthy oils have anti-inflammatory properties.
- Protein creates a sense of satiety, which means you will not be hunting many snacks between meals.

- Eliminating sugary foods and beverages will cause weight loss, giving you muscles that appear long and lean.
- Research indicates that the Paleo diet is heart-healthy[38,39] and reduces the risk of obesity.[40]

There are a few *drawbacks* of this diet:

- It is easy to consume more protein than necessary or eat too much of one food on the list. For example, if you are hungry and grab the can of nuts, you may be looking at the bottom of the can before you know it. Five thousand calories later, you are hating yourself.
- If you are athletic, carbohydrates are needed for high performance and sustained energy. Bread, spaghetti, and pancakes are not on the authorized food list.
- Because of elimination of dairy and grains, the diet may be deficient in calcium and vitamin D.[41]

Visit www.paleomagonline.com for information on modern day primal living.

Gluten Free

Gluten is a mixture of two proteins present in grains, especially wheat, barley, and rye, which gives dough its gluey texture.[42] Reaction to the gluten can manifest as either celiac disease or gluten sensitivity, which has separate clinical diagnoses.[43] It is estimated that 1 in 100 people has celiac disease and 6 in 100 have a gluten sensitivity. Elimination of gluten from the diet is the only cure.

- Celiac disease is an *autoimmune reaction* to eating gluten. It affects the lining of the small intestine (duodenum) and causes **villous atrophy**, which prevents nutrients from being absorbed by the body. (See Chapter 1, Digestion of Nutrients). Symptoms include abdominal bloating, chronic diarrhea, constipation, gas, stomach pain, and vomiting. Many times, the symptoms are confused with lactose intolerance and irritable bowel syndrome. The autoimmune response causes intestinal inflammation and potentially malnourishment.
- Gluten sensitivity is more like an *intolerance or allergy* to gluten. The reaction is time-limited and does not cause permanent damage.[44] Symptoms are similar to celiac disease, but the condition is different in that it does not cause damage to the small intestine. A biopsy of the small intestine confirms the presence or lack of celiac disease.

According to the Mayo Clinic Web site (www.mayoclinic.org), avoiding wheat takes some deliberate thought when you first begin the gluten-free diet. Some foods to avoid are common sense, like breads, cakes, pies, cereals, croutons, pasta, boxed rice mixes, potato, and tortilla chips. But others may surprise you like beer, communion wafers, French fries, salad dressings, and soups.

Of course, all the healthy foods are part of this diet like eggs, fish, shellfish, grass-fed meat, fresh vegetables and healthy seeds, and fats. Food manufacturers have jumped on the bandwagon and now keep grocery store shelves stocked with gluten-free choices. They make it easy to eat pizza and crackers, cookies, and breads and not suffer the annoying bloating and nausea caused by gluten.

Mediterranean Diet

The Mediterranean diet gets its inspiration from dietary patterns of Greece, Crete, Southern Italy, France, and Spain. It is strongly associated with decreased incidence of heart disease, diabetes, and cancer. What makes it unique from traditional diets is proportionally high consumption of legumes, fruits, vegetables, unrefined grains, olive oil, and wine. Yes, red wine, packed with resveratrol that has been shown to improve blood flow to the brain and keep the heart muscle flexible. Added in moderate amounts to the aforementioned staples are fish, specific dairy products like yogurt and kefir, and occasionally some red meat.[45]

The Mediterranean diet is low in saturated fat and high in fiber. Olive oil is the main fat in this diet, replacing butter and lard used in cooking. Seventy-five percent of all olive oil in the world comes from Italy, Spain, or Greece as olive trees are native to these countries. Olive oil has high amount of oleic acid, which has been shown to lower bad cholesterol (LDL) and homocysteine levels, both of which are heart protective.[46,47] Studies have also shown the diet has a positive effect on mood and cognition.[48]

FOOD SAFETY AND PREPARATION

Even though your kitchen may rival that of an interior showplace, it may not be fit for cooking. Clean floors, spotless countertops, and organized cupboards are not indicators of a kitchen that employs **safe food-handling** practices. We are unable to see, feel, or smell bacteria that contaminate our food. Keeping food safe for consumption depends on how it is stored, handled, and cooked. Eating food that contains harmful bacteria, toxins, parasites, viruses, or chemical contaminants can causes food-borne illness.

Campylobacter, *Salmonella*, *Listeria*, and *Escherichia coli* are the most common invaders. You do not have to eat a lot of contaminated food before you feel ill—you can become sick by eating just a few bites. Because food-borne illnesses resemble the common flu, many people are unaware it was the food that made them sick. Symptoms can appear about 30 minutes after eating or can take up to 3 weeks to manifest. It is estimated that up to 33 million people in the United States are sickened each year with a food-borne illness. To ensure that you are not part of this statistic, follow these four simple steps when handling or preparing food:

1. Clean
   a. Wash your hands for 20 seconds with hot, soapy water before and after handling food and after using the bathroom, playing with your pet, or changing diapers.

    b. Wash cutting boards, dishes, utensils, and countertops with hot, soapy water each time you prepare a new food for the meal. Food for Thought given below gives advice for handling cutting boards.

    c. Use disposable paper towels versus cloth towels, which can harbor bacteria.

    d. Clean liquids that spill in the refrigerator, including those that leak out of packaged lunchmeat and hot dogs.

2. Separate (do not cross-contaminate)

    a. Separate raw meat, poultry, and seafood from other foods in your shopping cart and refrigerator and on the counter.

    b. Designate separate cutting boards for food groups: one for cutting meat, another for chopping vegetables, and another for slicing bread.

    c. Wash anything that comes into contact with raw meats and their juices with hot, soapy water.

    d. Use one plate for raw meat, poultry, and seafood and another plate after they are cooked.

3. Cook

    a. Use a thermometer to determine that food is fully cooked.

    b. Cook roasts and steaks to 145°C, poultry to 180°C, and pork to 160°C.

    c. Fish is done when it flakes with a fork.

    d. Never use or eat ground beef that is still pink.

    e. Cook eggs until both the yolk and white are firm, and avoid recipes that call for raw eggs.

    f. Microwaved food should be hot throughout with no cold spots.

    g. Reheated food should be cooked to 165°C or boiled.

4. Chill

    a. Keep the temperature of your refrigerator at or below 41°C to slow the growth of bacteria.

    b. Refrigerate or freeze perishables, cooked food, and all leftovers within 2 hours and put a date on the container. Leftovers should be used within 3 to 5 days.

    c. Thaw food in the refrigerator, under cold water, or in the microwave—never on a counter at room temperature.

    d. Marinate all food in the refrigerator.

    e. Store leftovers in small shallow containers versus large containers for quick cooling.

    f. Do not overpack the refrigerator—cool air must circulate to keep food safe.

See Figure 11-4.

Remember: Clean, separate, cook, and chill

CLEAN   **SEPARATE**

CHILL   **COOK**

Figure 11-4   Keep food safe.

FOOD FOR THOUGHT   IS YOUR CUTTING BOARD SAFE?

- Use smooth cutting boards made of hard wood or plastic.
- Use one board for cutting meats and one for ready-to-eat foods such as vegetables, fruits, and bread.
- Boards should be free of cracks and crevices.
- Scrub boards with a brush in hot soapy water after use.
- Sanitize boards in the dishwasher or rinse in a solution of 1 teaspoon bleach in 1 quart of water.

Figure 11-5   Safe refrigerator and freezer temperatures.

Figure 11-5 illustrates safe refrigeration temperatures and the danger zone for food.

OTHER KITCHEN DANGERS

Other **kitchen dangers** include lead, microwave packaging, and insects and dirt:

- Lead leached from ceramic dishes into food and drink is the number one source of dietary lead. To reduce your exposure to lead, do not use ceramic or lead crystal containers to store food. Use them sparingly for serving.
- Microwaving can cause adhesives and polymers from the package to leach into food. If at all possible, do not use the package carton to heat your food; instead, use a microwave-safe dish.
- Wash the tops of cans before removing lids to eliminate dust and dirt from falling into the food.
- Avoid storing food in cupboards under the sink or where water can leak or drain. Insects and rodents are attracted to dark, damp places and can invade openings in packages.
- Keep dishcloths and sponges clean and dry. When wet, they harbor bacteria and promote bacterial growth.
- When washing dishes by hand, wash within 2 hours and air-dry so they are not handled when wet.
- If you have an infection or cut on your hands, wear rubber gloves and wash the gloves as often as bare hands.

- When thawing food in cold water, seal it in a watertight bag and submerge it in water, changing the water every 30 minutes.
- Food defrosted in the microwave should be cooked immediately.
- Do not buy frozen seafood if the package is open, torn, or crushed on the edges.

RELATE TO PATIENTS

Sticking to the tried-and-true food guidelines are the best place to start when recommending changes to your patient's eating patterns. Just as it is recommended that dental professionals only recommend products approved by the American Dental Association, we should suggest behaviors recommended by the Food Guidelines for Healthy Americans and the USDA MyPlate (or those from the patient's homeland). Stay current on food selections for healthy lifestyle diets like the Paleo, Mediterranean, gluten-free, or vegetarian diet to offer meaningful counseling for a healthy oral cavity. After collecting data and analyzing a food diary, do the following:

1. Compare the patient's food diary to suggestions made by MyPlate or other food guide that would be best suited to his/her diet and cultural considerations, and point out excesses and deficiencies.
2. Choose food guidelines best suited to your patient's diet, medical and cultural tendencies, and suggest ways to improve in areas of neglect.
3. Recommend 30 minutes of moderate exercise each day, and work with your patient to discover ways to incorporate more movement into the daily schedule.
4. Outline safe food-handling and preparation techniques to ensure your patient is keeping food safe to prevent food-borne illnesses.

CHAPTER
REVIEW

PRACTICE FOR PATIENTS

Patient #1

Your patient is a 19-year-old college student who has made the decision to eliminate animal food products from her diet. During her dental exam, you identify two new carious lesions. After quizzing her on foods consumed over the past 24 hours, it is revealed she has eaten a disproportionate amount of calories from simple sugars versus protein.

1. Write your explanation of the dangers of substituting carbohydrate-rich foods for the calories lost from eliminating protein-rich foods.
2. Calculate her daily protein needs based on a body weight of 126 lb.
3. List foods that can be included in her diet to ensure an adequate daily protein intake.
4. Write your explanation of how inadequate protein intake can affect the oral cavity.

Patient #2

Your patient is a 40-year-old man who is reevaluating his appearance. He recently started visiting the gym where he is working with a personal trainer to turn soft muscle into hard. To assist the process, he states he is on a high-protein diet and even supplements with protein shakes when he limits daily calories.

1. How much quicker will muscles respond to weight training when there is more protein available in the diet?
2. Would you expect to see any oral changes from the protein shake supplementation?

RELATE TO YOU

Assignment #1

1. Using the guidelines from around the world as example, invent a 10-point dietary guidelines to lead your family into a healthier lifestyle.
2. Explain the key differences between MyPlate for adults and for children.
3. Make a food pyramid or other shape to illustrate your family's current eating habits, including favorite foods cut from magazines.
4. Using your family's food plate, list some changes that should be made to follow the dietary guidelines you developed for your family.

Assignment #2

Visit www.MyPlate.gov and complete the information request to create a meal plan for yourself. Compare it with your current eating practice and determine if following the plan would be a healthier lifestyle change for you.

REFERENCES

1. Obesity and overweight. *World Health Organization Media Center Fact Sheet*; January 2015.
2. Sample CH, Martin AA, Jonea S, et al. Western-style diet impairs stimulus control by food deprivation state cues: implications for obesogenic environments. *Appetite* 2015;93:13–23.
3. Zeeni N, Dagher-Hamalian C, Dimassi H, et al. Cafeteria diet-fed mice is a pertinent model of obesity-induced organ damage: a potential role of inflammation. *Inflamm Res* 2015;64(7):501–512.
4. Reddy V, Sridhar A, Machado RF, et al. High sodium causes hypertension: evidence from clinical trials and animal experiments. *J Integr Med* 2015;13(1):1–8.
5. *Boost Your Memory by Eating Right*. Harvard Health Publications; August 2012.
6. Trans fat consumption is linked to diminished memory in working-aged adults. *American Heart Association Newsroom*; November 18, 2014.
7. Morris MC, Evans DA, Bienias JL, et al. Dietary fat intake and 6-year cognitive change in an older biracial community population. *Neurology* 2004;62(9):1573–1579.
8. Das PK, Panja D. Study of major factors developed among young swimmers during the practice session and competition causing interference of their performances. *J Indian Med Assoc* 2013;111(12):837–839, 844.
9. Brown CL, Halvorson EE, Cohen GM, et al. Addressing childhood obesity: opportunities for prevention. *Pediatr Clin North Am* 2015;62(5):1241–1261.
10. Zhang J, et al. Dietary patterns and their associations with childhood obesity in China. *Br J Nutr* 2015;113(12):1978–1984.
11. Braithwaite I, et al. Fast-food consumption and body mass index in children and adolescents: an international cross-sectional study. *BMJ Open* 2014;4(12).
12. Payab M, et al. Association of junk food consumption with high blood pressure and obesity in Iranian children and adolescents: the CASPIAN-IV Study. *J Pediatr (Rio J)* 2015;9(12):196–205.
13. Estrade M, et al. A qualitative study of independent fast food vendors near secondary schools in disadvantaged Scottish neighborhoods. *BMC Public Health* 2014;14:793.
14. Scully P, et al. Food and beverage cues in children's television programmes: the influence of programme genre. *Public Health Nutr* 2015;17:1–9.
15. Russell CA, Buhrau D. The role of television viewing and direct experience in predicting adolescents' beliefs about the health risks of fast-food consumption. *Appetite* 2015;92:200–206.
16. Schwartz J, Byrd-Bredbenner C. Portion distortion: typical portion sizes selected by young adults. *J Am Diet Assoc* 2006;106(9):1412–1418.
17. Kelley WM, Wagner DD, Heatherton TF. In search of a human self-regulation system. *Annu Rev Neurosci* 2015;38:389–411.
18. Slavin JL. The challenges of nutrition policymaking. *Nutr J* 2015;14:15.
19. Rowe S, et al. How experts are chosen to inform public policy: can the process be improved? *Health Policy* 2013;112(3):172–178.
20. Turconi G, Bazzano R, Roggi C, et al. Helping consumers make a more conscious nutritional choice: acceptability of nutrition information at a cafeteria. *Public Health Nutr* 2012;15(5):792–801.

21. American Cancer Society Guidelines on Nutrition and Physical Activity for Cancer Prevention. Last review January 11, 2012.

22. Leiter LA, et al. Identification of educational needs in the management of overweight and obesity: results of an international survey of attitudes and practice. *Clin Obes* 2015;5(5):245–255.

23. Nagle CM, et al. Cancers in Australia in 2010 attributed to inadequate consumption of fruit, non-starchy vegetables, and dietary fiber. *Aust N Z J Public Health* 2015;39(5):422–428.

24. Li YH, et al. Role of phytochemicals in colorectal prevention. *World J Gastroenterol* 2015;2(31):9262–9272.

25. Hermando RO, Rodriguez R. Nutrition and cancer. *Nutr Hosp* 2015;32(suppl 1):67–72.

26. Harvie M, Howell A, Evans DG. Can diet and lifestyle prevent breast cancer: what is the evidence? *Am Soc Clin Oncol Educ Book* 2015;35:e66–e73.

27. Manninen A. Metabolic effects of the very-low carbohydrate diets: misunderstood "villains" of human metabolism. *J Int Soc Sports Nutr* 2004;1(2):7–11.

28. Reid M, et al. Meeting the nutrient reference values on a vegetarian diet. *Med J Aust* 2013;199(4 suppl):S33–S40.

29. Chiu UF, et al. Cross-sectional and longitudinal comparisons of metabolic profiles between vegetarian and non-vegetarian subjects: a matched cohort study. *Br J Nutr* 2015;114(8):1313–1320.

30. Kahleova H, Pelikanova T. Vegetarian diets in the prevention and treatment of type 2 diabetes. *J Am Coll Nutr* 2015;34(5):448–458.

31. Beezhold B, Radnitz C, Rinne A, et al. Vegans report less stress and anxiety than omnivores. *Nutr Neurosci* 2015;18(7):289–296.

32. Rippe J, Angeloopoulos T. Fructose-containing sugars and cardiovascular disease. *Adv Nutr* 2015;6(4):430–439.

33. Sheiham A, James W. Diet and dental caries: the pivotal role of free sugars reemphasized. *J Dent Res* 2015;94(10):1341–1347.

34. Pawlak R, Lester S, Babatunde T. The prevalence of cobalamin deficiency among vegetarians assessed by serum vitamin B12: a review of literature. *Eur J Clin Nutr* 2014;68(5):541–548.

35. Naik S, et al. Daily milk intake improves vitamin B-12 status in young vegetarian Indians: an intervention trial. *Nutr J* 2013;12:136.

36. Koneswaran G, Nierenberg D. Global farm animal production and global warming: impacting and mitigating climate change. *Environ Health Perspect* 2008;116(5):578–582.

37. Brathwaite N. Obesity, diabetes, hypertension, and vegetarian status among seventh-day Adventists in Barbados: preliminary results. *Ethn Dis* 2003;13(1):24–29.

38. Pastore RL, Brooks JT, Carbone JW. Paleolithic nutrition improves plasma lipid concentrations of hypercholesterolemic adults to a greater extent than traditional heart-healthy dietary recommendations. *Nutr Res* 2015;35(6):474–479.

39. Boers I, et al. Favourable effects of consuming a Palaeolithic-type diet on characteristics of the metabolic syndrome: a randomized controlled pilot-study. *Lipids Health Dis* 2014;11:160.

40. Bligh HF, et al. Plant-rich mixed meals based on Paleolithic diet principles have a dramatic impact on incretin, peptide YY and satiety response, but show little effect on glucose and insulin homeostasis: an acute-effects randomised study. *Br J Nutr* 2015;113(4):574–584.

41. Jew S, AbuMweis SS, Jones PH. Evolution of the human diet: linking our ancestral diet to modern functional foods as a means of chronic disease prevention. *J Med Food* 2009;12(5):925–934.
42. Allen PJ. Gluten-related disorders: celiac disease, gluten allergy, non-celiac gluten sensitivity. *Peadiatr Nurs* 2015;41(3):146–150.
43. Lebwohl B, Ludvigsson JF, Green PH. Celiac disease and non-celiac gluten sensitivity. *Br Med J* 2015;351:h4347.
44. Elli L, Roncoroni L, Bardella MT. Non-celiac gluten sensitivity: time for sifting the grain. *World J Gastroenterol* 2015;21(27):8221–8226.
45. Eustruch R., Salas-Salvado J. Towards an even healthier Mediterranean diet. *Nutr Metab Cardiovasc Dis* 2013;23(12):1163–1166.
46. Hernaez A, et al. Olive oil polyphenols decrease LDL concentrations and LDL atherogenicity in men in a randomized controlled trial. *J Nutr* 2015;145(8):1692–1697.
47. Hernaez A, et al. Olive oil polyphenols enhance high-density lipoprotein function in humans: a randomized controlled trial. *Arterioscler Thromb Vasc Biol* 2014;34(9):2115–2119.
48. Lee J, et al. Switching to a 10-day Mediterranean style diet improves mood and cardiovascular function in a controlled crossover study. *Nutrition* 2015;31(5):647.

SUGGESTED READINGS

Campbell TC , Campbell TM II. *The China Study*. Dallas, TX: Benbella Books; 2006.
Zinczendo D. *Eat This Not That—The No-Diet Weight Loss Solution*. Pennsylvania: Rodale; 2012.

SUBSCRIBE TO: ONLINE HEALTH NEWS LETTERS

Nutrition Action Health Letter www.cspinet.org/nah
Tufts Health Letter www.tuftshealthletter.com
Berkeley Wellness Letter www.berkeleywellness.com
Harvard Health Letter www.health.harvard.edu/newsletters/harvard_health_letter
Mayo Clinic Health Letter www.healthletter.mayoclinic.com
Johns Hopkins Medicine Your Health Newsletter www.hopkinsmedicine.org

WEB RESOURCES

Rudd Center for Food Policy and Obesity www.uconnruddcenter.org
Cleveland Clinic Health www.my.clevellansclinic.org/health/service/newsletter
http://www.johnshopkinshealthalerts.com/alerts/nutrition_weight_control/ JohnsHopkinsNutritionandWeightControlHealthAlert_1150-1. html?st=email&s=ENH%20070919%20013
Partnership for Food Safety Education—Fight Bac!: Keep Food Safe From Bacteria www. fightbac.org
Dietary Guidelines for Americans http://www.health.gov/DietaryGuidelines/
Canada's Food Guide http://www.hc-sc.gc.ca/fn-an/food-guide-aliment/index_e.html
European Food information Council http://www.eufic.org/index/en/
Food Safety—Gateway to Government Food Safety Information www.foodsafety.gov
U.S. Food and Drug Administration www.fda.gov

American Dietetic Association www.eatright.org
Federal Citizen Information Center www.pueblo.gsa.gov
The Vegetarian Resource Group www.vrg.org
Atkins Diet and Low Carbohydrate Support (Canada) www.lowcarb.ca
Atkins Nutritionals www.atkins.com
Beyond Vegetarianism—Transcending Outdated Dogmas www.beyondveg.com
International Vegetarian Union www.ivu.org

FOR MORE INFORMATION ABOUT SAFE FOOD HANDLING AND PREPARATION

USDA's Meat and Poultry Hotline: 1-800-535-4555
FDA's Food

12

Reading Labels

Learning Objectives

> Real food doesn't have ingredients, real food is ingredients.
>
> *Jamie Oliver—Celebrity Chef*

- Outline the major points of the Nutrition Labeling and Education Act (NLEA)
- List nutrients that *must* be included on a food label
- Explain the meaning of daily value (DV) on a food label
- Describe how food ingredients are listed
- Give examples of FDA-approved health claims
- State five common mistakes when reading a food label
- Identify the number of calories per gram for carbohydrates, protein, fat, and alcohol
- Calculate the percentage of major nutrients in a food product and the amount of calories in one serving size

Key Terms

Curing
Daily Value
Food Preservatives
Genetically Engineered
GRAS
HFCS

Kilocalorie
MSG
NLEA
Organic
Nutrition Facts

INTRODUCTION

Over the course of a century, nutrients have been added to our food supply by manufacturers, often for disease prevention. Potassium iodide was added to table salt in the 1920s to reduce the incidence of goiters in thyroid disease. As early as the 1930s, milk has been fortified with vitamins A and D to prevent rickets and osteomalacia. In the 1940s, iron and B vitamins were added to bleached flour (which made bread) to keep the population healthy during wartime. With the increased production of convenience foods, as nutrients and flavor were lost, additives were incorporated to enrich the food and make it more palatable. This created a need for policies to assure that additives were safe for consumers.

The Federal Food and Drug Administration (FDA) is responsible for assuring foods sold in the United States are safe for consumption and properly labeled. The Federal Food, Drug, and Cosmetic Act and Fair Packaging and Labeling Act are the federal laws governing food products under FDA's jurisdiction.[1]

NUTRITION LABELING AND EDUCATION ACT

In 1990, the U.S. Food and Drug Administration (FDA) established the Nutrition Labeling and Education Act (NLEA) so consumers would know what was included in the food they purchased.[2] NLEA requires package labeling for all food except meat and poultry and is voluntary for raw produce and fish. Shoppers are able to determine ingredients, total calories, major nutrients, vitamins, and minerals in the container. The NLEA also sets guidelines for stating nutrient claims, such as *low fat* or *sugar-free*, and certain FDA-approved health claims, such as *lowers cholesterol*. All food labels are titled "Nutrition Facts" and information is organized in an identical format, allowing consumers to compare similar products to make the best choice.

In 2004, the Food, Drug, and Cosmetic Act amended the law to require listing of eight major food allergens on food labels. Over 160 foods have been identified to cause food allergies in sensitive people, but the eight that were required to list account for 90% of all food allergies. This applies to spices, flavorings, colorings, and other incidental additives. The following are identified as most predominant food allergies[2,3]:

1. Milk
2. Egg
3. Fish (bass, flounder, or cod)
4. Shellfish
5. Treenuts (almonds, pecans, Brazil nut, cashew, pistachio, and walnuts, to name a few)
6. Wheat
7. Peanuts
8. Soybeans

FOOD FOR THOUGHT — EXCEPTIONS TO FOOD LABELS

In 1994, food package labeling became law. The following foods are exceptions to that law and do not require food labels:

- Food served in hospital cafeterias, on airplanes, in vending machines, and at mall counters
- Bakery, deli, or candy store that serves ready-to-eat food prepared on site
- Food shipped in bulk
- Medical foods that are consumed to address the needs of certain diseases
- Coffee, tea, spices, or other nonnutritive foods
- Food served in restaurants, unless they make a health or nutrient claim on their menu, advertisement, or other notice

FOOD FOR THOUGHT — COKE! IT'S THE REAL THING! (OR MAYBE NOT)

Coca-Cola changed their recipe around 1970. Prior to that, public taste tests indicated their competitor's soda was preferred because of its sweeter taste. Coke began gradually substituting high-fructose corn syrup (HFCS) for sucrose as it was just as sweet but cheaper and would mean bigger profits for the corporation. As the recipe neared 100% fructose "New Coke" was born. Although Coca-Cola claimed the taste was new and improved, Coke aficionados disagreed. Many complained it left a bitter aftertaste in their mouths. Sales dropped and the company lost profits. Corporate leaders relented, and brought back "Classic Coke," which contained only 40% fructose compared with 100% fructose in "New Coke."

Today, discerning Coke fans can tell the difference in taste from bottling plants. One plant in Mexico uses 100% sucrose for a taste that is closest to original Coke. Next time you grab for a six pack of Coke, read the label and determine origin of bottling. Not all use the same recipe as most other countries use sucrose because it is more readily available in their region.

Here is an article related to the topic: Walker RW, Dumke KA, Goran MI. Fructose content in popular beverages made with and without high-fructose corn syrup. *Nutrition.* 2014;30(7–8):928–935.

(Prefer Pepsi to Coke?—Pepsi Throwback is also made with sucrose instead of HFCS.)

The majority of consumers read package labels, but most become confused while doing so.[3-5] And even though most consumers read the food label, information is being under-utilized.[6] Although labels are not meant to be tricky, they can be misleading if not read carefully. It is important to check food labels even if you are a routine shopper because just as the design of a food package can change, so can ingredients. Routine shoppers have a tendency to make the same food choices and repeatedly purchase the same brand of baked beans, boxed macaroni and cheese, or loaf of bread. Manufacturers can change ingredients at any given time, and unless the label is read and compared to other like products, there is no guarantee you are still making the best choice.

READING A NUTRITION FACTS LABEL

Reading and understanding the Nutrition Facts Label provides information you need to know to plan a balanced diet. There are many reasons for reading a label other than to know what ingredients the product contains or whether it is *rich* in certain nutrients. Individuals following a specific diet might need to know how much saturated/trans fats or carbohydrates/sugar a product has or how much protein and vitamins/minerals the food contains. For those who have a medical disorder or condition requiring avoidance of certain additives, constant review of labels is a must, for example, allergies to specific additives like peanut oil, sensitivities to colorants and flavoring agents, and need for sugar substitutes instead of sucrose.

Nutrition Facts contain several parts and under the NLEA, food manufacturers are *required* (by 2018) to provide daily values, based on a 2,000-calorie diet, for the following:

- Serving size and number of servings per container
- Total calories
- Total grams of fat (saturated and trans fats, polyunsaturated, and monounsaturated)
- Grams of cholesterol
- Grams of sodium
- Total carbohydrate (fiber and sugars)
- Protein
- Vitamin D
- Percentage of vitamin A as beta-carotene
- Calcium

- Potassium
- Iron
- Voluntary reporting of vitamins A and C
- Other added nutrients

Figure 12-1 provides an example of a typical food label.

Figure 12-1 Nutritional label for condensed tomato soup.

Example				
	Single serving	Percentage DV	Double serving	Percentage DV
Serving size	1 cup (228 g)		2 cups (456 g)	
Calories	250		500	
Calories from fat	110		220	
Trans fat	1.5 g		3 g	
Saturated fat	3 g	15%	6 g	30%
Cholesterol	30 mg	10%	60 mg	20%
Sodium	470 mg	20%	940 mg	50%
Total carbohydrate	31 g	10%	62 g	20%
Dietary fiber	0 g	0%	0 g	0%
Sugars	5 g		10 g	
Protein	5 g		10 g	
Vitamin A		4%		8%
Vitamin C		2%		4%
Calcium		20%		40%
Iron		4%		8%

Figure 12-2 Comparison of two label showing calculations for consuming two servings.

Serving sizes (listed at the top under the title) have long been an issue with nutritionists when a package that appears to be one serving may actually be two or two-and-a-half, as with a 20-oz soda.[7] When you eat a whole box of macaroni and cheese or a can of soup, it may be two servings, yet the information on the label is for one serving. That means all nutrient values should be multiplied by 2. Figure 12-2 compares value for two servings versus one. Visit www.fda.gov and enter food label in the search box. Several short instructional videos highlight how to read and understand calories and serving sizes. Also, there are several short videos on YouTube that can assist with understanding of food labels.

The percentage **Daily Value** (DV) column helps you figure how much of a nutrient you are getting from a food that contributes to your total daily intake. If a label has 25% of vitamin A, it means you have to accumulate 75% from other food the rest of the day to reach 100% of the recommended intake. Sodium, saturated fat, and sugars are the three nutrients you may want to keep track of to make sure you are not getting more than you need.

Calories per serving appear on the label under serving size. It is important to know how many calories per day you eat to compute your DV of nutrients. Although the labels are based on a 2,000-calorie diet, as explained at the bottom in the footnote, it is recommended that women in the age group of 35 to 70 restrict their diet to 1,600 to 1,800 calories per day, and men in the same age group consume 2,000 to 2,200 calories per day. Depending on whether you are male or female and active or sedentary, you may have to increase or decrease the rest of the day's nutrients. Computing the DV for nutrients would then require a good pair of reading glasses and a calculator.

Trans fats are the newest addition to Nutrition Facts labels. FDA estimates that the average person eats 4.7 lb of trans fats per year. A small amount of trans fat is naturally occurring in beef and dairy products, but most of the trans fat in our diets comes from infusing vegetable oils with hydrogen. Manufacturers began using hydrogenated fats about 20 years ago to prolong the shelf-life of their product. According to reports from Mayo Clinic, trans fats are actually worse for us than saturated fats because not only do they clog arteries but are also bad for cholesterol levels—increases low-density lipoprotein (LDL) level and lowers high-density lipoprotein (HDL) level, which protects the heart.

INGREDIENTS

Ingredients are listed in descending order of predominance. For example, on a loaf of bread, you would assume the first ingredient listed would be bread flour or beans on a can of green beans. Knowing what the first three ingredients are in a food product gives you a good idea of what you are eating. Two facts are very important to remember when looking at this section:

1. Sugar can be listed under other names on the label, and if all varieties were added together, it would equal the first ingredient. There are over 60 identified names for sugar that may appear on a label. Examples are sucrose, HFCS, agave nectar, beet sugar, brown sugar, cane juice, caramel, coconut palm sugar, corn sweetener, corn syrup, dextrin, dextrose, fructose, glucose solids, honey, invert sugar, maltodextrin, molasses, palm sugar, sorghum syrup, and treacle.
2. Partially hydrogenated oils are trans fats, which are more harmful to arteries than saturated fat. They can raise bad cholesterol and lower good cholesterol. Look for the words hydrogenated or partially hydrogenated on the ingredient panel.

FOOD ADDITIVES

FDA created the acronym **GRAS** to mean generally recognized as safe when referring to food additives. Substances can receive GRAS recognition either through scientific procedures or through experience of being safely used by significant numbers of consumers. Any new food additive that does not have a track record of safety must undergo scientific testing by experts before receiving approval by the FDA for use in food. Preservatives, sweeteners, flavorants, and colorants are all considered additives.

Individuals with food allergies or sensitivities may need to avoid certain additives, even though they have the GRAS distinction. Food allergies cause immune reactions like hives, vomiting, drop in blood pressure, and, in extreme cases, anaphylaxis shock. An intolerance (sensitivity) is more common than a true allergy and is not life threatening. Symptoms come on slower and could be headache, heartburn, or gas/bloating. The only way to know if the trigger appears in your food is to read the label. For a synopsis of the medical community's advice about artificial food additives, watch WebMD's video on Food Additives Effects on Kids.

Food Preservatives

Oxidation, heat, light, and bacterial contamination are some of the ways food products can spoil, but in reality, food begins to decay the moment it is harvested. **Food preservatives** have been used for hundreds of years to prevent the spoiling of food. To survive, ancient cultures invented ways to preserve their food for periods when it was not practical to hunt or gather. With weather conditions being unpredictable, it was prudent to have stored food to assure availability at all times. Drying and freezing were the first methods of preserving, and fermenting, pickling, canning soon followed. **Curing**, another form of preservation, uses salt or nitrates/nitrites and/or sugar to draw moisture out of meats and fruit. The following are common preservative chemicals identified on food labels today:

- Benzoates are found in both plants and animals. Sodium benzoate is used by manufacturers to prevent growth of microorganisms in food that contain acid: pickles, pickled relishes, fruit juice, and sodas. Although many people can consume benzoates without any problems, those who are sensitive to additives may have allergic reactions.
- Sorbates are prolific in our food supply. You will see it listed on the ingredient panel of labels for wine, jelly, syrup, bread, baked goods, cheese, and many other products. Serving as an antimicrobial preservative, it is added to many recipes to prevent the growth of mold.

- Sulfites can be dangerous for asthma sufferers. In the 1980s, restaurants soaked iceberg lettuce in sulfite solution to prevent wilting and rusting so it always appeared crisp and fresh on the plate. By 1986, the FDA banned the use of this preservative from fresh fruits and vegetables eaten raw (salad ingredients), but this dictate came only after multiple reported deaths. Sulfites are still found in potato chips, pre-cut potatoes, juice, packaged gravy mixes, canned vegetables, jam, baked goods, and many other food products. This chemical can cause asthma outbreak, tightness of the chest, and breathing difficulties for sensitive individuals and, if the reaction is severe, anaphylactic shock. The FDA reports that one out of every 100 people have allergic symptoms to sulfites, which can be listed as other names: sulfur dioxide, potassium bisulfite, potassium metabisulfite, sodium sulfite, sodium bisulfite, sodium metabisulfite, calcium sulfite, and others containing any mix of chemical names.
- Butylated hydroxyanisole (BHA) is an antioxidant intended to delay fats and oils from becoming rancid. Other foods that contain BHA are butter, cereal, potato chips, vending snack foods, bread, and chewing gum.
- Nitrates (and nitrites) are used to cure foods like ham, salami, many other lunch meats, bacon, sausage, hot dogs, jerky, and smoked salmon and give them their pretty pink color. It is added to inhibit the growth of the bacteria known to cause botulism. For years, nitrates were associated with an increase in gastric cancer, but this has since been disproven.[8,9] Vegetables and fruits naturally provide nitrite and nitrates to the body and are considered to be more beneficial than harmful to maintaining good health.[10]

Sweeteners

High-fructose corn syrup (HFCS), a sweet syrup made from corn starch, made its debut into our food supply in the mid-1970s, replacing the more expensive sucrose. HFCS can be made from rice, tapioca, wheat, potato, and cassava, but with the US's huge corn crop, corn is the primary source.

The switch from sucrose to HFCS steadily increased for about 20 years and then began to taper off around 1998. Today, HFCS accounts for 50% of nutritive sweeteners used in the United States but only 8% in the rest of the world.[11]

You will see HFCS on labels for a wide array of foods and products: sodas, fruit juice, cereal, yogurt, breads, candy, boxed stuffing mixes, bottled iced tea, eggos, ketchup, relish, cranberry sauce, ice cream, jellies, jams, miracle whip, lunch meat, crackers, cheese, cool whip, salad dressing, nutrition bars, baked goods, cough syrup, and Vicks VapoRub. It is a fructose-glucose sweetener that manufacturers prefer because it is easy to handle in its liquid form and remains heat stable during food processing. Although HFCS is chemically similar to table sugar, researchers hesitate to determine whether the body handles the two differently. Most current studies claim HFCS and sucrose are not significantly different, and increased consumption of calories from either HFCS or granular sugar causes weight gain.[12] One study found that there is an association between high consumption of soft drinks with HFCS and incidence of chronic bronchitis.[13]

For information on sugar substitutes like aspartame and saccharine, see Chapter 9.

Artificial Flavors

Monosodium glutamate (MSG), the salt of glutamic acid, is a flavor *enhancer* that intensifies the taste of soups, chicken broth, bouillon cubes, salty flavored snacks (chips crackers and nuts), lunch meat, ramen noodles, seasoned french fries, pasta sauce, frozen meals, salad dressings, and soy sauce, to name a few. Glutamic acid is a naturally occurring amino acid circulating in your body and in meat, fish, mushrooms, cheese, and tomatoes. The body metabolizes both (in the body and in food) renditions in the same way.

In spite of the scientific community declaring MSG safe for consumption, it has been at the center of controversy for several decades.[14,15] MSG has been notoriously accused of causing Chinese restaurant syndrome (1968) that elicits symptoms like headache (migraine), heart palpitations, tightness in chest, numbness or tingling, sweating, nausea, and dizziness.[15] An in-depth study was conducted by the FDA to determine legitimacy of complaints against MSG. Their final report recognizes that although a small percent of individuals may be sensitive to MSG, their symptoms are transient and non-life-threatening. The majority of scientific evidence concludes that MSG is a safe food additive.[16,17] For those who are sensitive to glutamates, be aware that MSG can be called by other names on a food label, soy extract, hydrolyzed yeast extract, and hydrolyzed vegetable protein, or just falls under the catch-all of "spices."

Artificial Colors

Food colorant can be liquid, powder, gel, or paste. When foods are processed for packaging, they may lose color from exposure to extreme sanitizing temperatures or light. Manufacturers correctly assume that consumers would prefer a vibrant color be associated with favorite flavors.

For example, green for lime, yellow for lemon, red for cherry, or purple for grape, you get the idea. The practice of adding color to food dates back to the Middle Ages when wine pigment and colored spices, like saffron, were used to improve the appearance of foods.

For over 39 years, scientists have been studying the effects of artificial food colorants on child behavior, particularly in relation to ADHD.[18-20] Currently, there is general consensus that more studies are needed before a definitive relationship can be concluded.[21,22]

In the United States, the following seven FD&C (approved for food, drugs, and cosmetics) colors are considered GRAS with three accounting for 90% of all used*:

- Blue #1 and #2
- Red #3 and #40*
- Yellow #5* and #6*
- Green #3

Two other colorants are permitted for specific circumstances: Citrus Red 2 to color orange peels and Orange B to add color to hot dog and sausage casings.

FOOD FOR THOUGHT LABELING FLAWS

Nutrition Facts labels allow for a 20% margin of error. This could make a huge difference when counting calories or watching for amounts of certain ingredients like sugar (carbs) and salt. The FDA does not have a process in place to audit accuracy of food labels and expects food manufacturers to self-enforce.

In a 2008 sampling of 300 labels, the audit discovered iron and vitamin A to be the least accurate. This bit of news might lead you to wonder if reading labels is worth your time. Read on before throwing the "baby out with the bathwater."

Another study in 2010 published in Journal of Consumer Affairs stated that a survey of 3,700 subjects 37 to 50 who were reading labels as part of their weight loss regimen (without exercising) were more likely to lose weight than those who did not read labels yet exercised. It appears there is some benefit to reading flawed labels.

Tamara Freuman. When Nutrition Labels Lie: Reading between the lines on nutrition labels. U.S. News and World Report: Health 2012 August.

HEALTH CLAIMS

Health claims are posted on the front of the food package for shoppers desiring a certain benefit from their food. The NLEA specifies which claims are allowed and the requirements the food has to meet to make that claim. See Tables 12-1 to 12-4 for information on FDA-approved health claims.

Table 12-1	Approved Nutrient-Related Health Claims
Nutrient	**Approved Claim**
Calcium and vitamin D	Calcium, vitamin D, and osteoporosis: adequate calcium throughout life, as part of a well-balanced diet, may reduce risk of osteoporosis
Dietary fat	Development of cancer depends on many factors. A diet low in total fat may reduce the risk of some cancers
Sodium	Diets low in sodium may reduce the risk of high blood pressure, a disease associated with many factors
Saturated fat and cholesterol	While many factors affect heart disease, diets low in saturated fat and cholesterol may reduce the risk of this disease
Fiber	Low-fat diets rich in fiber-containing grain products, fruits, and vegetables may reduce the risk of some types of cancer, a disease associated with many factors
Fruits and vegetables	Low-fat diets rich in fruits and vegetables may reduce the risk of some types of cancer, a disease associated with many factors.
Folate	Healthful diets with adequate folate may reduce a woman's risk of having a child with a brain or spinal cord defect.
Noncariogenic sweeteners	Sugar-alcohol does not promote tooth decay
Soy protein	25 g of soy protein a day, as part of a low in saturated fat and cholesterol diet, may reduce the risk of heart disease
Plant sterol	Foods containing at least 1.3 g of plant sterol a day, as part of a diet low in saturated fat and cholesterol, may reduce the risk of heart disease
Potassium	Diets containing certain foods that are a good source of potassium and that are low in sodium may reduce the risk of high blood pressure and stroke
Fluoride	Drinking fluoridated water may reduce the risk of dental caries

Adapted from FDA Food Labeling Guide Appendix C Health Claims.

Table 12-2	Trans Fat in Common Foods
Food	**Approximate Grams of Trans Fat**
Crackers	0.36 g per cracker
Pound cake	4.3 g per slice
Cream-filled cookies	1.9 g each
Microwave popcorn	5 g per half bag
KFC original recipe chicken dinner	7 g
Doughnuts	5 g each
Potato chips	3 g small bag
French fries	10 g medium serving
Maria Calendar's chicken pot pie	1.96 g
Mrs. Smith's apple pie	4 g each slice
Nabisco chips ahoy	1.5 g per 3
Stick margarine	2.8 g per tablespoon

Table 12-3	U.S. Food and Drug Administration (FDA) Requirements to Meet Health Claims
Health Claim	**Requirements to Meet**
Fat-free	0.5 g of fat per serving or less
0 g trans fat	<0.5 g of trans fat per serving
Low fat	3 g of fat per serving or less
Less fat	25% less fat than original recipe
Light (fat)	50% less fat than original recipe
Saturated fat-free	0.5 g of saturated or trans fat per serving or less
Cholesterol-free	2 g or less saturated fat/serving and <2 mg cholesterol per serving
Low cholesterol	2 g or less saturated fat/serving and <20 mg cholesterol per serving
Reduced calorie	25% fewer calories than original recipe
Low calorie	40 calories or less per serving
Light (calories)	One third fewer calories than original recipe
Extra lean	5 g fat or less, 2 g saturated fat or less, 95 mg cholesterol/100 g serving of meat, poultry, or seafood
Lean	10 g fat or less, 4.5 g saturated fat or less, 95 mg cholesterol/100 g serving of meat, poultry, or seafood
High fiber	5 g or more per serving
Sugar-free	0.5 g or less per serving
Sodium-free (salt-free)	0.5 g or less per serving
Low sodium	140 mg or less per serving
Very low sodium	35 mg or less per serving
Heart healthy	Low in saturated fat, cholesterol, sodium

Table 12-4	Meanings of Health Claims
Health Claim	**Meaning**
Healthy	Low in fat, saturated fat, cholesterol, and sodium and has at least 10% DV of protein, iron, calcium, fiber, and vitamins A and C
Good source of, more, added	10% more DV of given nutrients than original recipe
High, rich in, excellent source of	20% or more of the given nutrient per serving
Less, fewer, reduced	25% less of given nutrients than original recipe
Low, little, few, low source of	Frequent consumption of food will not exceed DV

DV, daily value.

SPECIALIZED CLAIMS

Organic

To earn the distinction of **organic** on a label, the United States Department of Agriculture (USDA) states a farmer must prove the food was produced in a way that was good for the earth. According to the USDA Web site on Organic Agriculture, organic processors preserve natural resources, use only approved materials, do not use genetically modified ingredients, and keep non-organic food separate from organic food. Each year, farmers must undergo an inspection and present an updated farm plan to prove their practices meet the organic labeling standards. Food grown on organic farms must be nurtured without synthetic pesticides, fertilizers, antibiotics, hormones, or genetic engineering (GE).

Organic food products usually cost more than non-organic counterparts because the process is more labor intensive and requires more time from field to market. There are fewer growing opportunities during a season and harvests can be smaller.

100% Natural

Sometimes, the terms 100% Natural and *organic* are mistakenly used to mean the same thing. The FDA *does not sanction* the use of 100% Natural but *does not object* as long as the product *does not contain* artificial colors, flavors, and preservatives. 100% Natural does not necessarily mean the food product is good for you because it could be loaded with sugar and fat. Empty calorie foods can be all natural but bad for your diet and contribute very little to your daily nutrient requirements. An example is when many years ago, 7-Up soda was marketed as 100% Natural, and although it may have had natural flavorings, it was not the most nutritious choice in beverage.

No Antibiotics

The FDA allows the claim of *no antibiotics* on packages of meat, poultry, and milk if the producer provides proof the animals were raised without using antibiotics to keep them healthy while growing. Approximately 11 million kg of antibiotics are fed to US livestock each year. In a USDA-funded study conducted at the University of Minnesota, scientists found antibiotic residue in plants that were grown using manure excreted by animals that were fed antibiotics. This means that organic farmers can only use the manure from livestock that were not fed antibiotics, adding to the reasons why organic produce costs more.

No Hormones

According to the FDA Web site on Meat and Poultry Labeling Terms, *hormones are not allowed in raising hogs or poultry.* However, this health claim *is allowed* on packages of beef. Cattle ranchers insert hormone pellets behind the ear which eventually dissolve. Dairy cows that receive hormone injections under the skin produce greater quantities of milk. However, if dairy producers provide scientific proof the animals were raised without administering hormones, they too can use the label. Food products with this label cost more than their counterparts because it takes longer to get the product to market. Hormones can cause a rapid growth cycle, which means less time between birth and slaughter, and that means feed costs are greatly reduced.

Genetically Engineered

Genetic engineering (GE) also known as genetic modification (GM) is the process of isolating a segment of an organism's DNA and deliberately inserting it into another similar organism for a more desirable outcome.[23] GE is the same concept as cross breeding animals and grafting plants for a better product. Growers of produce and ranchers of livestock have been *engineer*ing changes to their food products for thousands of years for many reasons: better flavor and texture, resistance to insect damage and disease, higher crop yield, or larger size. The most common GM crop is corn with 88% of our growing crops genetically engineered. Other GE crops include cotton, soybeans, potatoes, papaya, squash, and apples. Genetically engineered crops are also used to make other food products like HFCS, canola oil, mayonnaise, and snack foods, just to name a few. Regulated by the FDA, growers of genetically engineered crops must submit proof to the organization that all their growing practices meet food safety regulations. For more information on GMOs read: Consumer Info About Food from Genetically Engineered Plants on the FDA Web site: www.fda.gov.

COMMON MISTAKES WHEN READING LABELS

There are five common mistakes made when reading labels.

1. Not reading serving sizes.[4] A can of soup is usually two or two-and-a-half servings, so all values must be multiplied accordingly.
2. Forgetting that all label values are based on a 2,000-calorie diet. If you eat fewer or more than 2,000 calories, an adjustment must be made.
3. Thinking *reduced fat* or *reduced sodium* on the label means the food is low fat or low sodium. All it means is that the food has 25% less fat or sodium. If the amount of either was high to begin with, reducing by 25% would not make much of a difference.
4. Thinking the percentage of DV is the percentage of calories. If the DV is 20%, it means you have consumed 20% of the recommended nutrient for the day.
5. Assuming the amount of sugar on a label is all added sugar. If one of the ingredients naturally has sugar, such as an orange, the amount of sugar includes what the ingredient naturally brings to the product.

FOOD ENERGY = CALORIES

The word **kilocalorie**, shortened to kcal, is the correct way to refer to the energy produced by food and expended by our bodies, although it is more commonly referred to as *calorie*. Most food has a calorie value, or the ability to provide energy. Knowing how many calories per gram a nutrient provides is the first step in figuring nutrient (instead of doing the) calculations. The following are calorie values of three major nutrients plus alcohol:

- Carbohydrates: 4 cal/g
- Protein: 4 cal/g
- Fat: 9 cal/g
- Alcohol: 7 cal/g

CALCULATIONS

When working with numbers, you have to use similar values to multiply or divide. This means to find percentage of calories, and both numbers have to be calories. One cannot be grams and the other calories.

To compute the number of calories from grams:

1. Find the number of grams of the nutrient.
2. Multiply by 4 for carbohydrate or protein, or 9 for fat.
3. Your answer is the number of calories generated from the nutrient.

Example:

If there are 32 g of carbohydrate: 4×32 g = 128 calories.
If there are 14 g of fat: 9×14 g = 126 calories.

Fat is the primary nutrient that is restricted in daily diets, and the one that is usually factored from a label to determine if the food product is a healthy choice. To keep track of how much fat you have in your diet, computing the percentage of calories that come from fat in a food will help you decide if it is something you want to include in your meal.

1. Find the total number of calories for a serving size.
2. Find the total number of calories from fat.
3. Divide the calories from fat by the total calories and multiply by 100 to get a percentage.
4. If it is more than 30%, it is probably not a good choice.

RELATE TO PATIENTS

Reading labels is a learned skill. Teaching your patient how to read labels and how the information can work to improve the food choices can have a great impact on long-term health. The following are some suggestions when teaching your patients this important tool for food selection:

1. Suggest that they bring in labels from the following:
   a. Packages of their favorite foods
   b. Packages of similar foods for comparison
2. Calculate a healthy range for calories consumed daily, taking into consideration the following factors:
   a. Age
   b. Body size
   c. Desired weight
   d. Activity level

3. Identify the parts of the label for them:
   a. Serving size: point out that some containers have more than one serving size.
   b. Total calories per serving and those from fat.
   c. DV of nutrient values.
   d. Ingredients: instruct about hidden sugars and trans fats
   e. Footnote: values are based on a 2,000-calorie diet.
4. Explain the meaning of certain health claims.
5. Identify which nutrients are most important to your patient and explain how to obtain the percentage contained in a serving size.
6. Review common mistakes when reading labels.

CHAPTER
REVIEW

 PRACTICE FOR PATIENTS

At your patient's recare visit, *two* new root caries were discovered. As part of their treatment plan, you asked him to complete a 3-day diet diary. Assessment of his diet revealed he ate on average four bowls of instant apples and cinnamon oatmeal. You asked him to bring in the box to compare labels with whole grain Quaker oats. Here is what you found:

Ingredients of whole grain Quaker oats:
   Whole grain rolled oats

Ingredients of apples and cinnamon instant oatmeal:
   Whole grain rolled oats, sugar, dehydrated apples (treated with sodium sulfite), cinnamon, salt, calcium carbonate, natural flavors, citric acid, guar gum, oat flour, ferric phosphate, pyridoxine hydrochloride, riboflavin, vitamin A, thiamin mononitrate, folic acid, and one of the B vitamins.

1. What advice would you give to him after reading the Nutrition Facts labels?
2. Highlight the most healthy ingredients and use another color to highlight ingredients that should be avoided to reduce dental caries.

RELATE TO YOU

The following values were taken directly off food labels. Practice computing calories and amount of major nutrients:

1. If one serving of baked beans has 260 calories and the label says there are 2 g of fat per serving, how many calories are from fat?
2. If one serving of Toaster Strudel has 350 calories and 140 of those calories are from fat, what percentage of the Toaster Strudel is fat?
3. If one cup of Cranapple juice has 160 calories with 30 g of carbohydrates, what percentage of the calories are carbohydrates?
4. There are 1.5 g of protein in one serving of Campbell's beef and potato soup. The can has two servings but you eat the whole can. How many grams of protein have you consumed?
5. If one serving of turkey breast has 60 calories and the label says that there are 1.5 g of fat per serving, how many calories are from fat?
6. If one serving of turkey breast has 60 calories with 13.5 of those calories being fat, what percentage of the turkey breast is fat?
7. If one cup of Instant Breakfast has 250 calories with 30 g being carbohydrates, what percentage of the Instant Breakfast is carbohydrate?
8. Compare labels for Campbell's and Healthy Choice chicken noodle soup. Which contains the most sodium per serving?

REFERENCES

1. Porter DV, Earl RO. *Food Labeling: Toward national uniformity.* National Academy of Medicine 1992.
2. U.S. Food and Drug Administration. *Guidance for Industry: A Food Labeling Guide.* Available at: www.fda.gov. Revised January 2013
3. Duffy D. Ingredient labeling laws. *OLR Research Report.* June 2008.
4. Azman N, Sahak S. Nutritional label and consumer buying decision: a preliminary review. *Procedia Soc Behav Sci* 2014 May;130:490–498.
5. Cowburn G, Stockley L. Consumer understanding and use of nutrition labelling: a systematic review. *Public Health Nutr* 2005;8(1):21–28.
6. Zhang Y, Kantor MA, Juan W. Usage and understanding of serving size information on food labels in the United States. *Am J Health Promot* 2016;30(3):181–187.
7. Miller LM, Cassady DL. The effects of nutrition knowledge on food label use. A review of the literature. *Appetite* 2015;92:207–216.
8. Butler A. Nitrites and nitrates in the human diet: carcinogens or beneficial hypotensive agents? *J Ethnopharmacol* 2015;167:105–107.

9. Milkowski A, et al. Nutritional epidemiology in the context of nitric oxide biology: a risk-benefit evaluation for dietary nitrite and nitrate. *Nitric Oxide* 2010;22(2):110–119.

10. Hord NG, Tang Y, Bryan NS. Food sources of nitrates and nitrites: the physiologic context for potential health benefits. *Am J Clin Nutr* 2009;90:1–10.

11. White J. Straight talk about high-fructose corn syrup: what it is and what it ain't. *Am J Clin Nutr* 2008;88(6):1716S–1721S.

12. Duffey K, Popkin B. High-fructose corn syrup: is this what's for dinner? *Am J Clin Nutr* 2008;88(6):1722S–1732S.

13. DeChristopher LR, Uribarri J, Tucker KL. Intake of high fructose corn syrup sweetened soft drinks is associated with prevalent chronic bronchitis in US adults, ages 20-55. *Nutr J* 2015;14:107.

14. Singh M. Fact or fiction? The MSG Controversy. *Digital Access to Scholarship at Harvard.* 2005. Accessed September 2016.

15. Xiong J, Branigan D, Li M. Deciphering the MSG controversy. *Int J Clin Exp Med* 2009;2(4):329–336.

16. Geha RS, et al. Review of alleged reaction to monosodium glutamate and outcome of a multicenter double-blind placebo-controlled study. *J Nutr* 2000;130(4S suppl): 1058S–1062S.

17. Walker R, Lupien J. The safety evaluation of monosodium glutamate. *J Nutr* 2000;130(4S suppl):1049S–1052S.

18. Oplatowska-Stachowiak M, Elliott CT. Food colours: existing and emerging food safety concerns. *Crit Rev Food Sci Nutr* April;2015:0

19. Schab DW, Trinh NT. Do artificial food colors promote hyperactivity in children with hyperactive syndromes: a meta-analysis of double-blind placebo-controlled trials. *J Dev Behav Pediatr* 2004;25(6):423–434.

20. Weiss B. Synthetic food colors and neurobehavioral hazards: the view from environmental health research. *Environ Health Perspect* 2012;120(1):1–5.

21. Arnold LE, Lofthouse N, Hurt E. Artificial food colors and attention-deficit/hyperactivity symptoms: conclusions to dye for. *Neurotherapeutics* 2012;9(3):599–609.

22. Kleinman RE, et al. A research model for investigating the effects of artificial food colorings on children with ADHD. *Pediatrics* 2011;127(6):1575–1585.

23. Evans EA, Ballen FH. *A synopsis of US Consumer Perception of Genetically Modified (Biotech) Crops.* Gainesville, FL: EDIS FE934, Food and Resource Economics Department, Florida Cooperative Extension Service, Institute of Food and Agriculture Sciences, University of Florida; 2013.

BOOKS

Stefanie Sacks. *What the Fork Are You Eating?* New York: Penguin; 2014.

OTHER READING

Landrigan P, Benbrook C. GMOs, herbicides and public health. *N Engl J Med* 2015;373: 693–695.

PART V

Food for Growth

13

Nutrient Needs for Development and Maintenance of Oral Structures

> The nitrogen in our DNA, calcium in our teeth, the iron in our blood, the carbon in our apple pies were made in the interiors of collapsing stars. We are made of starstuff.
>
> *Carl Sagan, Astronomer and Author*

Learning Objectives

- Relate how a well-formed craniofacial complex can impact future oral health
- Explain the difference between pre-eruptive and posteruptive nutrition
- Define critical period of development and explain the need for good maternal nutrition
- Give examples of oral manifestations caused by nutrient deficiencies during critical period of development
- List nutrients necessary for proper tooth calcification
- Identify the nutrient necessary for development of healthy epithelial tissue and salivary gland function
- List nutrients that assist with wound healing
- Discuss the role fluoride plays pre-eruptively and posteruptively, and explain the significance of ingestion of too much fluoride during the critical period of development

Key Terms

Craniofacial Complex
Critical Period
Dysphagia

Maternal Nutrition
Pre-eruptive
Posteruptive

319

INTRODUCTION

A well-educated, well-informed dental clinician can determine by a quick glance around the oral cavity whether a patient has been well nourished during three phases of life: fetal development, pre-eruption of permanent teeth, and posteruption of permanent teeth. The oral cavity is a treasure trove of information regarding past and present nutritional choices and habits.

The importance of the craniofacial complex cannot be overemphasized. Composed of the cranium and everything in it—dentition, oral tissues, and bones of the face—it allows us to communicate with the world. Craniofacial bones and tissue are arranged in a way that allows the body to hear, taste, speak, see, express emotions, and signals the brain when pain is felt or there is a need to act on something.[1]

Maternal nutrition should be emphasized as it plays a pre-eminent role in the future of healthy oral structures. The critical period of development is the time during which the growth environment has the greatest impact on the developing embryo.[2,3] The presence or absence of specific nutrients during fetal craniofacial development can make the difference between health and disease of soft and hard structures. In the pre-eruptive stage, mineralization of primary teeth usually begins around the 3rd month of pregnancy, a time when the woman may not even know she is pregnant. At birth, crowns of *primary* teeth are almost completely formed, and by the age of 1 year, calcification of the crowns of *permanent* teeth is complete. Well-formed, well-calcified tooth structure can reduce the incidence of dental caries later in the life.

Presence or lack of other nutrients can make the difference between high-functioning salivary glands or those that are atrophied and produce little saliva. It also can make the difference between periodontal tissues that are resistant to bacterial invasion or those that have a tendency to pocket formation.

Although we have no control over the nutrition habits of our biological mothers, posteruptively, we can learn to develop healthy nutritional habits to countereffect any deficiencies resulting from poorly formed hard and soft structures.

FOOD FOR THOUGHT WHAT TEETH CAN REVEAL

In 2012, a skeleton was discovered under a parking lot in Leicester, England. Researchers from the British Geological survey and University Leicester determined through DNA testing that it was the body of King Richard III who was the last king to die in battle: Battle of Bosworth in 1485. He was buried on the grounds of Grey Friars, a Franciscan Monastery, which was razed in 1538 and the real estate was redeveloped multiple times over the centuries. Using chemical isotope analysis of two teeth, femur, and rib, researchers determined King Richard III's diet included primarily foods considered a luxury at that time: freshwater fish, exotic birds (swan, crane, and heron), and copious amounts of wine. Isotope analysis examined amount of carbon, nitrogen, and oxygen in each bone, and the higher levels of nitrogen in the rib suggested the rich diet was eaten later in life. An important point made by the discovery and analysis is that nutrients from foods we eat are incorporated into our bodies. The dictum isn't necessarily food in and all food out. Nutrients consumed in food become for the most part a significant part of our bodies.

NUTRIENTS NEEDED TO *DEVELOP* HEALTHY ORAL STRUCTURES (PRE-ERUPTIVE)

Entering pregnancy well nourished is the first gift a mother can give her child as her state of health, while growing the fetus, can impact hard and soft oral tissue development. Deficiencies in certain vitamins and minerals can affect the quality of tooth calcification and put the child at risk for enamel hypoplasia, salivary gland atrophy, and crowded dentition.[4,5]

Most obstetricians prescribe prenatal vitamins to assure optimal prenatal nutrition, even if the diet is adequate. Prenatal vitamins differ from standard adult vitamins in that they contain more folic acid and iron. They are not meant to replace a well-chosen healthy diet but rather to supplement—just in case.[5,6]

A good prenatal vitamin should contain the following nutrients:

400 mcg of folic acid
400 IU vitamin D
200 to 300 mg calcium
70 mg vitamin C
3 mg thiamine (B_1)
2 mg riboflavin (B_2)
20 mg niacin (B_3)
6 mcg Bc
10 mcg vitamin E
10 mg zinc
17 mg iron
150 mcg iodine

Pre-eruptive Nutrient Need

Nutrient	Purpose	Deficiency
Vitamin A	Formation of mucous-secreting cells of the salivary glands and helps with the normal formation of enamel and dentin.	Abnormal formation of enamel and dentin and contributes to the formation of cleft lip and/or palate and abnormal formation of salivary glands.
Vitamin D	Aids with the calcification of all hard tissues—bone, enamel, dentin, and cementum. Contributes to developing immunity.	Causes enamel or dentin hypoplasia.
Vitamin K	Aids with blood clotting time.	Prolonged clotting time.
B complex	Builds healthy oral tissues.	Neural tube defects. (There has been much research about the relationship between lack of folic acid during fetal development and neural tube defects. Although there is evidence folic acid supplementation prevents congenital heart defects, there is still debate about its prevention of cleft lip and palates.)[7–10]
Vitamin C	Helps with formation of bone and teeth as well as formation of all connective tissues.	Irregular formation or absence of dentin.
Calcium, magnesium, phosphorus	Mineralization of enamel, cementum, and bone.	Hypocalcification of enamel.
Fluoride	Incorporates into the developing tooth structure to strengthen mineralizing tissues.[11]	Calcified structures are weak, porous, and open for attack against acid destruction. Dental fluorosis, which is manifested by intrinsic staining and appears as parchment white spots in its mildest form and dark brown porosities in its most severe form.
Iodine	Needed for the development of the brain and nervous system.	Causes stunted physical growth, deafness, and mental challenges.

Nutrient	Purpose	Deficiency
Iron	Used for synthesis of hemoglobin.	
Protein	Needed during formation of maxilla, mandible, and periodontal tissues and forms the matrix for enamel and dentin.	Deficiency slows the development of bone and tooth structure, which results in crowded and rotated teeth posteruptively. (See Figure 13-1.) Crowded and rotated teeth lend themselves to increased caries susceptibility.

Figure 13-1 Pre-eruptive protein deficiency causes narrow palate and crowding. (Photo courtesy of Bob Sconyers and Kevin Brown.)

NUTRIENTS NEEDED TO *MAINTAIN* HEALTHY ORAL STRUCTURES (POSTERUPTIVE)

Cell renewal is happening in your body as you read this. Your body's innate wisdom functions like clockwork, replacing tissue cells at a predetermined rate. There are about 75 trillion body cells, and each has its own life span. Rate of replacement can be weekly (blood and epithelial cells) or last a lifetime (brain). Continually including nutrient dense foods in the diet will keep the immune system in optimal working order, which assists the body in building healthy replacement cells and fighting off invading organisms.[12]

A *poorly* nourished body with a *poorly* functioning immune system leaves the host vulnerable to all disease processes including those that affect the oral cavity. Diseased epithelial sulci provide opportunity for invading bacteria to pass through and destroy connective tissue. Not only will a host with a poorly functioning immune system fail to fight off bacterial invaders, but healing is also delayed allowing rapid progression of periodontal disease.

Nutrient	Purpose	Deficiency
Vitamin A	Maintains epithelial tissues and keeps the salivary glands working. It also maintains the integrity of the sulcular epithelium. Assists in healthy immunity.	Causes salivary glands to atrophy, reducing the amount of saliva available to the oral cavity. Can also hyperkeratinize normally thin, mucous membranes. Periodontal tissues can appear hyperkeratinized or hyperplastic with a tendency to chronic gingivitis and pocket formation. (See Figure 13-2.)
Vitamin D	Helps repair diseased bone. Supports protective activity of immune function.	Deficiency causes osteomalacia in adults and loss of lamina dura, as seen on dental radiographs. A deficiency results in an overall lack of mineralization of bone and cementum.
Vitamin K	Aids with blood clotting time.	Deficiency causes prolonged clotting time.
Vitamin C	Helps with maintenance of healthy collagen, which includes dentin, pulp, cementum, alveolar bone, periodontal fibers, blood vessels, gingival nerves, and periodontal ligament. Maintains the integrity of blood vessels and assists with phagocytosis. Helps with iron absorption and keeping the immune system healthy.	Causes the deficiency disease of scurvy. Oral appearance of scurvy mocks advanced, acute periodontal disease. Gingival tissues appear dark red to purple, spongy, and hemorrhagic; teeth are mobile; and breath is fetid. Its diagnosis is unusual in developed countries, but it is seen on rare occasions.
B complex	Maintains healthy oral tissues. B_6, B_{12}, and folic acid support activity of immune cells	B_1 Causes deficiency disease of beriberi. Can manifest as an increase in the sensitivity of oral tissues. The tongue exhibits a burning sensation, and there is a general loss of taste. B_3 Causes the deficiency disease of pellagra. Affects the tongue causing it to be sore, red, and swollen. Pain with eating and swallowing accompanies the symptoms. B_2 Affects the tongue, causing it to be inflamed. Causes angular chelosis and a greasy, red, scaly lesion resembling a butterfly shape around the nose.

Nutrient	Purpose	Deficiency
		B_{12} Causes the deficiency disease of pernicious anemia. Tongue appears bright red, smooth, and burns. Folacin Causes burning tongue and bright red oral mucosa, angular cheilosis, gingivitis, and frequent oral lesions. (Deficiency of many B vitamins causes tongue papilla to atrophy, giving it a bright/dark red and smooth/shiny appearance. See Figure 13-3.)
Calcium, phosphorus, magnesium	Calcium and phosphorus are needed in abundance for calcification and remineralization of hard tissues and need vitamin D to help with absorption.	Could precipitate alveolar bone loss.
Copper	Works with zinc, iron, and selenium to support healthy immune function. Keeps bone, blood vessels, and nerves healthy and assists with iron absorption.	Decreased immunity.
Fluoride	Fluoride offers protective benefits against dental caries. Offsets detrimental effects to teeth with oral delivery of fluoride by using fluoridated toothpaste daily.	Detrimental if too much or too little is ingested during the critical period of development of permanent teeth (age group of 6 months to 2.5 years). Deficiency during this period can result in the teeth that are more susceptible to dental caries, and excess can result in enamel fluorosis.
Iron	Needed for synthesis of hemoglobin and to maintain healthy immune system.	Causes glossitis and **dysphagia** (difficulty swallowing). The papilla of the tongue becomes atrophied and appears shiny, smooth, and red. (See Figure 13-3.) It causes mucous membranes to appear ashen gray, as with anemia; it also can cause the occurrence of angular cheilitis.
Iodine	Needed for healthy thyroid function.	
Selenium	Works with iron, copper, and zinc to support optimal immunity. Assists with making antioxidants.	Decreased immunity.

(continued)

Nutrient	Purpose	Deficiency
Zinc	Needed for wound healing and healthy immune function.	Deficiency causes delay in wound healing and the epithelium of the tongue to thicken, which would decrease the sensation of taste.
Protein	Used to build, repair, and maintain tissues.	Deficiency slows tissue healing and causes degeneration of periodontal connective tissues (periodontal ligament, bone, and cementum).

Figure 13-2   Vitamin A deficiency causes chronic gingivitis. (Photo courtesy of Bob Sconyers and Kevin Brown.)

Figure 13-3   Iron and vitamin B deficiencies cause atrophied papillae on the tongue and angular cheilitis. (Photo courtesy of Bob Sconyers and Kevin Brown.)

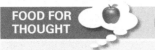

FOOD FOR THOUGHT   MORE ON FLUORIDE

Fluoride is a nutrient of utmost interest to the dental community. It is a unique nutritive substance in that it can be detrimental if too much or too little is ingested during the critical period of growth and in the age group of 6 months to 2.5 years when permanent teeth are developing. Too little fluoride during this period can result in the teeth being more susceptible to dental caries, and too much during this period can result in enamel fluorosis. There is an optimal level of ingestion that falls somewhere between too much and too little, but there are many factors to consider and various avenues of delivery that make it difficult to control: community water supply, fluoridated toothpaste, fluoride content in food and beverages, amount consumed, and stage of tooth development during consumption. Visit the American Dental Association website to learn more about their position on fluoride, recommended water levels, and supplementation schedule: http://www.ada.org/public/topics/fluoride/facts/fluoridation_facts.pdf

Pre-eruptively, it incorporates into the developing tooth structure to strengthen mineralizing tissues.[11] Posteruptively, it continues to offer protective benefits against dental caries.

If there is a **deficiency** of fluoride in the diet during tooth development:

- You can offset detrimental effects to teeth with oral delivery of fluoride by using fluoridated toothpaste daily.

If there is an **excess** in the diet:

- It has topical protective effects against dental caries, and excess is excreted.

ENVIRONMENTAL INFLUENCE ON TOOTH DEVELOPMENT

Some environmental substances, that if either ingested or inhaled during the *pre-eruptive* stages of tooth development, can have a *future* negative impact on caries resistance and tooth aesthetics.

- Research conducted on school-aged children established a direct relationship between high blood levels of lead and high incidence of dental caries. Children in urban areas had higher lead content in enamel than those living in rural areas.[13]
- Cotinine, a by-product of nicotine, has a direct relationship with increased caries in children exposed to second-hand smoke. Also, smoking

increases cavity-causing bacteria; therefore, when parents who smoke kiss their children, they transfer the bacteria from their mouths to the child's.[14,15]

- Tetracycline causes permanent intrinsic tooth staining if ingested during tooth development. Pediatricians have discouraged prescribing the medication to pregnant women and infants since 1970s, but the effects can still be seen in some older dental patients whose teeth were affected by the drug.[16]
- High levels of naturally occurring fluoride in drinking water causes unsightly dental fluorosis, a condition that manifests as permanently brown mottled enamel. Patients who drink well water should have the mineral content checked yearly to assure that the fluoride level is safe (www.cdc.gov: Community Water Fluoridation, FAQS for Dental Fluorosis).

RELATE TO PATIENT

Consider the current state of oral tissues: do oral deficiencies/lesions have a pre-eruptive or posteruptive origin? Encourage patients to visit www.choosemyplate.gov and design a diet plan that is specific for their needs

If your patient is pregnant:

- Encourage use of prenatal vitamins.
- Explain how lack of certain nutrients will impact the child's teeth and periodontal structures.
- Inform that primary teeth are developing and need adequate calcium, magnesium, and phosphorus and vitamin D to build strong and resistant enamel.
- Give examples of foods rich in calcium; magnesium; phosphorus; vitamins D, A, C; and protein.
- Inform that vitamin A is needed to build healthy periodontal tissues and salivary glands

If periodontal disease is present:

- Inform of the need to choose a well-balanced diet rich in vitamins and minerals and how nutrient-dense foods support periodontal health.
- Inform that protein, zinc, and vitamin C assist with repair of soft tissues.
- Explain how vitamin A assists with epithelial repair (cells turn over every 3 to 4 days).
- Explain the importance of keeping the immune system healthy so the "host" is resistant to periodontal disease: give examples of specific foods that contain immunity-boosting nutrients. Give examples of foods rich in immune-boosting nutrients.

If caries are present:

- Inform that calcium, magnesium, and phosphorus help with recalcification. Give examples of foods rich in these nutrients.
- Explain how vitamin A assists in production of good salivary function and the importance of ample saliva in caries prevention.
- Inform of the need to remineralize enamel with fluoride on a daily basis using fluoridated toothpaste. Explain that tea and other foods may have naturally occurring fluoride for added benefit. Give examples of cariostatic foods and detriment of frequent carbohydrate consumption (see Chapter 9).

CHAPTER
REVIEW

 PRACTICE FOR PATIENTS

The last patient of the morning, a 35-year-old female, is new to your practice and presents for initial assessment. Her last dental visit was 6 years ago, and she had a "deep cleaning" and a few fillings replaced at that time. Her chief complaint today is sore, bleeding gums.

Medical history is unremarkable.

Extraoral examination reveals the following:

- Angular cheilitis
- Few facial moles
- Infected bilateral ear piercing
- Wearing of contacts

Intraoral examination reveals the following:

- Smooth, red tongue
- Amalgam tattoo buccal of mandibular left first molar
- Aphthous ulcer on labial near mandibular central incisors

Gingival examination reveals the following:

- Generalized marginal redness
- Heavy bleeding upon probing

Dental examination reveals the following:

- Past and present dental caries
- Impacted third molars
- Maxillary and mandibular anterior crowding

Based on the initial assessment information, comment on probable:

1. Maternal nutrition during fetal development
2. Pre-eruptive nutrition
3. Posteruptive nutrition

RELATE TO YOU

Consider the state of your dentition and oral structures then answer the following:

- Do you believe enamel on your teeth was well calcified during development?
- Have you benefited from fluoride posteruptively?
- Do you manufacture adequate saliva to keep oral tissues healthy?
- Are you, as a host, well nourished?

REFERENCES

1. National Institute of Dental and Craniofacial Research. *Chapter 2: The craniofacial complex.* Accessed September 2016.
2. Farraz-Pereira KN, Toscano AE, Manhaes-de-Castro R. Effect of early undernutrition on masticatory morphophysiology: review of the literature. *Arch Oral Biol* 2013;58(11):1735–1743.
3. Touger-Decker R, Mobley C, Epstein J. Chapter 2: Pregnancy, child nutrition, and oral health. In: *Nutrition and Oral Medicine.* 2nd ed. New York: Humana Press; 2014.
4. Tanaka K, Miyake Y, Sasaki S, et al. Dairy products and calcium intake during pregnancy and dental caries in children. *Nutr J* 2012;11:33.
5. Dean SV, et al. Preconception care: nutritional risks and interventions. *Reprod Health* 2014;26:11
6. Czeizel A, Banhidy F. Vitamin supply in pregnancy for prevention of congenital birth defects. *Curr Opin Clin Nutr Metab Care* 2011;14(3):291–296.
7. Gildestad T, et al. Folic acid supplements and risk for oral clefts in the newborn: a population-based study. *Br J Nutr* 2015;114(9):1456–1463.
8. Kelly D, O'Dowd T. Use of folic acid supplements and risk of cleft lip and palate in infants: a population-based cohort study. *Br J of Gen Pract* 2012;62(600):e466–e472.

9. Bailey L, Berry R. Folic acid supplementation and the occurrence of congenital heart defects orofacial clefts, multiple births, and miscarriage. *Am J of Clin Nut* 2005;81(5);1213–1217.

10. Houston M. Taking folic acid at start of pregnancy seems to lower risk of cleft lip and palate. *Br Med J* 2012;345:e4614

11. Maturo P, Costacurta M, Cocimo R. Fluoride supplements in pregnancy, effectiveness in the prevention of dental caries in a group of children. *Oral Implantol* 2011;4(1–2): 23–27.

12. Maggini S, Wintergerst ES, Beveridge S, et al. Selected vitamins and trace elements support immune function by strengthening epithelial barriers and cellular humoral responses. *Br J Nutr* 2007;98(suppl 1):S29–S35.

13. Pradeepp K, Hegde A. Lead exposure and its relation to dental caries in children. *J Clin Pediatr Dent* 2013 Fall;38(1):71–74.

14. Huang R, Li M, Gregory R. Nicotine promotes streptococcus mutans extracellular polysaccharide synthesis, cell aggregation and overall lactate dehydrogenase activity. *Arch Oral Boil* 2015;60(8):1083–1090.

15. Tanaka K, et al. Association of prenatal exposure to maternal smoking and postnatal exposure to household smoking with dental caries in 3-year old Japanese children. *Environ Res* 2015;143(pt A):148–153.

16. Vijayasree V. Tetracycline-induced discoloration of deciduous teeth: case series. *J Int Oral Health* 2014;6(3):115–119.

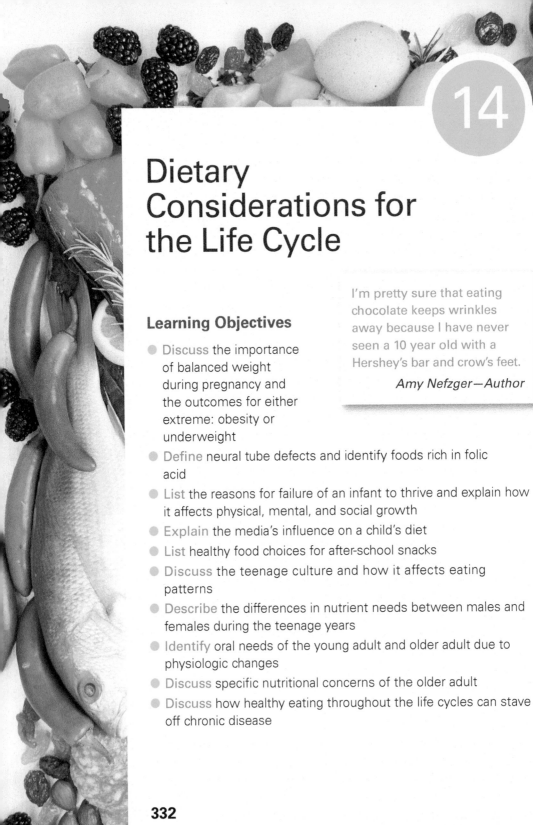

14

Dietary Considerations for the Life Cycle

> I'm pretty sure that eating chocolate keeps wrinkles away because I have never seen a 10 year old with a Hershey's bar and crow's feet.
>
> *Amy Nefzger—Author*

Learning Objectives

- Discuss the importance of balanced weight during pregnancy and the outcomes for either extreme: obesity or underweight
- Define neural tube defects and identify foods rich in folic acid
- List the reasons for failure of an infant to thrive and explain how it affects physical, mental, and social growth
- Explain the media's influence on a child's diet
- List healthy food choices for after-school snacks
- Discuss the teenage culture and how it affects eating patterns
- Describe the differences in nutrient needs between males and females during the teenage years
- Identify oral needs of the young adult and older adult due to physiologic changes
- Discuss specific nutritional concerns of the older adult
- Discuss how healthy eating throughout the life cycles can stave off chronic disease

Key Terms

Failure to Thrive
Gastroesophageal Reflux Disease
   (GERD)
Lactose Intolerant
Micronutrient Malnutrition
Pica

Pregnancy Myths
Premature
Prenatal
Protein Energy Malnutrition
Neural Tube Defect

INTRODUCTION

Good nutrition is vital for growth and health on the life continuum. Your body requires the same basic nutrients your entire life span, but the recommended *quantities* for each vary as physiologic needs change with aging.

General information on what to include in your diet to remain healthy can be found in Chapters 1 to 7. *This chapter* includes highlights of those recommendations and how the diet relates to the oral cavity at a specific point in the growth continuum.

As we age, we need less of certain nutrients and more of others. Paying attention to and feeding your body what it needs throughout the life cycle will contribute to keeping you physically and mentally fit well into advanced years.

Stages of the life cycle can be divided in many different ways depending on the topic being discussed. For the purpose of this chapter, the following stages will be used to discuss oral changes and suggested food selections for optimal oral health (see Figure 14-1):

- Prenatal—fetal
- **Infant**—birth to 12 months
- **Toddler**—1 to 4 years
- **Child**—5 to 12 years
- **Teenager**—13 to 19 years
- **Young adult**—20 to 50 years
- **Older adult**—51 years and older

PRENATAL

Ideally, a woman thinking of or wishing to conceive should prepare her body by practicing good nutrition months before actual conception. Unfortunately, many women are unaware of their pregnancy in the first few months. If a mother remains overweight or underweight throughout pregnancy, it increases her chance of medical complications. Aiming for optimal weight and health before conception, during pregnancy, and after delivery will give the child the greatest start in life.[1,2]

Figure 14-1 Stages of the human life cycle.

- Obesity increases the mother's chance of developing life-threatening diseases for herself and fetus. There is an increased incidence of hypertension, diabetes, preeclampsia, and prolonged delivery for the mother and congenital central nervous system malformations for the fetus. Obese mothers frequently have vitamin D deficiency, which means the child she delivers will be deficient in Vitamin D also.[3,4]
- A pregnant mother who is severely underweight during pregnancy can be anemic and experience early delivery of a low birth weight baby.[5,6]

Foods rich in calcium, phosphorus, and vitamin D are important in the expectant mother's diet for her growing baby's healthy tooth formation. Tooth development begins as early as the sixth week after conception, and calcification of the primary dentition begins at 4 months in utero. Formation (not calcification) of many of the permanent teeth begins by the time of birth. Table 14-1 charts tooth development for primary and permanent dentition.

A woman planning on becoming pregnant should make sure there are plenty of folate-rich foods in her diet or take a supplement containing at least 400 µg of folic acid. Visit www.cdc.gov for good advice on planning ahead. If a woman consumes adequate amounts of folic acid in her diet prior to conceiving, it can help prevent **neural tube defects**.[7-9] Below are examples of neural tube defects:

Table 14-1	Tooth Development
Tooth	**Time of Formation**
Primary incisors	4–5 months in utero
Primary molars	5–6 months in utero
Permanent central incisors	3–4 months
Permanent lateral incisors	10–12 months (3–4 months mandible)
Permanent canine	4–5 months
Permanent premolars	1.5–2.5 years
Permanent first molars	At birth
Permanent second molars	2.5–3 years

- Spina bifida: embryonic failure of fusion of one or more vertebral arches
- Malformation of the brain and skull
- Anencephaly: absence of bones of the cranial vault and cerebral and cerebellar hemispheres
- Encephalocele: gap in the skull with herniation of the brain

Following are examples of folate-rich foods:

Dark-green leafy vegetables
Citrus fruit and juices
Fortified cereal
Broccoli
Asparagus
Legumes
Beans
Peas
Nuts

There are two well-known **"pregnancy myths"** that continue to exist in spite of a body of scientific research refuting them:

1. A pregnant woman must eat enough for two
2. Mothers lose one tooth for every child

Although the mother is eating to nourish herself and the baby, the body requires only an extra 300 cal/day beginning in the 4th month until delivery. The pregnant woman should try not to waste those 300 calories on simple carbohydrates and should consider including the following:

- Extra protein for fetal tissue synthesis
- Calcium for bone mineralization

- Foods rich in all the B complex vitamins for increase in energy metabolism
- Fluids for the 25% increased need to support increase in maternal blood volume

Visit www.nlm.nih.gov; Medline Plus: Pregnancy and Nutrition for the details on "extra calories" needed during pregnancy.

Many people still believe that a mother can lose "one tooth per child" because the growing baby draws calcium from the mother's teeth. There is no scientific evidence to support this theory, but there is a correlation between motherhood and periodontal disease, due to stress. Visit www.niams.nih.gov: *Pregnancy, Breast-feeding, and Bone Health* for a detailed explanation of how the growing fetus gets enough calcium to build a strong skeleton. If a mother loses teeth during pregnancy, it is usually due to preexisting decay and corresponding pain. If the mother has sufficient calcium in her diet, there will be plenty of calcium available for the growing fetus. Early in the pregnancy, hormones cause an increase in calcium absorption and storage in the mother's body. If calcium is deficient in the diet, it may be taken from bones, where it is stored for rapid fetal bone growth during the third trimester (but not from the teeth.)

Women can experience specific food cravings during two times in their lives: perimenstrually and prenatally.[10,11] For hundreds of years, pregnant women report loss of taste for foods once relished and that other foods smell bad and are no longer desired. Pregnancy cravings and aversions due to altered sense of taste and smell are not supported by research and require further study to report a connection.[12] However, while pregnant, eating patterns may seem very different and your patient may have preferences for certain foods. For compliance with your counseling suggestions, consider pregnant patient diet nuances.

Some pregnant women report symptoms of pica—a condition where a person will crave and eat nonnutritive substances like ashes, dirt, or laundry detergent. In one recent study of pregnant women, 30% reported chewing on ice (which indicates iron deficiency), and another 30% reported consuming fruit with salt.[13,14] In another study, 57% reported eating clay and/or dirt.[15] Pica is usually an indication of iron or other mineral deficiency but is not contingent on pregnancy. Both males and females of any nondeterminate age have reported this condition.

It takes about 40 weeks for a fetus to fully develop; about 10% of births are premature with the infant being born before the 37th week of gestation. With premature birth, organs are not completely formed requiring the infant to stay in neonatal intensive care unit until it is determined that they are functioning properly. Breast-feeding is preferred for preterm babies as it is higher in protein and rich in nutrients.[16] Many premature infants will have delayed eruption patterns or teeth that erupt with enamel defects. Enamel formation begins around the 14th week in utero, and any growth disruption can alter the laying down of enamel.[17]

INFANT

Infancy is a time of tremendous growth—weight usually triples by the first birthday. There are two important facts to learn about this time period:

Intestinal absorption is inefficient.
Renal function is immature.

With this in mind, infant nutrition must be specialized. Breast milk and infant formula both contain all the nutrients necessary for this time of rapid growth and should be provided exclusively for infants aged 4 to 6 months. A 9-year study on the relationship between breast-feeding and dental caries revealed children who are breastfed for less than 6 months have a higher incidence of caries in primary teeth than infants breastfed more than 6 months.[18] Read the World Health Organization's view on Infant and Young Child Feeding at www.who.int. Here, they state a belief that over 800,000 children's lives could be saved by breast-feeding the first 2 years of life. According to WHO:

"Breast feeding improves IQ, school attendance, and is associated with higher income in adult life."

Breast milk, commercial infant formula, and cow's milk can vary in nutrient composition. Nutrient intake from cow's milk is low in vitamin E, iron, and linoleic acid and high in sodium, protein, and potassium. The higher protein content in cow's milk taxes kidneys, and iron content is low, which causes iron absorption issues later in life. Pediatricians do not recommended cow's milk until after the age of one.[19]

Solid foods should be introduced into the diet one at a time so that possible allergies can be identified. By the age of 1 year, the immature motor development allows the infant to attempt to feed himself or herself with a spoon or grab a cup, and the diet changes to include more variety.

Around the age of 6 months, the first primary teeth erupt into the oral cavity. See Figure 14-2: Calcification of primary and permanent dentition at 6 months of age. Parents should be counseled on cleaning the newly erupted teeth with soft baby toothbrushes or cloths.

Information should be provided on the dangers of putting the infant to bed with a bottle propped in their mouth. Early childhood caries (ECC) is of epidemic proportions and can be prevented by feeding the baby before putting them to bed (see Chapter 9).[20]

Sometimes, infants do not exhibit rapid growth expected in this stage of the life cycle. When infants **fail to thrive**, weight is not proportional to height, which ranks them in the bottom third or below of standard growth charts. They appear much smaller than infants of same sex and age and their physical, mental, and social skills are underdeveloped. It is well known that when a mother withholds her affection and nurturing touch, her baby will fail to thrive. But many times, the cause of failure

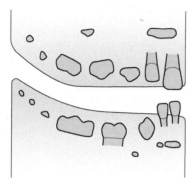

Figure 14-2 Calcification of primary and permanent dentition at 6 months of age. (*Pink* is primary, and *blue* is permanent.)

to thrive is multifactorial and combines medical, emotional, psychosocial, and nutritional issues.

Medical causes are many: chromosome abnormalities, defective organs (heart and lung) that affect oxygen flow throughout the body, thyroid or other hormone deficiency, brain damage, cerebral palsy, metabolic disorders, low birth weight, chronic infections, and parasites.[21,22]

Nutritional-related causes can be nutrient malabsorption, poor eating habits, gastric reflux, and lack of digestive enzymes. Visit www.nlm.nih.gov for more in-depth information on failure to thrive.

TODDLER

Toddlers are moving from a fluid diet to one that consists of more solid foods. This is the time for parents to set a good example, because eating habits learned as a toddler can last a lifetime.[23] Many toddlers become *picky eaters*, due to decrease in appetite since rate of growth has dropped. Appetites will be erratic, but toddlers should not be forced to eat when they are not hungry as it can lead to childhood obesity. Parents can strategically interest toddlers in food, setting a course for healthy eating throughout life.[24,25]

It is not uncommon for toddlers to request the same foods for lunch and dinner in the same day or for 5 days in a row. Because their calorie requirement has decreased, it is important for parents to guide their food choices to get the most nutrients from food. Snacking is an important part of the diet at this stage, so it is important to provide nutritious snack food versus snacks detrimental to teeth, such as acidic soda and fermentable carbohydrates.

Children have a tendency to develop eating patterns similar to their parents. If fast food is a staple in the family diet, now is the time to teach children to make healthy food choices. Milk or water instead of soda, and a salad instead of French fries will go a long way in fostering healthy eating habits in later life cycle stages. Eye–hand coordination is improving, and toddlers want to feed themselves. Mealtime can be messy, but it is important to let the child develop the movements necessary for independent feeding.

FOOD FOR THOUGHT   SENSORY SNACKS

Toddlers enjoy the sensory effects of food. Healthy snack suggestions for food to hold in hands:

- Sliced apples, pears, peaches, and grapes
- Slivers of carrots or celery with dip
- Bagels topped with peanut butter, smashed fruit, or cream cheese
- Soft taco rolls filled with leftover meat
- Cheese strips or cubes
- Yogurt pops
- Small crustless sandwiches
- Popcorn
- Peanut butter or cheese on crackers
- English muffin pizzas
- Tortillas with bean dip or hummus

Protein energy malnutrition (PEM) is one of the leading causes of childhood mortality in developing countries. Marasmus and kwashiorkor are two examples of PEM and are seen in instances where children are starving. A child suffering from marasmus appears emaciated with very thin limbs and lack of muscle definition. Kwashiorkor is similar to marasmus except the belly is distended giving the child a pot-bellied appearance. Extreme lack of protein causes an osmotic imbalance, which leads to *edema* or swelling of the gut. Both conditions develop after weaning when the child's diet does not have enough protein to meet requirements for growth.[26]

SCHOOL-AGE CHILD

The school-age child continues to form a lifelong relationship with food. Although the brain is the same size as an adult, the liver—where glucose is stored—is only about half as big. To maintain a steady blood glucose level, children need to eat more frequently—about every 4 hours. When children are not able to eat, their brains are depleted of glucose, which makes concentration in school difficult.

Food takes on social, emotional, and psychological implications. Preference for comfort foods can last a lifetime, and other food choices may take on reward significance. Rewarding a child with sweets can be a hard habit to break later in life.[27] We have all seen the entire little league ball team ordering ice cream after winning their game.

The appetite of school-age child is usually very good, with snacks making up the majority of the daily calories. Snacks provide the child with calories needed to maintain high energy levels. At this stage, children enjoy most foods, but as one can imagine, vegetables are not at the top. Vitamin/mineral supplements are very important as a backup to an inadequate diet.

Children can be ravenous after school and head toward the refrigerator as soon as they walk in the door. Stocking up on ready-to-eat *healthy* snacks is a smart fix for their hunger.

Target advertising of low-nutrient foods to young children can contribute to childhood obesity.[28] If the child self-feeds on convenience foods, their choices will be high in fat, sugar, and salt and low in fiber.[29] If the majority of a child's daily calories are from fast food, their bodies will become deficient in major nutrients.[30] Parents should discourage daylong grazing and beverage sipping and establish regular family eating times to reduce both the caries potential of the diet and excess caloric intake.[31] According to a Harvard Health Publication of the Harvard Medical School: *Distracted Eating May Add to Weight Gain*, meals should be eaten away from the TV, and electronics should not be welcome at the dinner table.[32] A study by AC Nielsen, Co., states that 66% of American families watch television as they eat dinner. For a child, this factors out to 20,000—30-second TV commercials per year. When a child who is already overweight views a food advertisement on TV, their food intake is increased by at least 100%. If parents are at all concerned about their child keeping a healthy weight, they should monitor hours spent in front of the television and make sure it is off at mealtime.

For good oral health, an increase in calcium is needed at this age to support exfoliation of primary teeth, eruption of permanent teeth, and a growth spurt in long bones. A diet rich in calcium, phosphorus, and vitamin D should be continued for healthy development of bones and teeth.

Females will require more iron as menstruation begins. This is also a time when they become aware of their body image. Parents should use caution with their own projection of body image, because this can influence how a growing young woman feels about her own body.

TEENAGERS

Teenagers make the least healthy food choices of any life cycle group. Their diets are influenced by everyone and everything: peer pressure, acne control, muscle building, and weight control. According to the Centers for Disease Control (CDC) and Prevention Nutrition and Health of Young People Web resource, youths 2 to 18 years of age consume 40% of their daily calories from six sources: soda, fruit drinks, dairy desserts, grain desserts, pizza, and whole milk, all loaded with added sugar and solid fats.

The teenage years are a period of very rapid physical growth, second only to infancy, and also of intense stress and change. Hormonal changes affect every body organ, including the brain.[33] About half of adult bone structure is deposited during adolescence and the other half over a spread of 10 years. Nutrient and energy needs are greatly accelerated. Calcium-rich diets are recommended to keep pace with bone growth.

More responsibility is added to teenagers' lives as they obtain driver's licenses, begin dating, and work part-time jobs. Their busy lifestyles can dictate when, where, and what they eat. Unfortunately, their food selection usually does not meet their increased energy needs. Teenagers' favorite foods have been identified as hamburgers, pizza, fried chicken, Tex-Mex, French fries, spaghetti, ice cream, orange juice, and soda. Sodas replace milk and fruit juice, which causes inadequate calcium intake. Teenagers today drink twice as much soda as milk, whereas the opposite was true 20 years ago.

Males drink an average of 22 ounces (almost three cans) of regular soda each day.
Females drink an average of 14 ounces (almost two cans) of regular soda each day (CDC).

Of primary concern in replacing milk with soda is that phosphoric acid in sodas can demineralize enamel and subsequently cause dental caries (see Chapter 9).

Skipping breakfast and eating outside the home are common practices. According to the American Dietetic Association, 50% teenaged males and 65% females routinely skip breakfast.[34]

This is also an age when nutrient requirements differ for males and females. Females have reached their maximum linear growth and begin to increase their percentage of body fat. This is also the time when for storing calcium for peak bone mass and to stave off osteoporosis in later years. Males, on the other hand, are building up to their maximum linear growth and begin to develop more bone and muscle mass: a 15-year-old male can consume 4,000 calories each day just to maintain his current weight. More calories should be added for the extra energy needs. Table 14-2 compares the difference in growth and nutrient needs between males and females.

Both genders place tremendous importance on body shape and image during the teenage years. Females may worry they are not thin enough and males may worry they are not as muscular as they should be. The roots of many eating disorders begin at this stage and, if allowed to progress, can be a lifelong battle to remain mentally and physically healthy (see Chapter 15).

Table 14-2	Growth and Nutrient Needs for Males and Females	
Males	**Females**
Maximum linear growth is reached by age 15	Maximum linear growth is reached by age 13
Eat twice as much as females of same age	Interested in achieving a slender figure through calorie reduction
2,500 calories for ages 11–14	2,200 calories for ages 11–18
4,000 calories for ages 15–18	Need more iron because of monthly blood loss

Orthodontics and bleaching/whitening are important to this age group as they explore ways to express their self-image. Peer pressure during the teenage years can be intense. Behaviors that may seem hip, trendy, and the norm for the peer group can lead to regret later in life. Smoking and drug abuse are of dental concern with 35% of high school students reporting some use of tobacco and 2.3 million 12 to 17 year olds abuse of at least one controlled prescription drug.[35,36] Developing an addiction to tobacco or drugs can be hard to shake and if continued into adulthood will cause detrimental oral changes.[37] Research has established a direct cause and effect relationship between smoking, drug abuse, poor oral health, and malnutrition with periodontal disease and dental caries.[38,39] The sooner substance abuse is identified, the better the chance of successful intervention.

Consider the following factors for your teenage patients' diet influence:

- Rate of very rapid growth.
- Typically consume unhealthy diet.
- Nutrient needs for males and females differ.
- Females need more calcium and iron.
- Males have an increase in all major nutrient needs.
- Food choices are influenced by peers.
- Heightened awareness of body shape.

YOUNG ADULTHOOD

Twenty-first century adults are very busy people. Lunch is usually eaten away from home, many meals are skipped, and dinner is prepared as quickly as possible.[40] It is a time of multiple stresses and multitasking: raising children, managing a home, and keeping track of both household and work schedules. In spite of all this *busyness*, nutrient needs are reduced. There is a gradual slowing of metabolic rate that goes unnoticed at first, but emerges into consciousness somewhere around the age of 45. Adults will notice they may eat less and still gain weight and squint to bring written words into focus. Decline in organ function begins around the age of 30 and progressively declines over the years.[41-44] The adult will notice subtle changes in texture, color, and amount of hair as well as a *loosening* of the skin. Internal organs are also going through gentle changes in function. All five senses begin to diminish, some more noticeably than others: ability to see and hear slowly fades and can make reading labels and recipes difficult. Inability to taste well may lead to over seasoning. The thirst mechanism begins to diminish, which can cause dehydration.[45]

Evidence of chronic diseases may start to manifest—diabetes, cardiovascular disease, and hypertension to name a few. After years of improper nutrition or perhaps bad genes, young adults can no longer say "It won't happen to me." The average age of diabetes II diagnosis is late 40s and 30 to 50 years for hypertension. According to the American Heart Association Heart Disease and Stroke Statistics, one out of every three adults has one or more types of cardiovascular disease. Visit the American Heart Association's Web site at http://www.americanheart.org/ and type in statistics 2015 in the query box for current information on incidence.

Many young adults begin to complain of digestive irregularities such as lactose intolerance and gastric reflux disease. Both disorders can take away the pleasure of eating and limit choices in food.

- **Lactose intolerant** means that small intestines no longer produce the enzyme lactase that breaks apart lactose in dairy products. If the small intestines cannot process lactose, it passes on to the colon where bacteria metabolize it for a gaseous result. Lactose intolerance may be part of the natural aging process for certain individuals, which means their diet can no longer include dairy products as a source of calcium, magnesium, and phosphorus. For others, culture and genetics dictates occurrence; Latinos, Asians and American Indians are more prone to being lactose intolerant.[46] Those who are lactose intolerant will experience nausea, bloating, and abdominal pain anywhere from 30 minutes to 2 hours after eating some form of dairy product. Total elimination of all calcium-rich dairy foods is unhealthy for the skeleton and muscle function so finding another food source or daily supplement is vital to maintain good health.

- **Gastroesophageal reflux disease (GERD)** occurs when digested food/bile is allowed to backwash into the esophagus, because of malfunctioning sphincter between the lower esophagus and upper portion of the stomach. The acidic contents irritate the lining of the esophagus causing significant burning sensation. If left untreated, it can potentially cause narrowing of the esophagus, ulcerous sores, or cancer.[47] Those who smoke, are obese, are pregnant, have a hiatal hernia, or have a medical condition that causes the stomach to empty slower (Diabetes) are prone to GERD.[48] Prescriptions and over-the-counter medications can offer some relief, and weight control and eating smaller meals reduce number of episodes. Foods that can worsen the condition are alcohol, chocolate, fatty fried food, citrus, garlic, onions, mint, tomatoes, and anything spicy.

As an older adult, oral changes will parallel overall body changes. If proper oral hygiene has not been a routine practice, devastation from periodontal disease and dental caries is present: bone loss, multiple missing, and/or restored teeth. Xerostomia becomes a concern as the aging process causes mucosa to be less lubricated, thirst mechanism diminishes, and practicing polypharmacy is common. Dry mouth equals poor saliva, which can equal dental caries in enamel and on roots. Decrease in manual dexterity and impaired senses lead to an increase in bacteria in the mouth exposed from recession. Adult patients should be reminded of the importance of thorough daily oral hygiene, including foods that stimulate saliva, and the use of home fluoride for sensitive and exposed root surfaces. When providing diet counseling, be sensitive to self-reported diet adjustments due to discomfort.

OLDER ADULT

Current medical technology and development of new medications has led to extension of life expectancy. Babies born in 1900 would live on average to 50: a baby born today can expect to live to 81 (www.nia.nih.gov).

Immunizations, good nutrition and clean drinking water contributed to reduction in disease, infection, and death at a young age. The global increase in centenarians is expected to rise 10-fold by 2050. Odds of living to 100 are 1 in 50 for females living in Sweden and Japan.

It is not uncommon for a person who has reached the age of 80 to have a biologic age of a 60-year-old, and *vice versa*. Depending on genetics, life experiences, and ability to resist disease, our bodies age at different rates.[49] Good nutrition plays an important role in keeping the body free from disease and the dentition healthy. You can read suggestions on healthy eating after 50 on the National Institute on Aging's Web site (www.nia.nih.gov). As we age, calorie intake should *decrease* to accommodate *decrease* in energy needs. Unfortunately, many find the opposite to be true as they *sit more* and *eat more*.

FOOD FOR THOUGHT   LIVING PAST 100

Scientists are tracking people from an increasing number of *Blue Zones*—areas of the world that have high concentrations of centenarians (people who live past 100 years)—to determine if there are specific or unique life habits that support longevity. The Blue Zone Project funded by National Geographic has identified nine common lifestyle characteristics among residents in the zones:

The Power Nine-Reverse Engineering Longevity:

1. They moved naturally—environments nudged them to move without thinking about it.
2. They knew their purpose—worth up to 7 years of extra life expectancy.
3. They downshifted—remembered their ancestors, prayed, and napped.
4. They ate until their stomachs were 80% full.
5. Beans, soy, and lentils are the cornerstone of their diets.
6. They all drank alcohol moderately and regularly.
7. They all belonged to a faith group—attending faith-based service is worth 4 to 14 years life expectancy.
8. They put their families first.
9. They created a social circle of supportive friends.

In his book, Healthy at 100: The Scientifically Proven Secrets of the World, John Robbins states that "although we are living longer in an industrialized world, we are getting sicker at a younger age." The Blue Zones highlighted in his book were all rural villages where the people survive on diets of whole fresh foods indigenous to the area. Village centenarians exercise daily by walking instead of driving; automobiles and public transportation are not available to them. Extended families provide emotional support, and their work is predominantly stress-free. Most Blue Zones revere their elders and allow them to work and be productive all their years. Chronic diseases are nonexistent; there are no signs of diabetes, hypertension, cancer, or autoimmune diseases. For more information on Blue Zones and to see if there is one near you, visit the *Blue Zones Projects* at www.bluezones.com. See Figure 14-3: The Power 9.

Figure 14-3   The Power 9.

The older adult group is different from those previously mentioned in that biologic age varies widely with chronological age. Many physiologic changes happen as the body ages[50]:

- Reduction in bone density increases risk for osteoporosis.
- Loss of lean body mass (sarcopenia) can lead to gain in body fat.
- Basal metabolic rates decrease.
- Energy requirement per kg of body weight is reduced.
- Loss of cognitive function.
- Deteriorating vision.
- Decrease in gastric acid production limits absorption of iron and vitamin B_{12}.
- Decrease in saliva production causes foods to stick to teeth or become difficult to swallow (dysphagia).
- Slowing of gastrointestinal motility (peristalsis) may cause constipation.
- Loss of teeth may lead to changes in ability to chew, which leads to change in food choices.
- Weight loss can lead to ill-fitting dentures.
- Decrease in sensations may lead to burning of delicate oral tissues from spicy foods.
- Decrease in taste and smell may cause someone to eat food that is spoiled.
- Decrease in immune function.

The natural aging effects on the body combined with medical conditions and medications generate negative outcomes for the state of dental health in the elderly. A decrease in cognition further compounds the lack of adequate oral care. Decrease in manual dexterity and impaired senses may result in greater plaque retention and more oral disease over time.

Many elderly patients will report polypharmacy—taking multiple medications, most of which cause salivary gland hypofunction (xerostomia). Eating with a very dry mouth becomes uncomfortable. Foods will stick to teeth and soft tissues, allowing spicy foods to burn unlubricated mucosa. Each bolus of chewed food might seem to "stick" going down. This can lead to eliminating dry, sticky, and crunchy foods and adding soft, bland items to the diet.

With a higher incidence of root caries and periodontal disease at this stage, good nutrition is very important to maintain a healthy dentition. Loss of teeth makes chewing difficult, and the elimination of crunchy foods with meals minimizes the flow of good saliva reducing good buffering effects of sodium bicarbonate, calcium, and phosphorus. Those who suffer from tooth loss or wear dentures do not have the powerful grinding force of a natural dentition and may prefer a bland soft diet to one that includes crunchy fibrous foods. The following list includes some common psychosocial reasons for poor eating habits of the elderly:

- Economics: fixed incomes mean a greater percentage of the elderly at poverty level, with failing health and high medical bills (polypharmacy can be expensive).
- Psychological: apathy and depression cause decreased appetite and loss of interest in food.

FOOD FOR THOUGHT   COMMON QUESTIONS ON AGING

Here are some common questions on the relationship between nutrition and longevity:

1. Is there such a thing as an antiaging diet? There is a body of evidence emerging that indicates low-caloric regimens and exercise may counteract aging.[51] Phytochemicals have been proven to extend life span in animals but studies on adults are lagging. Visit the National Institute on Aging (www.nih.gov) for most current research on diet and aging.[52]

2. Can modifying the diet prevent or delay onset of cognitive decline of Alzheimer's? Presently, there is no cure for the disease so focus is intense on prevention. There is consensus among researchers that nutritional excess and deficit are associated with Alzheimer's but direct cause and effect remains illusive.[53] The Mediterranean diet may have promise.[54,55] Japan and Mediterranean countries have lower incidence of the disease so examination of their diets makes sense. There is a direct correlation between disease progression and intake of certain foods: red meat, saturated fats, and alcohol. Antioxidants, fish, low glycemic vegetables and fruits, and moderate amounts of red wine have been shown to decrease oxidative stress related to the Alzheimer's disease.[56]

- Side effects of medication and social factors (inability to drive and living alone); most of their friends may have passed on.
- Eating meals out frequently: meet in groups at fast-food restaurants for socialization and to take advantage of senior discounts.

Research is ongoing to determine why the immune system slows down and weakens as we age, causing delayed response to healing and repair of the body.[57-59] To maintain healthy oral tissues throughout the life cycle, it is important to include nutrient-dense foods to prevent **micronutrient malnutrition**, which is caused from dietary deficiency of vitamins and minerals.

Indigent and older adult diets have a tendency to be deficient in quantity and variety of food. Individuals who lack good nutrients in the diet or the ability to absorb nutrients from food are more vulnerable to infections and disease processes. Micronutrients missing from a limited-variety diet include zinc, selenium, iron, calcium, antioxidants (vitamins A, C, E), vitamin D, folic acid, and vitamin B_6. Maintaining a strong immune system is important in keeping oral tissues healthy throughout the life cycle. Visit http://www.choosemyplate.gov/older-adults for suggestions on Eating Healthy after 50.

RELATE TO PATIENTS

Pregnancy

- Prenatal vitamins are a good idea, even if pregnancy is just a consideration.
- Around the fourth month of pregnancy, increase daily calorie intake by 300 but include extra protein, calcium, and other nutrient-dense foods.
- Get at least 400 μg of folate in the diet or through supplementation to reduce chance of neural tube defects.
- Increase fluid intake.
- Avoid caffeine, alcohol, tobacco, and any drug not prescribed by a physician—all pass through the placental barrier and affect the growing child.
- Minimize processed foods from the diet—many have artificial additive and it is not well known how these affect the growing child.
- Take adequate iron to avoid iron deficiency anemia.
- Assure adequate calcium, phosphorus, and vitamin D intake for good calcification of the child's teeth.

Infancy

- If formula is made with distilled or bottled water that does not contain fluoride, ask the pediatrician if fluoride supplementation is needed.
- Primary teeth are beginning to erupt into the oral cavity. Prevent ECC by not putting the infant to bed with a bottle. Fluid pools around teeth, causing dental caries.
- Use water to quench thirst and occasionally juice—acidic pH contributes to ECC.
- The crowns of permanent teeth are in a stage of calcification—adequate calcium, phosphorus, and vitamin D are required.

Toddlers

- Have suggestions for healthy snacks readily available when counseling.
- Consider level of income and availability of foods.

School-Age Child

- Avoid using food as punishment, reward, or consolation.
- There is a tendency for the school-age child to choose soda over milk—this practice should be discouraged for a healthy dentition.
- Involve children in meal preparation; they are more apt to eat what they cook.
- Encourage family mealtime with all electronics turned off.

Teenagers

- Appeal to their body image, such as muscular development.
- Praise good food choices and ignore the others.
- Encourage healthy and cariostatic snacks—cooked meats, nuts, cheese, milk, fruit, peanut butter, and popcorn.
- Young women should begin storing a surplus of calcium in their bones—counsel on incorporating more calcium in the diet.

Young Adult

- Between 30 and 40, resorption of existing bone begins to exceed formation of new bone, resulting in a net loss of bone—assure good sources of daily calcium in the diet.
- Bone loss occurs for both males and females and continues throughout the rest of life. Osteoporosis is the result of excessive bone loss.
- Encourage developing an interest in cooking family meals from fresh ingredients. Involve children in the cooking process.

Older Adult

- Increase protein and fiber intake.
- Decrease fat intake.
- Recommend a senior vitamin/mineral supplement.
- Ensure adequate calcium intake to avoid osteoporosis.
- Multiple medications can alter how the body absorbs vitamins and minerals.
- Increase low-impact exercise, which will resist bone resorption for prevention of osteoporosis.
- May avoid fluid intake due to incontinence or nocturia.

CHAPTER REVIEW

 PRACTICE FOR PATIENTS

Patient #1

1. Your patient asks your opinion on after-school snack ideas for their school-age child that will not contribute to dental caries; what suggestions would you give them?
2. Give an example of a healthy snack for each of the following age groups:
   - Toddler
   - School-age child
   - Teenager
   - Adult
   - Elderly
3. What nutrition advice would you give a pregnant patient to assure her unborn child develops strong and healthy teeth?
4. Your grandparents are invited for dinner. Create a nutrient-dense meal suitable for their age group.

Patient #2

A 77-year-old woman lives alone in a mobile home park. Medications include baby aspirin, warfarin, and Inderal. The doctor has also prescribed calcium supplements but she often can't afford them. Her fixed income allows $75/week for groceries.

1. Describe factors of consideration regarding oral health and nutrition for this patient.
2. What advice would you give her regarding nutrition and calcium? How does it benefit her health?
3. Make a list of calcium-rich foods.
4. Find a community resource that could assist with the calcium supplement.
5. What education would you provide regarding exercise?

RELATE TO YOU

Assignment #1

Watch the second episode of a four-part documentary (on Netflix) called *Cooked*. Relate to your own experience of cooking with family.

1. As a young adult, do you understand the value of preparing your own food or that which you serve your family? Name two ways it affects those who eat the home cooked meal.
2. Share a family recipe that has been handed down over generations and explain the significance of it.
3. How is a meal prepared from a treasured family recipe different from prepackaged food from the grocery store?

Assignment #2

Think back to when you were in high school and name your favorite snack; why did you choose that particular food?

1. Read the label on the package of your favorite high school snack. Is it a healthy choice? If not, why?
2. If the snack is unhealthy, what would you replace it with today that is more nutrient dense?
3. Are there any foods that you ate as a teenager that you no longer eat today?
4. How does your favorite snack today compare with your favorite food as a teenager?

Assignment #3

1. Obtain an informational brochure on the nutrient content of foods served at two of your favorite fast-food restaurants.
   a. Compare the fat, cholesterol, carbohydrates, and sodium for your favorite selections at each restaurant.
   b. Is one choice better than the other?
   c. How could you boost the nutrient content of your selection and at the same time reduce fat and sodium?
   d. What would you suggest to improve the selections of a client who frequents fast-food restaurants?

Name of Restaurant		
Nutrient	First Selection	Second Selection
Saturated fat		
Total fat		
Cholesterol		
Carbohydrate		
Sodium		

REFERENCES

1. Yan J. Maternal pre-pregnancy BMI, gestational weight gain, and infant birth weight: a within-family analysis in the United States. *Econ Hum Biol* 2015;18:1–12.
2. Deputy NP, Sharma AJ, Kim SY, et al. Prevalence and characteristics associated with gestational weight gain adequacy. *Obstet Gynecol* 2015;125(4):773–781.
3. Kennedy NJ, et al. Maternal abdominal subcutaneous fat thickness as a predictor for adverse pregnancy outcome: a longitudinal cohort study. *BJOG* 2016;123(2):225–232.
4. Lee KK, et al. Maternal obesity during pregnancy associates with premature mortality and major cardiovascular events later in life. *Hypertension* 2015;66(5):938–944.
5. Wohl ML, Gur E. Pregnancy inn anorexia nervosa—an oxymoron that has become reality. *Harefuah* 2015;154(7):456–459.
6. Hoellen F, et al. Does maternal underweight prior to conception influence pregnancy risks and outcome? *In Vivo* 2014;28(6);1165–1170.
7. Atta CA, et al. Global birth prevalence of spina bifida by folic acid fortification status: a systematic review and meta-analysis. *Am J Public Health* 2016;106:159.
8. Al Rakaf MS, et al. Patterns of folic acid use in pregnant Saudi women and prevalence of neural tube defects—results from a nested case–control study. *Prev Med Rep* 2015;2:572–576.
9. Santos LLM, et al. Prevention of neural tube defects by the fortification of flour with folic acid: a population-based retrospective study in Brazil. *Bull World Health Organ* 2016;94(1):22–29
10. Orloff NC, Hormes JM. Pickles and ice cream! Food cravings in pregnancy: hypotheses, preliminary evidence, and directions for future research. *Front Psychol* 2014;5:1076.
11. Hill AJ, Cairnduff V, McCance DR. Nutritional and clinical associations of food cravings in pregnancy. *J Hum Nutr Diet* 2016;29:281–289.
12. Cameron EL. Pregnancy and olfaction: a review. *Front Psychol* 2014;5:67.
13. Ayeta AC, Cunha AC, Heidelmann SP, et al. Nutritional and psychological factors associated with the occurrence of pica in pregnant women. *Rev Bras Ginecol Obstet* 2015;37(12):571–577.
14. Rabel A, Leitman SF, Miller JL. Ask about ice, then consider iron. *J Am Assoc Nurse Pract* 2016;28(2):116–120.
15. Santos AM, et al. Pica and eating attitudes: a study of high-risk pregnancies. *Matern Child Health J* 2016;20(3):577–582.
16. Schanler RJ, Shulman RJ, Lau C. Feeding strategies for premature infants: beneficial outcomes of feeding fortified human milk versus preterm formula. *Pediatrics* 1999;103:1150–1157 (current as of 2007).

17. Zaidi I, Thayath MN, Singh S, et al. Preterm birth: a primary etiological factor for delayed oral growth and development. *Int J Clin Pediatr Dent* 2015;8(3):215–219.
18. Hong L, et al. Infant breast-feeding and childhood caries: a nine-year study. *Pediatr Dent* 2014;36(4):342–347.
19. American Academy of Pediatrics Policy Paper. The use of whole cow's milk in infancy. *Pediatrics* 1992;89:1105–1109.
20. Colak H, Dulgergil CT, et al. Early childhood caries update: a review of causes, diagnoses, and treatments. *J Nat Sci Biol Med* 2013;4(1):29–38.
21. Wright C. Identification and management of failure to thrive: a community perspective. *Arch Dis Child* 2000;82:5–9.
22. Cole SZ, Lanham JS. Failure to thrive: an update. *Am Fam Physician* 2011;83(7):829–834.
23. Birch L, Savage J, Ventura A. Influences on the development of children's eating behaviours: from infancy to adolescence. *Can J Diet Pract Res* 2007;68(1):s1–s56.
24. Nicklaus S. The role of food experiences during early childhood in food pleasure learning. *Appetite* 2016;104:3–9.
25. Fangupo LJ, et al. Impact of an early-life intervention on the nutrition behaviors of 2-yr-old children: a randomized controlled study. *Am J Clin Nutr* 2015;102(3):704–712.
26. Lu J, et al. Using food as reinforcer to shape children's non-food behaviour: the adverse nutritional effect doubly moderated by reward sensitivity and gender. *Eat Behav* 2015;19:94–97.
27. Scheinfeld N, et al. *Protein-energy malnutrition.* 2015. Accessed on Medscape News and Perspective, September 2016.
28. Tarabashkina L, Quester P, Crouch R. Food advertising, children's food choices and obesity: interplay of cognitive defences and product evaluation: an experimental study. *Int J Obes (Lond)* 2016;40(4):581–586.
29. Ustjanuskas AE, Harris JL, Schwartz MB. Food and beverage advertising on children's websites. *Pediatr Obes* 2014;9(5):362–372.
30. Ohri-Vachaspati P, Isgor Z, Rimkus L, et al. Child-directed marketing inside and on the exterior of fast-food restaurants. *Am J Prev Med* 2015;48(1):22–30.
31. Park S, Li R, Birch L. Mothers' child-feeding practices are associated with children's sugar-sweetened beverage intake. *J Nutr* 2015;145(4):806–812.
32. Harris J, Bargh J. The relationship between television viewing and unhealthy eating: Implications for children and media interventions. *Health Commun* 2009;24(7):660–673.
33. Berenbaum SA, Beltz AM, Corley R. The importance of puberty for adolescent development: conceptualization and measurement. *Adv Child Dev Behav* 2015;48:53–92.
34. Marlatt KL, Farbakhsh K, Dengel DR, et al. Breakfast and fast food consumption are associated with selected biomarkers in adolescents. *Prev Med Rep* 2015;3:49–52.
35. Ragan DT. Peer beliefs and smoking in adolescence: a longitudinal social network analysis. *Am J Drug Alcohol Abuse* 2016;42(2):222–230.
36. Awgu E, Magura S, Coryn C. Social capital, substance use disorder and depression among youths. *Am J Drug Alcohol Abuse* 2016;42(2):213–221.
37. Shetty V, et al. Dental disease patterns in methamphetamine users: findings in a large urban sample. *J Am Dent Assoc* 2015;146(12):875–885.
38. Moon JH, Lee JH, Lee JY. Subgingival microbiome in smokers and non-smokers in Korean chronic periodontitis patients. *Mol Oral Microbiol* 2015;30(3):227–241.
39. Bergstrom J. Smoking rate and periodontal disease prevalence: 40-year trends in Sweden 1970–201. *J Clin Periodontol* 2014;41(10):952–957.

40. Larson N, Neumark-Sztainer D, Laska MN, et al. Young adults and eating away from home: associations with dietary intake patterns and weight status differ by choice of restaurant. *J Am Diet Assoc* 2011;111(11):1696–1703.

41. Sehl M, Yates E. Kinetics of human aging. Rates of senescence between ages 30 and 70 years in healthy people. *J Gerontol A Biol Sci Med Sci* 2001;56(5):B198–B208.

42. Nair KS. Aging muscles. *Am J Clin Nutr* 2005;81(5):953–963.

43. Bean B. Composite study of weight of vital organs in man. *Am J Phys Anthropol* 1926;9:293–317.

44. Maninnii TM. Organ-o-penia. *J Appl Phys* 2009;106(6):1759–1760.

45. Kenney WL, Chiu P. Influence of age on thirst and fluid intake. *Med Sci Sports Exerc* 2001;33(9):1524–1532.

46. Swagerty D, Walling AD, Klein RM. Lactose intolerance. *Am Fam Physician* 2002;65(9):1845–1850.

47. Herbella FA. Pratti MG. Gastroesophageal reflux disease: from pathophysiology to treatment. *World J Gastroenterol* 2010;16(30):3745–3749.

48. Pluta RM, et al. Gastroesophageal reflux disease. *JAMA* 2011;305(19):2024.

49. Mitniski AB, et al. Frailty, fitness and late-life mortality in relation to chronological and biological age. *BMC Geriatr* 2002;2:1.

50. Culross B. *Nutrition: meeting the needs of the elderly*. Gerontology Update. Aug/Sept 2008;7. ARN Network.

51. deCabo R, et al. The search for antiaging interventions: from elixirs to fasting regimens. *Cell* 2014;157(7):1515–1526.

52. Si H, Liu D. Dietary antiaging phytochemicals and mechanisms associated with prolonged survival. *J Nutr Biochem* 2014;25(6):581–591.

53. Guftafson DR, et al. New perspectives on Alzheimer's disease and nutrition. *J Alzheimers Dis* 2015;46(4):1111–1127.

54. Safouris A, et al. Mediterranean diet and risk of dementia. *Curr Alzheimers Res* 2015;12(8):736–744.

55. Van de Rest O, et al. Dietary patterns, cognitive decline, and dementia: a systematic review. *Adv Nutr* 2015;6(2):154–168.

56. Lara HH, et al. Nutritional approaches to modulate oxidative stress that induce Alzheimer's disease. Nutritional approaches to prevent Alzheimer's disease. *Gac Med Mex* 2015;151(2):245–251.

57. Dato S, Bellizzi D, Rose G, et al. The impact of nutrients on the aging rate: a complex interaction of demographic environment and genetic factors. *Mech Ageing Dev* 2016;154:49–61.

58. Griffin SO, et al. Burden of oral disease among older adults and implications for public health priorities. *Am J Public Health* 2012;102(3):411–418.

59. Chandra RK. Nutrition and the immune system: an introduction. *Am J Clin Nutr* 1997;66(2):460S–463S.

BOOKS

Castle J, Jacobsen M. *Fearless Feeding: How to Raise Healthy Eaters from High Chair to High School*. San Francisco CA: Jossey-Bass; 2013.

Robbins J. *Healthy at 100: The Scientifically Proven Secrets of the World*. Ballantine Books; New York, 2008.

Weston Price DDS. *Nutrition and Physical Degeneration*. 8th ed. Price-Pottenger Nutrition Foundation; Lemon Grove, CA 2014.

Nutritional Counseling

Eating Disorders

Today I will not eat a thing
I will run till my legs feel the sting
I might chew and then spit
Maybe swallow a bit
This action will not a pound bring

Limerick of the day. Hmmmmm....lime-rick. Cilantro lime rice, chicken lime soup, lemon-lime icee. I'm so hungry. When is the last time I ate? I had a boiled egg (75 cal) for breakfast yesterday and ran for 30 minutes (burn = 100 cal). STOP IT! You are stronger than this. You are better than them. Thin = beautiful, fat = ugly. Do you want to be like the rest of the losers? Go get the distraction box. Put the CD in and dance to Buddy Holly. My mind just won't shut off thinking about food ☹

Learning Objectives

- List the most commonly diagnosed eating disorders
- Differentiate between anorexia nervosa and bulimia nervosa
- Explain the psychology behind binge eating
- Advise individuals with eating disorders on good dental self-care practices
- Identify physical and oral signs of eating disorders
- Discuss the etiology of eating disorders
- Understand what constitutes the best dental treatment plan to repair oral destruction
- Use effective communication techniques when treating individuals with eating disorders

Key Terms

Anorexia Athletica
Anorexia Nervosa

Binge Eating Disorder (BED)
Body Dysmorphic Disorder

Bulimia Nervosa
Disordered Eating
Diabulimia
Emotional Triggers
Lanugo

Orthorexia Nervosa
Perimolysis
Pica
Purging
Russell's Sign

INTRODUCTION

An eating disorder is the pink elephant in the room anytime friends and family gather to share a meal. It affects 1 in 10 so chances are someone you know and/or love is afflicted. Eating disorders are not the same as being on a diet or being careful with what you eat but rather a mental illness that must be treated. If the disease is left unchecked, it can lead to organ damage and, if severe, eventually death. Although treatment may be successful, the person who suffers may spend the rest of their lives equating food with numbers, resisting the urge to purge, or feeling guilty for eating too much. Eating disorders are not contagious like a cold or flu, nor are they temporary stages of **disordered eating**. A person with disordered eating may share some common behaviors with eating disorders, but the level and frequency are less severe. For example, someone with disordered eating may skip an occasional meal, perhaps binge when under stress, or use various purging techniques, but the behavior is not sustained and does not have serious physiologic consequences. Frequent dieting is an example of disordered eating and conscious effort may need to be employed to prevent it from morphing into a true eating disorder. See Table 15-1 Difference between a Diet and Eating Disorder.

Table 15-1	Difference between Dieting and Eating Disorders
Diet	**Anorexia**
Temporary change in eating habits	Mental illness causes change in lifestyle
Set a goal for finite amount of weight loss	Bottomless pit—continual quest to weigh less and less
Feel guilty for going off the diet but rapidly moves beyond the feeling	Chest crushing guilt leads to self-punishment for eating more than desired
Going to the gym is social and fun	Exercise used as punishment
The scale is a tool to measure progress. May measure weight once a day or a few times a week	The scale can be either friend or foe, depending on weight registering. Weighs self multiple times in a day
Exercise is moderate	Exercise is excessive and usually exceeds amount of calories taken in
Cheating is allowed occasionally	Meals are carefully planned, calories counted, and there is never any cheating

(continued)

Table 15-1	Difference between Dieting and Eating Disorders (*continued*)
Diet	Anorexia
Self-esteem is gained through multiple avenues	Self-esteem is related to ability to lose weight
Recognize what looks healthy	Unwillingness to maintain a normal healthy weight
Realistic self-image perception	Distorted perception of the body
Concerned about disease prevention	Health is not a goal nor of concern
Thoughts about dieting are momentary	Not eating disrupts life and becomes all consuming

INCIDENCE

According to the National Eating Disorders Organization (www.nationaleatingdisorders.org), the figures of those afflicted are staggering: 70 million worldwide, including 30 million in the United States. Two thirds of those afflicted in the United States are young and female in the age group of 15 to 24. The remaining third are males, children, and elderly. Numbers don't lie. This is an epidemic of global proportion and success of treatment hinges on bringing the insidious secret into the open. Healing begins when the person struggling realizes it is not a disordered eating pattern but rather an eating disorder. Once the truth is accepted, they can begin an emotionally painful healing process.

ETIOLOGY

The etiology of eating disorders is not black and white. Many factors may contribute to the start of the disorder and others will sustain it. Emotional triggers are in great abundance: fear of growing fat as a body goes through puberty, after childbirth, or menopause; loss of control over life situations like death of a loved one or drastic life changes; guilt over not being perfect; ill-defined sense of self; obsession with beautiful celebrities and the wish to emulate them; thoughts of distorted body image and preoccupation with plastic surgery; and stress and anxiety. It is also common for eating disorders to be coupled with other psychological issues like substance abuse, anxiety, and depression. A combination of biological, psychological, and social factors can contribute:

Biological

- Genetic predisposition. Studies involving twins who were raised in separate households indicate that there is a strong genetic link to eating disorders.[1]
- Studies using MRI imaging on patients with anorexia indicate change in global architecture (neural activity throughout the brain), which may be linked to abnormal representations of body size and hunger.[2]

- Dysfunction in the hormone ghrelin—found to be lower in obese subjects causing impairment in smell and increased in subjects with anorexia.[3]
- Low serotonin and dopamine levels in the binge eaters. Mounting research indicates bulimia and binge eating (both involving massive consumption of carbohydrates) may be another manifestation of depression. The brain's frantic desire to acquire sugar to release serotonin—the body's natural "feel good" drug—causes binging.[4]

Psychological

- Negative emotions influence eating patterns in all eating disorders.[5]
- High percentage of individuals with eating disorders suffer with mood and anxiety disorders.[6]
- Feelings of loneliness have a negative impact and increases chances for eating disorders.[7]
- Anger levels are higher in those with eating disorders than those without.[8]
- Low self-esteem and shame are predominant in those with eating disorders.[9]
- Individuals with eating disorders have a tendency to dislike and misperceive their body shapes.[10,11]
- Childhood sexual abuse plays a role in the emergence of eating disorders.[12,13]

Social

- Internalization of media's perception of beauty can influence eating disorders. Marketing advertisement depicts people with thin bodies enjoying life, perhaps more so than average or overweight people. As children, we are exposed to promotional campaigns and products putting preference for thin bodies over what is realistic.[14–16]
- Difficulty with family relationships may lead to eating disorders.[17,18]
- Difficulty socializing and being assertive are positively related to eating disorders.[19]
- Victims and perpetrators of bullying are at increased risk for eating disorders.[20]
- Social media has a powerful influence over youth. The Internet is saturated with diet and fitness information on websites touting *fitspiration* and *thinspiration*. Visitors to these websites are mostly young females, using content as major source for current health trends.[21]

The following are facts referenced on the website of National Association of Anorexia Nervosa and Associated Disorders (ANAD):

- 80% of American women are dissatisfied with their appearance.
- The average American woman is 5 ft 4 in. tall and weighs 140 lb. Compare that to the average American model, who is 5 ft 11 in. tall and weighs 117 lb.
- Most fashion models are thinner than 98% of American women.
- 81% of 10-year-olds are afraid of being fat.
- 51 % of 9- and 10-year-olds feel better about themselves if they are on a diet.

- 91% of college women attempt to control their weight through dieting.
- 95% of all dieters will regain their lost weight in 1 to 5 years.
- Forty billion dollars is spent on dieting and diet-related products each year.

| FOOD FOR THOUGHT | HOW TO DETERMINE IF YOU ARE AT RISK FOR AN EATING DISORDER? |

Visit the following websites for free online surveys/screenings to determine if you or someone you know have or are at risk for an eating disorder:

www.nationaleatingdisorders.org—National Eating Disorder Association
http://psychcentral.com/quizzes/eat.htm—Psyc Central's Eating Attitudes Test
http://eatingdisorder.org/eating-disorder-information/online-self-assessment/—
    Center for Eating Disorders

The SCOFF Questionnaire is frequently used by health care professionals to determine if an eating disorder exists. It was devised by Morgan, Reid, and Lacy in 1999 and is still used today.

SCOFF is an acronym that stands for Sick, Control, One stone, Fat and Food.
SCOFF questions on the survey:

- Do you make yourself **S**ick because you feel uncomfortably full?
- Do you worry that you have lost **C**ontrol over how much you eat?
- Have you recently lost more than **O**ne stone (14 lb) in a 3-month period?
- Do you believe yourself to be **F**at when others say you are too thin?
- Would you say that **F**ood dominates your life?

Honest answers to these five questions will reveal whether the disorder exists or someone is merely at risk.

MAJOR CATEGORIES

Eating disorders are listed as "mental disorders" by the National Institute of Mental Health and are included in the Diagnostic and Statistical Manual of Mental Disorders (DSM 5). Collectively, they are defined as abnormal eating patterns that ultimately affect physical or mental health. Here are the major categories:

1. Anorexia nervosa (AN)
2. Bulimia nervosa (BN)
3. Binge eating disorder (BED)
4. Other specified feeding or eating disorders (OSFED)

Even though not all those referred to specialists for assessment will score within range for eating disorders, there are many who score in subclinical ranges for AN and bulimia.[22]

ANOREXIA NERVOSA

Anorexia nervosa literally means nervous lack of appetite. It is mainly a disease that develops in young females shortly after puberty or during adolescence when the body begins to change. Its characteristic self-imposed severe caloric restriction that stimulates gross weight loss stems from a distorted attitude toward food. Anorexics appear painfully thin; yet even though they look like skin on a skeleton, some think they look fat (Figure 15-1). Others are more self-aware and know they are thin but have strong resolve to continue with weight loss. For both thought groups, food is the enemy, and creative starvation strategies are imposed. Anorexics establish distractors allowing them to redirect sensations of hunger. A few examples are dancing to music, cleaning a closet, spending time on social media including proanorexia sites, and studying in the library. Anorexics are brilliant in calculating calories in and calories out (eating/exercising). Ultimately, self-imposed starvation takes a physical toll. If left untreated, an electrolyte imbalance can cause cardiac arrest = death.[23-25] Figure 15-2 lists physiologic changes of AN.

Most anorexics are very secretive and will exhibit behaviors to conceal their starvation tactics to avoid comments or questions: denial that there is a problem, wearing clothing that makes them appear of normal weight, lying about eating habits, and avoidance of being weighed or putting rocks or other heavy items in their pockets before stepping on a scale if someone is watching. They establish rituals—mash their peas, cut everything on the plate into tiny pieces, push it around, and pile one bite under another. You will see them chewing, but some will spit the food into a napkin. They will lie and say they just ate pizza with a friend or say they are busy when invited to a restaurant. (If you didn't see it, it didn't happen.)

Proanorexic websites exist to support anorexics in food restriction efforts, thus preventing them from talking about their disorder with family and professionals who can actually help.[26]

FOOD FOR THOUGHT   EATING DISORDER WEBSITES

For a glimpse into the mind of an anorexic or bulimic, Google pro ana for a list of websites created by individuals with and for eating disorders. You will find blogs, recipes, pictures, YouTube videos, and a lot of other information in support of eating disorders. Visit www.community.livejournal.com/proanorexia to read live-time comments of anorexics and bulimics.

Figure 15-1   Distorted Vision of an Anorexic.

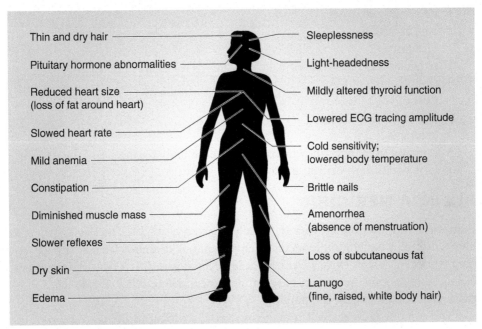

Thin and dry hair

Pituitary hormone abnormalities

Reduced heart size
(loss of fat around heart)

Slowed heart rate

Mild anemia

Constipation

Diminished muscle mass

Slower reflexes

Dry skin

Edema

Sleeplessness

Light-headedness

Mildly altered thyroid function

Lowered ECG tracing amplitude

Cold sensitivity;
lowered body temperature

Brittle nails

Amenorrhea
(absence of menstruation)

Loss of subcutaneous fat

Lanugo
(fine, raised, white body hair)

Figure 15-2 Signs and symptoms of anorexia nervosa.

Signs and Symptoms of AN

- Terrified of gaining weight
- Making excuses for not eating meals
- Cooking for others then not eating any of the food
- Overusing diuretics and laxatives—can take up to 20 times the recommended dose in a day
- Low self-esteem—may feel like they do not deserve to eat
- Excessive exercising calculated to burn more calories than consumed
- Striving for perfection
- Food rituals like cutting everything into small bites
- Pushing food around the plate
- Chewing food then spiting it out concealed in a napkin
- Drinking a large volume of water before eating
- Distorting self-image—seeing pockets of fat where there are none
- Connecting self-worth to ability to lose weight
- Very knowledgeable about caloric content of foods
- Wearing baggy clothes to cover up thinness or wearing inappropriate clothing for the season (wearing a coat in summer)
- Fatigue and muscle weakness
- Irregular or absence of menstruation (amenorrhea)

- Fainting or dizziness
- Pale complexion (pallor)
- Headaches
- Irregular heartbeats (abnormally slow means the heart muscle is changing)
- Cold hands and feet
- Loss of bone mass
- Electrolyte imbalance
- Insomnia
- Presence of **lanugo**—downy hair to keep the body warm
- Low potassium—cardiac arrest

BULIMIA NERVOSA

Individuals with **bulimia** nervosa are usually of average weight. The classic symptom of this disease is binging on food and then purging. A diagnosis is made if binging/purging occurs at least twice a week for at least 3 months. It is a cycle of overeating, feeling guilty about overeating, purging, and then feeling relief. Figure 15-3 illustrates the cycle of binging and purging.

The amount of food used to binge can vary according to the perception of the person who suffers from this disorder. For some, eating one cookie may be binging, and for others, it may be eating two whole packages of cookies, a whole pizza, and a half-gallon of ice cream in one sitting. **Purging** is not only vomiting but also can be use of laxatives and/or enemas, excessive exercising, fasting, and use of diuretics and/or diet pills. Vomiting with the help of the first two fingers down the throat is the most reported means of purging. Many times, a callous will develop on the fingers used to help purge as they rub against the central incisors. This is called **Russell's sign** after British psychiatrist Gerald Russell who first defined callused knuckles as a sign of purging. Oral effects of purging are erosion on lingual of maxillary anterior teeth

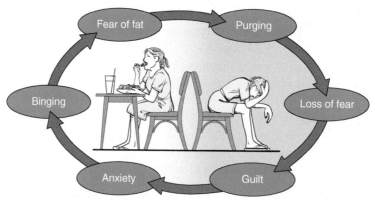

Figure 15-3 Binging and purging cycle.

A   **B**

Figure 15-4 **A:** Enamel erosion on lingual of maxillary anteriors. **B:** Enamel erosion of lingual of maxillary posteriors. (Photos courtesy of Dr. Richard Foster, Jamestown, NC.)

(enamel is smooth, thin and appears darker than on facials) and ditched out posterior fillings (looks like an instrument gouged along the margins). See Figure 15-4A, B for examples of erosion on maxillary anterior and posterior lingual. Most bulimics are women and the disease is not checked by culture and nationality as it has made its way into homes around the world. Bulimia is common in baby-boomer females aged 35 years and older who are struggling with the pressures of a career, aging, and the narrow view of the media-hyped symbol of beauty. The disease crosses generations as children learn from mothers who struggle with self-image issues, and there is a very high incidence of bulimia among college students.[27-29]

Some precipitants of binging episodes include anxiety, stress, threat of physical harm, disruption in relationships, boredom, and societal pressure.

Signs and Symptoms of BN

- Binge eating
- Visits to bathroom immediately after eating
- Frequent vomiting
- Misuse of laxatives and diuretics
- Use of diet pills
- Fasting
- Depression
- Excessive exercising

- Avoiding restaurants and planned social meals
- Broken blood vessels in eyes
- Fatigue
- Muscle weakness
- Irregular heartbeats
- Dizziness
- Headaches
- Dehydration
- Amenorrhea
- Electrolyte imbalance and low blood pressure
- Chest pains
- Stomach ulcers and gastric ruptures during binging
- Edema in hands and feet
- Dental caries—unaesthetic appearance of teeth

According to ANRED Web site (Anorexia Nervosa and Related Eating Disorders: www.ANRED.com), 50% of people who have anorexia begin to incorporate purging into their weight-loss regime. Table 15-2 compares symptoms of AN and BN.

Table 15-2	Symptoms of Anorexia and Bulimia	
Symptom	**Anorexia**	**Bulimia**
Weight loss	×	
Weight fluctuation		×
Secretive eating		×
Binge eating		×
Fasting	×	×
Food obsession	×	
Use of laxatives	×	×
Use of diuretics	×	×
Use of diet pills	×	×
Purging		×
Heavy exercising	×	×
Wear inappropriate clothing	×	
Uncomfortable around food	×	
Frequent checking of weight	×	
Psychological depression	×	×

Table 15-2	Symptoms of Anorexia and Bulimia (*continued*)	
Symptom	**Anorexia**	**Bulimia**
Low self-esteem	×	×
Withdrawn	×	
Guilt	×	×
Perfectionistic	×	
Physical fatigue	×	×
Always cold	×	
Broken vessels		×
Swollen glands	×	×
Muscle weakness	×	×
Lanugo	×	
Amenorrhea	×	×
Menstrual irregularities	×	×
Dizziness	×	×
Fainting	×	
Dehydration	×	×
Pallor	×	
Headaches	×	×
Dry skin and brittle hair	×	
Shortness of breath	×	×
Irregular heartbeats	×	×
Constipation	×	×
Low blood pressure	×	×
High blood pressure		×
Electrolyte imbalance	×	×
Chest pains		×
Gastric problems		×
Edema	×	×
Loss of bone mass	×	
Insomnia	×	
Anemia	×	×
Low potassium	×	
Cardiac arrest	×	×
Abrasions on index and middle finger		×
Death	×	×

FOOD FOR THOUGHT PERIMOLYSIS

Perimolysis refers to decalcification of teeth from exposure to gastric acid in those with chronic vomiting. Although other health concerns may cause this to happen, it is often seen in bulimics in orthodontia. If your patient wears braces and starts to show severe weight loss, monitor for eating disorder and educate accordingly.

Psychiatry Investig 2015;12(3):411–411.

BINGE EATING DISORDER

Binge eating is the most common of all eating disorders, affecting more individuals than all the other disorders combined. There is no mistaking a binge eater. They eat a great amount of food in a short period of time, usually by themselves. They eat until they are uncomfortably full, many times when they are not even hungry, and end up feeling disgusted, depressed, and guilty for eating so much. The difference between the bulimic binging and the binge eater is that a binge eater does not purge. Excess calories consumed end up making them obese. Obesity further complicates their life by adding risk for associated diseases. According to the ANAD (www.Anad.org), female-to-male ratio is lower for males: 5 million women and 3 million men. Treatment for BED may be complicated due to comorbidity of mood and anxiety disorders.[30,31] Mindfulness-based treatment for BED has shown some success.[32,33]

Signs and Symptoms of BED

- Obesity
- Diabetes
- High blood pressure
- High cholesterol
- Osteoarthritis
- Decreased mobility
- Shortness of breath
- Heart disease
- Liver and kidney problems
- Cardiac arrest
- Death

FOOD FOR THOUGHT PICKING AND NIBBLING

"Picking and nibbling" (P&N) throughout the day are common for all three eating disorders: anorexics report P&N 34.3%, bulemics 57.6%, and binge eaters 44%. P&N are unplanned eating events and occur throughout the day. What they nibble on and how much vary by disorder, but the point is well made that regular eating patterns, breakfast, lunch, and dinner, are not well established in their lives.

Int J Eat Disord 2013;46(8).

OTHER SPECIFIED FEEDING OR EATING DISORDERS

- **Anorexia athletica:** frantic exercising and fanatic about weight and diet. Time may be taken from school or work to exercise. People with this disease are rarely satisfied with physical achievements and move from one challenge to the next.
- **Body dysmorphic disorder:** excessively concerned about appearance and magnifies flaws. People with this body dysmorphic disorder may undergo multiple unneeded plastic surgeries.
- **Orthorexia nervosa:** excessive focus on eating pure or superior food. People with orthorexia nervosa usually obsess over what to eat and where to obtain it.
- **Pica:** craving and eating nonfood items such as dirt, laundry detergent, cigarette butts, clay, chalk, paint chips, cornstarch, baking soda, coffee grounds, glue, toothpaste, and soap. Pica may accompany a developmental disorder such as autism, mental retardation, or brain injury.
- **Diabulimia:** when someone with diabetes I deliberately reduces/manipulates prescribed levels of insulin to lose weight. Increased health risks include hyperglycemia, severe dehydration, diabetic ketoacidosis, and possibly stroke, coma, and death.

TREATMENT

Current treatment strategies include medicating with antidepressants and other moderating drugs and both psychiatric and nutritional counseling. Dental restorative therapy is often part of total care. The earlier the treatment begins, the greater chance for permanent success. Advanced and persistent cases require hospitalization for 2 or 3 months, and if truly stubborn, the patient will be "tubed" with a nasogastric tube to force feed nutrients. Unfortunately, about 20% of those afflicted with eating disorders will succumb to death, making it the highest mortality rate for a mental illness (www.nationaleatingdisorders.org).

FOOS FOR THOUGHT — EATING DISORDER MORTALITY RATES

Mortality rates for those diagnosed with an eating disorder are:

- 4% for AN
- 3.9% for bulimia
- 5.2% for eating disorder not otherwise specified

There is a high suicide rate for anorexia and bulimia, more so in those exhibiting high exercise rates.[34,35]

HOW CAN YOU HELP?

First of all, understand there is tremendous shame and guilt when you have an eating disorder. If you know a friend or relative with an eating disorder, be honest and tell them of your concern in a loving and supportive way. Find a time and place to open the discussion away from the presence of food. Be gentle in your approach. Let them know of your suspicions and worry for them early on. Do not wait until the disease has wreaked havoc physically, mentally, and dentally. If they do not admit it, do not push. Just let them know you are there if they need you. Encourage them to seek professional care, but do not pressure them.

DENTAL CONSIDERATIONS

Each disorder may have distinct oral manifestations, and oral discomfort will eventually lead the patient to the dental office.[36] (See Table 15-3.) Since the dental auxiliary is the person most likely to take the medical/dental history and provide the first oral examination, he or she may also be the first to identify the disease. Dental auxiliaries usually are not regarded as people of authority or as threatening to the patient and, because of this, may be the perfect choice as confidant. Counseling and treatment for the specific eating disorder are not among the dental professional's responsibilities, but restoring oral problems and prevention of oral complications caused by the disease are both necessary and expected.[37]

Treatment for all eating disorders involves medical intervention, psychological help, and nutritional counseling. The sooner an eating disorder is diagnosed and treatment begins, the more successful the intervention. Antidepressants are usually prescribed once weight has been stabilized.

Dental care is part of the recovery program. Oral effects of gastric acids and binging on cariogenic foods are usually the impetus for a visit to the dental office. Pain from erosion, dentinal sensitivity, and caries can get intense. Comprehensive dental treatment is usually postponed until behavior is changed so that tooth damage does not continue. Choice in restorative dental treatment depends on mental health status and the severity of damage to the teeth.

- Composites, overlays, crowns, and veneers can restore the teeth, depending on the severity of erosion.
- Fluoride and sodium bicarbonate rinses can prevent further sensitivity and enamel demineralization.
- Restoring the teeth to a more aesthetic appearance helps increase self-esteem.

Table 15-3	Dental Treatment Concerns of Eating Disorders
Eating Disorder	**Dental Treatment Concerns**
Anorexia Nervosa	Anemic gingival tissues
	Appears emaciated and undernourished
	Chapped lips
	Dry brittle skin and nails
	Avoidance of eye contact
	Lanugo on the face
	Low blood pressure
	Low metabolic rate—always cold to the touch
	Orthostatic hypotension
Bulimia Nervosa	Brittle enamel
	Broken blood vessels in eyes
	Chronic sore throat
	Chapped lips
	Decalcified enamel from exposure to gastric acids (perimolysis)
	Dentinal sensitivity
	Edema in the hands and feet
	Enamel erosion—especially on maxillary lingual
	Extruded and ditched amalgam restorations
	Erythematous oral tissues and red palate
	Irregular heartbeat
	Low blood pressure
	Moderate to severe dental caries
	Oral pain
	Swollen parotid glands—"chipmunk cheeks"
	Unaesthetic appearance of teeth
	Xerostomia
Binge Eating Disorder	Decreased mobility
	High blood pressure
	High cholesterol
	High incidence of diabetes
	Shortness of breath
	Obesity

Reparative Dental Treatment

Aesthetic Restorations

- Crowns
- Composites
- Veneers

Home Care Instructions

- Wait 30 minutes after purging before brushing
- Rinse with sodium bicarbonate after purging
- Use a fluoride mouthwash before retiring for the night

Treatment for Sensitivity

- Use a toothpaste for sensitive teeth
- Use a commercially available desensitizing agent such as Protect, Seal and Protect, Duraflor, Pain-Free, etc.

RELATE TO PATIENTS

The patient usually initiates a dental visit because of dental erosion, sensitivity, or aesthetic problems. The role of dental professional in treating patients with eating disorders is as follows:

- Case finding and referring to a medical professional
- Restoring dental and oral tissues
- Prevention

It is important to realize that a patient may relapse, so establishing regular recall visits to monitor dental care may prevent further damage. When counseling patients with an eating disorder, take care in how you word instructions.[38] Their self-esteem is usually fragile, and if they perceive the visit as not going well, they will discontinue treatment. Avoid placing blame or shame and using accusatory statements. Give simple solutions to their dental problems. Express continued support, even if they have a relapse. Home care instructions should include the following:

- Rinse with water and baking soda or magnesium hydroxide after vomiting.
- Use home fluoride rinses before retiring for the night.
- Postpone toothbrushing for 30 minutes after purging—this allows saliva to remineralize enamel.
- Limit intake of acidic beverages.
- Avoid sticky, sweet foods between meals.
- Suck on sugar-free chewing gum or sugar-free hard candies (lemon balls) to stimulate saliva.

Educate about the oral effects of purging:

- Ditched amalgams
- Enamel erosion
- Sensitivity
- Irregular incisal edges
- Discolored teeth

CHAPTER
REVIEW

 PRACTICE FOR PATIENTS

A new patient presents to your office with the chief complaint of sensitive teeth. Upon close oral examination, you discover several areas of enamel erosion, especially on the lingual of maxillary anteriors. Other findings include angular cheilitis, mild generalized gingivitis, facial nevi, and two occlusal dental caries. You suspect your patient is bulimic.

1. Are all of the findings related to the eating disorder?
2. How would you manage notifying the dentist of your suspicions?
3. Write out a script of what you would say to your patient during patient education.

 RELATE TO YOU

1. Write out what you would say to a patient whom you suspect may be bulimic because of enamel erosion on the linguals of the maxillary anterior teeth and ditched posterior amalgam fillings.
2. If the client admits to bulimic purging, what would you suggest as prevention for further oral problems?
3. Research local eating disorder clinics and treatment centers. Make a notecard of addresses and phone numbers for client referral to be accessed when needed.

REFERENCES

1. Suisman J, et al. Genetic and environmental influences on thin-ideal internalization. *Int J Eat Disord* 2012;45(8):942–948.
2. Geisler D, et al. Abnormal functional global and local brain connectivity in female patients with anorexia nervosa. *J Psychiatry Neurosci* 2016;41(1):6–15.
3. Fernandez-Aranda F, et al. Smell-taste dysfunctions in extreme weight/eating conditions: analysis of hormonal and psychological interactions. *Endocrine* 2016;51(2):256–267.
4. Jimerson D, et al. Low serotonin and dopamine metabolite concentrations in cerebrospinal fluid from bulimic patients with frequent binge episodes. *Arch Gen Psychiatry* 1992; 49(2):132–138.
5. Naumann E, et al. On the role of sadness in the psychopathology of anorexia nervosa. *Psychiatry Res* 2014;215(3):711–717.
6. Meng X, D'Arcy C. Comorbidity between lifetime eating problems and mood and anxiety disorders: results from the Canadian Community Health Survey of Mental Health and Well-being. *Eur Eating Disord Rev* 2015;23(2):156–162.
7. Levine M. Loneliness and eating disorders. *J Psychol* 2012;146:243–257.
8. Saldana E, et al. Anger as comorbid factor for interpersonal problems and emotional dysregulation in patients with eating disorders. *Actas Esp Psiquiatr* 2014;42(5):228–233.
9. Kelly A, Vimalakanthan K, Carter J. Understanding the roles of self-esteem, self-compassion, and fear of self-compassion in eating disorder pathology: an examination of female students and eating disorder patients. *Eat Behav* 2014;15(3):388–391.
10. Espinoza P, Penelo E, Raich R. Disordered eating behaviors and body image in a longitudinal pilot study of adolescent girls: what happens 2 years later? *Body Image* 2010;7(1):70–73.
11. Vossbeck-Eisebusch A, et al. Overestimation of body size in eating disorders and its association to body-related avoidance behaviour. *Eat Weight Disord* 2015;20(2):173–178.
12. Molinari E. Eating disorders and sexual abuse. *Eat Weight Disord* 2001;6(2):68–80.
13. Moulding N. It wasn't about being slim: understanding eating disorders in the context of abuse. *Violence Against Women* 2015;21(12):1456–1480.
14. Rodgers R, McLean S, Paxton S. Longitudinal relationships among internalization of the media ideal, peer social comparison, and body dissatisfaction: implications for the tripartite influence model. *Dev Psychol* 2015;51(5):706–713.
15. Te'eni-Harari T, Eyal K. Liking them thin: adolescents' favorite television characters and body image. *J Health Commum* 2015;20(5):607–615.
16. Giordano S. Eating disorders and the media. *Curr Opin Psychiatry* 2015;28(6):478–482.
17. George M, Fairchild AJ, et al. Marital conflict in early childhood and adolescent disordered eating: emotional insecurity about the marital relationship as an explanatory mechanism. *Eat Behav* 2014;15(4):532–539.
18. Neumark-Sztainer D, et al. Family meals and disordered eating in adolescents: longitudinal findings from project EAT. *Arch Pediatr Adolesc Med* 2008;162(1):17–22.
19. Raykos B, et al. Interpersonal problems across restrictive and binge-purge samples: data from a community-based eating disorders clinic. *Eat Behav* 2014;15(3):449–452.
20. Copeland W, et al. Does childhood bullying predict eating disorder symptoms? A prospective, longitudinal analysis. *Int J Eat Disord* 2015;48(8):1141–1149.
21. Boepple L, Thomson J. A content analytic comparison of fitspiration and thinspiration websites. *Int J Eat Disord* 2016;49(1):98–101.
22. Touchette E, et al. Subclinical eating disorders and their comorbidity with mood and anxiety disorders in adolescent girls. *Psychiatry Res* 2011;185(1–2):185–192.

23. Nakai Y, et al. Relationship between duration of illness and cardiac autonomic nervous activity in anorexia nervosa. *Biopsychosoc Med* 2015;9:12.
24. Sidiropoulos M. Anorexia nervosa: the physiological consequences of starvation and the need for primary prevention efforts. *Mcgill J Med* 2007;10(1):20–25.
25. Westmoreland P, Krantz M, Mehler P. Medical complications of anorexia nervosa and bulimia. *Am J Med* 2016;129(1):30–37.
26. Mulveen R, Hepworth J. An interpretive phenomenological analysis of participation in a pro-anorexia internet site and its relationship with disordered eating. *J Health Psychol* 2006;11(2):283–296.
27. Elran-Barak R, et al. Anorexia nervosa, bulimia nervosa, and binge eating disorder in midlife and beyond. *J Nerv Ment Dis* 2015;203(8):583–590.
28. Walker M, et al. Facebook use and disordered eating in college-aged women. *J Adolesc Health* 2015;57(2):157–163.
29. Mangweth-Matzek B, Hoek H, Pope H. Pathologic eating and body dissatisfaction in middle-aged and older women. *Curr Opin Psychiatry* 2014;27(6):431–435.
30. Davis C. The epidemiology and genetics of binge eating disorder (BED). *CNS Spectr* 2015;20(6):522–529.
31. Schreiber L, Odlaug B, Grant J. The overlap between binge eating disorder and substance use disorders: diagnosis and neurobiology. *J Behav Addict* 2013;2(4):191–198.
32. Godfrey K, Gallo L, Afari N. Mindfulness-based interventions for binge eating: a systematic review and meta-analysis. *J Behav Med* 2015;38(2):348–362.
33. Katterman S, et al. Mindfulness meditation as an intervention for binge eating, emotional eating, and weight loss: a systematic review. *Eat Behav* 2014;15(2):197–204.
34. Kostro K, Lerman JB, Attia E. The current status of suicide and self-injury in eating disorders: a narrative review. *J Eat Disord* 2014;2:19.
35. Crow SJ, et al. Increased mortality in bulimia nervosa and other eating disorders. *Am J Psychiatry* 2009;166:1342–1346.
36. Aranha A, Eduardo C, Cordas T. Eating disorders part II: clinical strategies for dental treatment. *J Contemp Dent Pract* 2008;9(7):89–96.
37. Kavitha P, Vivek P, Hegde A. Eating disorders and their implications on oral health-role of dentists. *J Clin Pediatr Dent* 2011;36(2):155–160.
38. Hague A. Eating disorders: screening in the dental office. *J Am Dent Assoc* 2010;141(6):675–678.

WEB RESOURCES

National Association of Anorexia Nervosa and Associated Disorders www.anad.org
American Academy of Child Adolescent Psychiatry www.aacap.org
Academy for Eating Disorders www.aedweb.org
American Dietetic Association www.eatright.org
National Eating Disorders Association www.nationaleatingdisorders.org
National Institute of Mental Health www.nimh.nih.gov
The American Psychiatric Association www.psyc.org
National Eating Disorder Information Centre of Canada www.nedic.ca
National Centre for Eating Disorders in United Kingdom www.eating-disorders.org.uk
Eating Disorder Referral Information Center www.edreferral.com
Overeaters Anonymous www.overeatersanonymous.org
Boosting Body Image at Any Weight www.bodypositive.com

Nutritional Counseling

> Advice is like cooking-you should try it before you feed it to others.
>
> *Croft Pentz—Author—1001 Things Your Mother Told You*

Learning Objectives

- Understand the limitations of *dental* nutritional counseling
- Identify a patient who would benefit from nutritional counseling
- Discuss ways to incorporate nutritional counseling into a dental appointment
- Explain where nutritional counseling fits into the treatment plan
- Identify assessment findings that would indicate the need for nutritional counseling
- Choose the best diet inventory for the patient's situation
- Demonstrate nondirect counseling techniques to elicit the best compliance
- Offer well–thought-out suggestions to improve diet to keep the oral environment healthy

Key Terms

Direct Approach
Dysphagia
Nondirect Approach
Nutritional Referral
Open Body Language
24-Hour Recall

3-Day Diet Diary
7-Day Diet Diary
Nutritional Counseling
Computerized Diet
   Assessment

INTRODUCTION

"Do as I say, not as I do." Will this be your mantra when counseling patients for better nutritional habits? Aligning your own eating habits with sound nutritional practice is highly recommended before you start dispensing advice to patients. Dental hygienists and assistants occupy perceived positions of leadership, and there is no better way to build trust in patients than leading by example. People trust when they know advice is genuine. According to Robert Hurley, author of The Decision to Trust: How Leaders Can Create High Trust Companies, the following actions will create trust in patients:

1. Show that your interests are the same.
2. Demonstrate concern for others.
3. Deliver on your promises.
4. Be consistent and honest.
5. Communicate frequently, clearly, and openly.

Design counseling sessions around these five suggestions to elicit better compliance in changing poor eating habits.

The Academy of Nutrition and Dietetics recommends collaboration between dietetic and dental professionals to promote overall health as well as disease prevention and intervention. As research continues to establish solid links between oral and nutritional health, both professions must encourage their members to screen, educate, and refer to each other for total patient health.[1]

It makes perfect sense for dental hygienists and assistants to educated patients on the relationship between nutrition and a healthy mouth, but state laws and licensure regulations restrict the source of nutritional advice for *general medical* conditions to be the domain of a registered dietitian (RD). An RD can also be a registered dietician nutritionist (RDN), but use caution when selecting professionals. Anyone can self-designate as a "nutritionist," which does not require a certain level of education or regulated credentials.

Before you begin nutritional counseling in the dental office, it is wise to understand the difference between what is expected of dental professionals and what is considered beyond the scope of practice. Dental nutritional counseling's purpose is to prevent or minimize dental disease and should be the goal in discussing food and diet changes with patients. Becoming involved in a patient's weight loss or recommending a diet for a specific medical condition is beyond the scope of practice and is better left to physicians or registered dietitians (RD or RDN).[2]

What do dental patients know? Most fail to recognize the relationship that nutritional status and eating habits have with their dental health. They do not really understand that what, when, and how they eat can affect their oral health. When asked, your patient may express a vague or simplistic understanding that sugar causes cavities, but how diet relates to the health of the soft tissues and periodontium is not common knowledge. Teaching the interrelationship between diet and oral health can be as beneficial to the patient and as rewarding to the dental professional as teaching good home care.

Asking a patient to make a change in their eating habits is not as easy as it sounds. If you examine your own diet and strive for change, you can empathize with your patient's struggle. Prochaska's Transtheoretical Model of Change clearly states that each of us adopts change at our own pace, and there must be a reason and certain motivational level for the process to be successful.[3] Ascertain where your patient is on the 5-point scale (Precontemplation, Contemplation, Preparation, Action, and Maintenance) to assist you in the educational process. Knowing if your patient is thinking about changing eating habits, working on change, or have tried and given up allows you the ability to choose words that will move them to the next level. If they are contemplating a change, your words will serve as the seeds to get them started. If they admit to working on a change or have tried and given up, words of encouragement and problem solving may be just what they need to try again. Open the conversation by simply asking if they are aware of what their eating habits are doing to their teeth and oral structures.

WHO CAN BENEFIT FROM DIETARY COUNSELING?

Almost everyone can benefit from learning something new and receiving information that can help improve life. But certain groups are more at risk for nutritional deficiencies that cause or exacerbate dental disease. Knowing which groups to target can ensure that you are helping those with definite need. The following is a list of groups who can benefit from dental nutritional counseling:

- Elderly
  - The elderly are at high risk for dental caries because of salivary gland hypofunction and increased consumption of simple sugars. Buying food on a fixed income and preparing meals for one person are also complicating factors. Many are on multiple medications, which cause xerostomia and need to learn how to bring more saliva into the mouth.
- Teenagers
  - Peer pressure for females to be thin or males to be muscular can create unusual eating habits. Convenience and fast foods are staples in the teen diet, and a balance in food choices may be lacking. Fast food, snacks from vending machines, and skipping regular meals are predominant in this group.

- Single and Independents
  - People responsible only for themselves may spend little time on meal planning and preparation. Convenience takes high priority. When asked, they will say that it is not worth the effort to cook for just one. Remind them that cooking for *more* than one means they won't have to cook the next day or two. What could be easier than that?
- Adults who diet
  - Specialty diets should raise concerns. The grapefruit diet causes enamel erosion, and the Atkins diet eliminates all carbohydrates, including the healthy fiber-rich carbohydrates that are part of a balanced diet. Explaining the benefit of MyPlate's food groups, creates better awareness of the connection between a balanced diet and oral health
- Patients with change in dental health
  - New or recurrent caries can be a result of poor snack or meal choices. An increase in soda consumption and developing a new habit of sucking on hard candy can be devastating to enamel. A new diagnosis of periodontal disease is the perfect opportunity to explain how a nutrient-poor diet can exacerbate oral infection.
- Infants, toddlers, and school-aged children
  - Prevention of dental caries is of high importance in this group. Always counsel in the presence of whoever does the grocery shopping and meal preparation. Giving examples of healthy snacks versus cariogenic snacks is a must. Educating about cariostatic foods can benefit everyone in the household.

NUTRITIONAL COUNSELING AS PART OF PATIENT TREATMENT

In the Current Dental Terminology (CDT) catalog, Nutritional Counseling (code D1310) is listed under Preventive Services. Unfortunately, there is no third party compensation for this procedure. It falls into the same black hole as fluoride treatments or sealants for patients older than 14 years, which means to provide at the patient's expense. Because time equals money in the dental practice, the clinician may want to provide nutritional counseling during an appointment scheduled for another compensated procedure. Do not confuse an insurance company's lack of compensation for lack of importance. Preventive nutritional counseling is just as important during dental treatment as is reinforcing good home care.

The need for dental nutritional counseling is evaluated during the data collection phase of treatment. Procedures included in the data collection phase are as follows:

1. Medical/dental history
2. Vital signs
3. Intraoral/extraoral examination

4. Gingival examination
5. Periodontal Screening and Recording (PSR)/periodontal chart
6. Dental chart
7. Radiographs
8. Nutritional counseling

Clues to look for in the information obtained during data collection include the following:

- New or recurrent caries
- Tooth loss
- Skin lesions
- Atrophied lingual papillae
- Burning tongue
- Pale or gray mucosa
- Angular cheilitis
- Greasy scaly skin around nose
- Inadequately functioning salivary glands
- Difficulty chewing or swallowing
- Ill-fitting dentures
- Sores under appliances
- Loss of lamina dura
- Polypharmacy (multiple medications)
- Erythemic marginal and attached gingiva
- Report of dietary change without physician supervision

If any of the above positive findings are discovered during data collection, the next step would be to explain the need for nutritional counseling to patients. Give patients a reason for wanting to participate. Explaining the relationship between positive assessment findings to their diet is a great place to start. Initiating an open dialogue about food and snack selection gives the clinician insight into their eating habits. Once patients realize the connection between their diet and oral concern, their willingness for further investigation usually leads to informed consent. Patients have to be prepared and ready to make a change. Just as telling someone they need to quit smoking does not always cause the desired effect, neither will telling a patient to change their eating habits. Buy-in comes before willingness to change.

COLLECTING DIET INFORMATION

There are many well-designed nutritional counseling forms on which to collect diet information; some have different layouts, but all will get you to the same end. If your office does not have any forms or you are unhappy with the ones you have, most dental and dental hygiene schools are very willing to share what they currently use. If your school or office is open to trying new ideas, visit the website of the school of choice and navigate through the forms. You can also visit the section at the end of this book to see if the nutritional counseling forms and instructions will work for you. Complete a set on yourself first to get an idea of what you are asking of patients and how much time it takes to complete the process.

If it is determined that a patient can benefit from nutritional counseling and gives *consent* to participate, the next step is to gather information about eating habits from a diet diary. There are several types of diet diaries to choose from:

- 24-hour recall
- 3-day food record
- 7-day food diary
- Computerized diet assessment

The **24-hour recall** works best if desiring a quick inquiry of a patient's eating habits. Simply ask the patient to list all the foods consumed in a 24-hour period, including serving size and time of day consumed. Ask if it is a typical sample, and if not, ask what would make it typical. This can be accomplished while providing other treatment, while waiting for the dentist to give an examination, or after the dental charting. Although a form to record everything eaten in the course of a day is informative, quick target questions can be asked to determine the cariogenic potential of the diet if there are new carious lesions or erosion. If a patient reports sucking on breath mints or hard candy or sipping on four Diet Cokes in a day, you have probably discovered the source of new caries.

1. Do you drink either regular or diet soda or sweet tea?
2. Do you regularly drink fruit juice or sports drinks?
3. Do you suck on breath mints or hard candy?
4. Do you snack during the day, if so, how often?
5. Are the snacks usually sweet or sticky in nature?
6. Do you snack when you watch TV, play video games, and study?
7. Do you eat a lot of citrus fruits or drink citrus juices?
8. How many times a day do you brush and floss?

Use a highlighter to emphasize all sugar-laden foods eaten during meals or snacks. A second different-colored highlighter can be used to indicate foods high in saturated or trans fats. The color adds an important visual that can impact their awareness.

The **3- or 7-day diet diaries** are for a more in-depth study and should include at least 1 day of the weekend. This would require the patient to keep track of the food consumed on a daily basis. Forms should be explained and given to the patient to complete at home and returned at the end of the week. After analyzing the content, appoint the patient for a one-on-one counseling session where deficiencies can be explained and suggestions for improvements made. (See the Navigate 2 Advantage Access site for completed examples and instructions.)

The **computerized diet assessment** is more general than dental related but is good for analyzing the nutrient content of food. There are several online programs that are helpful if a particular nutrient deficiency is suspected. A good starting place is at www.choosemyplate.gov; patients can customize a diet based on age, height, weight, and activity level.

UNDERSTANDING BARRIERS TO EATING WELL

Before counseling the patient, it is best to consider their lifestyle and determine if there are any barriers to eating well. Sometimes, poor food choices are made for reasons other than lack of education. Certain lifestyle factors are beyond a patient's control, and to discount them may set both you and your patient up for failure. Be sure to inquire about daily eating patterns and ask open-ended questions about any concerns. When you have your answers, imagine yourself in their shoes, and ask what you would do to improve eating habits. Provide suggestions that you are sure will fit into their lifestyle; otherwise, you will be wasting a great opportunity to improve your patient's oral health.

- Many times, job schedules dictate odd hours of eating.
- If patients live alone, does it make sense to prepare a three-course meal?
- Income plays a huge role in where a person shops and foods they choose. They may consider organic produce and quality cuts of meat too expensive.
- Often single parents make choices as to whether they take a sick child to the doctor or dentist or buy food for the family for a week.
- Students in professional programs attend school from 9 AM to 5 PM and also try to work and study the remainder of the day.
- Convenience can be the single most important factor in choosing foods for busy families. Suggesting food choices that require time to prepare will fall on deaf ears. If they frequent fast-food restaurants, teach how to recognize and choose healthy items from the menu.
- And you can't rule out that your patient may prefer the taste of sweet or fast food to more wholesomely prepared food. Countless children have said that their mother's hamburgers taste funny compared to fast-food hamburgers.

COUNSELING TECHNIQUES

When providing one-on-one counseling, there are basically two techniques or interactions:

- The **direct approach** is when you are the dictator and the patient plays a passive role. This is the most *ineffective* method because it is human nature to put

Figure 16-1 Direct counseling approach. (Photo courtesy of Bob Sconyers, Wauchula, FL.)

up a defense when being told what to do. The directive to quit eating chocolate will fall on deaf ears every time. Figure 16-1 shows the patient in a passive role. The clinician is more like a dictator.

- With the **nondirect approach**, the patient is in control and the clinician's role is that of facilitator. This is also referred to the patient-centered technique. It demonstrates respect for what the patient already knows about his or her diet and nutrition and allows for the patient's input and personal preferences. Change is more apt to happen via this method. Figure 16-2 shows the patient actively engaged in the discussion.

Effective communication is a learned skill. The following are a few tips to make the counseling session more effective:

- Be nonjudgmental of current eating habits, likes, and dislikes.
- Let the patient know you are listening by engaging in good eye contact and nodding your head. Provide feedback as to what you understood them to say.
- Use **open body language**—no crossed arms, looking down, tapping pencils, swinging legs, or looking around.

Figure 16-2   Nondirect counseling approach. (Photo courtesy of Bob Sconyers, Wauchula, FL.)

- Offer encouragement.
- Sandwich criticism between two positive statements.
- Avoid finger pointing.
- Turn off or turn down the radio and block out external noises.

SETTING THE STAGE

Figures 16-3 shows an example of a staged counseling setting. Use both artificial and real examples of serving sizes, incorporating favorite foods that were documented on the diet diary. Be sure to display radiographs, oral photos, and oral education visual aids to help personalize and emphasize your counseling session.

It is best to counsel your patient in a place that does not invoke anxious feelings. Sitting at a table or counter is better than sitting in the treatment chair.

Seat patients at eye level and provide a surface where you can spread out their counseling forms and write, if necessary. Use the redireference card on the Navigate 2 Advantage Access site as you provide information about healthy eating, snacks, and effect of foods on the oral cavity. The following Food for Thought lists examples of visual aids.

Figure 16-3 Staging. (Photo courtesy of Bob Sconyers, Wauchula, FL.)

FOOD FOR THOUGHT   USING VISUAL AIDS

Your brain is an image processor, not a word processor.
According to Haig Kouyoumdjian, PhD, in his posting Learning Through Visuals on the Psychology Today website, July 20, 2012, effective use of visuals can decrease learning time, improve comprehension, enhance retrieval, and increase retention. Here are some examples of visuals that can enhance your diet counseling sessions:

- Laminated redireference card
- Food props that indicate appropriate serving sizes
- Empty boxes and bottles of favorite foods for reading labels
- Stuffed animal people to engage children
- Colorful Pyramid Guides to capture and keep attention focused

- Patient radiographs and completed dental and periodontal charting
- Oral hygiene aids to demonstrate proper plaque removal and interdental cleaning
- Copy of the Guidelines for Americans (or other guidelines) for reference
- Written changes patients have agreed to work on
- Written suggestions on how to make those changes

When counseling patients, there are two important considerations to keep in mind:

- If you counsel children, the parent has to be present.
- If you counsel a dependent person, the person responsible for his or her diet and preparing and serving his or her food must be present.

After the diet diary is returned and you have reviewed it, ask yourself the following relative questions:

(See expanded step-by-step suggestions on the Navigate 2 Advantage Access site).

1. Did the patient meet the serving suggestions for the food groups in MyPlate or other food guide (small or inactive people at the lower end and large or active at the upper end)?
2. Did the patient follow all points of the Dietary Guidelines chosen for them?
3. Did the patient minimize the minutes of acid attack each day?
4. Did the patient include one crunchy food per meal?
5. Did the patient include foods rich in nutrients that keep the periodontium healthy?

When diet changes are indicated

- Keep it simple.
- Make small changes.
- Offer no more than two suggestions at a time.
- Let the patient choose which two changes they want to work on.

When offering suggestions, consider the following:

- Be consistent with current food habits, cultural influences, and regional preferences.
- Consider foods in season.
- Consider cost of food and patient's ability to pay for it.
- Make suggestions for choosing healthy meals at restaurants.
- Suggest changes to reduce cariogenic potential of diet.

FOOD FOR THOUGHT — EATING NON-FOOD ITEMS

What if the patient is eating nonfood items? Recording the unusual....
Don't be surprised if strange items are listed on the diet diary.

Pica is defined in medical textbooks as the habit of eating any nonfood items. Pica is Latin for Magpie as Magpies are nondiscerning and eat anything in front of them. Examples are glass, dirt, clay, glue, balloons, cotton balls, stones, pieces of bricks, sheetrock, ashes, insects, chalk, paper, soil, hair, comet cleanser, soap, crayons, cigarette butts, and just about anything else you can think of. This disorder is more than chewing on pencils, ice, or hair. Those who suffer with this eating disorder chew, swallow, and many times digest the item, absorbing elements and chemicals into their bodies. Consuming nonfood items with no nutritive value may take the place of nutrient-based foods.

Many times, the practice begins as a toddler when everything goes into the mouth as they explore and get to know their world. Later in life, it can be a result of a mineral deficiency such as zinc, calcium, and iron. Once the deficiency is mitigated, the disorder disappears.

Pica is practiced in some cultures for medicinal purposes. An example is Nigerians who eat clay to help with diarrhea. In one study of pregnant Hispanics, it was discovered that one-third expectant mothers were eating dirt, ashes, or clay. They believed that if they didn't serve their craving for nonfood items, it would lead to miscarriage. Unless the disorder leads to poisoning or bowel obstruction, the doctor may never know.

Sometimes, pica will lead to problems with the dentition. Chewing on hard items such as stones and bricks can cause attrition and breakage of teeth. A medical referral is necessary to accompany any dental treatment plan put in place.

So will you ever see nonfood items appear on a diet diary? You just never know, and don't be surprised if you do.

Advani S, et al. Eating everything except food (PICA): a rare case report and review. J Int Soc Prev Community Dent 2014;4(1):1–4.

WHEN TO REFER

Identifying the name of a respected physician or registered dietician in your community will serve you well when it is determined that a patient's nutritional counseling needs are beyond the scope of your practice and a **nutritional referral** would be in their best interest. If possible, introduce yourself to health care providers you will be referring to and explain your goals for future referrals. Open up a discussion of how nutrition plays a specific role in oral hygiene treatment and explain that a referral will be made when you suspect a disease process (other than caries and periodontal disease) is the result of poor nutrition.

When you believe a patient could benefit from a nutritional referral to a professional, discuss oral findings and their relationship with systemic disease. Make sure the patient understands the relationship of their food choices and your concerns about their oral disease and how it contributes to other health concerns. This will lay the foundation for understanding that your referral to a doctor or nutritionist will further improve their overall well-being. The usual channel of referral is from doctor to registered nutritionist. The following list is are examples of reasons to recommend a patient visit their doctor for nutritional advice:

- Improving heart health
- Suspected diabetes
- **Dysphagia**—difficulty swallowing
- Eating disorders
- HIV/AIDS
- Malnutrition
- Osteoporosis

RELATE TO PATIENTS

1. If a specific major nutrient deficiency or excess is discovered, such as protein, carbohydrates, or fats, include the suggestions for increasing the nutrient in the patient's diet listed at the end of those respective chapters.

2. If counseling to reduce cariogenicity of the diet, suggest limiting eating events to three times a day. Reduce snacking unless required for pregnancy or a medical condition.

3. If a patient snacks, recommend fresh fruits, vegetables, popcorn, nuts, turkey slices, yogurt, or cheese strips.

4. Cariogenic foods such as retentive starches and sugary foods/liquids should be consumed with meals. If addicted to soda's caffeine, do not take away but recommend drinking with a meal.

5. When oral hygiene does not follow a meal or snack, suggest that the patient end the eating event with a dairy product, such as cheese or milk, or rinse thoroughly with water.

6. Discourage eating snacks before bed, unless followed by thorough brushing and flossing.
7. Include at least two to four servings of dairy products per day or a calcium supplement.
8. Drink water between meals (instead of soda or sweet tea) and with snacks.
9. The protein and fat in meats cannot be metabolized by oral bacteria, so they have no impact on caries risk.
10. Cheese eaten at the end of a meal prevents pH from falling into the critical range.
11. Reinforce eliminating snack foods perceived as highly retentive.
    - Cookies
    - Crackers
    - Dry cereal
    - Potato chips
    - Caramels, jelly beans, and milk chocolate deliver high levels of sugar to bacteria immediately after the foods are consumed, but only for short periods of time.
12. Educate about the rate of oral clearance, approximately 30 minutes for liquids and 60 minutes for solid.
    - Process of dilution and elimination of food debris from the oral cavity: normal salivary flow has a caries preventive effect by gradually diluting and removing carbohydrates from the mouth.
    - If meals or snacks are frequent, the calcium and phosphorus in saliva will not have a chance to remineralize the teeth between eating events (20 minutes on either side of a meal), and a net demineralization results.
13. Suggest eating foods that stimulate saliva production. Eaten with a meal, they promote the buffering of acids produced by bacteria and clear food from the oral cavity.
    - Celery, carrots, raw broccoli and cauliflower, green pepper sticks
    - Sugar-free candy and gum
    - Apples and pears
14. Inform about foods that raise the salivary pH back to basic pH 7.
    - Cheese
    - Chicken
    - Pork
    - Beef
    - Fish

- Dairy products
- Chewing gum with xylitol

15. Educate on the physical forms of carbohydrates.
    - Liquid forms: fruit juice, sports drinks, coffee and tea if sugar is added, and soft drinks are in an acidic medium, which further demineralizes teeth.
    - Softening of enamel can occur in as little as 1 hour.
    - Diet sodas lower salivary pH and can demineralize tooth surfaces, independent of bacterial acid production.

16. More suggestions:
    - Replace diet and regular sodas with tea—unsweetened is best or add artificial sweetener (or fruit juice or water, if patients do not need caffeine).
    - Increase dairy products with yogurt, milk in cereal, or cheese added to a sandwich.
    - Switch to whole grains gradually by combining breads—one piece of white, one piece of whole wheat—for a sandwich, with the white bread toward the tongue.
    - Gradually switch from whole milk to skim by drinking 2%, then 1%, then 0.5%, and finally skim milk.
    - Try mixing whole milk with 2% at first.
    - Vegetable and fruit juice is an excellent way to increase fruits and vegetables in the diet.
    - Select large pieces of fruit or take a larger portion of vegetables to increase serving size to equal to two for each eating event.
    - Try mixing white and brown rice. Start with two tablespoon of brown rice per cup of white and gradually increase the ratio until brown rice predominates.
    - Do not eliminate sweets if they are wanted; just eat them with meals.
    - Try a healthy salad with dinner for crunchy food. The fiber will go a long way.
    - Cereal is a quick way to increase grains and dairy products—and it is fortified.
    - Frozen vegetables purchased in bags (do not forget to shake) are great for microwaving.
      - Most people have a tendency to eat the same foods for days, but vegetables in bags allow you to choose something different every day.
      - Just take out what you need and put the bag back in the freezer.

CHAPTER REVIEW

 PRACTICE FOR PATIENTS

Patient Role Play

You are an 18-year-old college freshman living away from home for the first time. While home for a holiday break, you present for your 6-month recare appointment and are surprised to learn you have several areas of decalcification. Since you have never had a restoration before, this news makes you sit up and take notice. You ask a million questions about how this happened and what you can do to prevent the areas from progressing.

Clinical Concerns

- Generalized gingivitis.
- Several areas of decalcification at the gingival third on the facials of maxillary anteriors and buccals of mandibular posteriors.
- Oral hygiene is somewhat effective but is not practiced on a daily basis.

Diet Information

24-Hour diet recall reveals:

- Patient is a soda sipper.
- Meals are eaten in the campus cafeteria or occasionally a restaurant off campus.
- Diet is reasonably balanced with foods chosen from all categories on the pyramid.
- Snacks are available in vending machines, and sodas are kept in a small room refrigerator.

Counseling Advice

- Explain the relationship between decalcification and dental caries.
- Discuss drinking sodas throughout the day and their detrimental effect on teeth.
- Explain potential acid production and teach how to compute.
- What recommendations would you make to improve the nutritional value of food choices?

(For more practice scenarios, visit the Navigate 2 Advantage Access site.)

RELATE TO YOU

Complete a diet analysis on yourself using the forms provided in the form section of this book. Follow the instructions for completion, analysis, and counseling. Take the following notes in a small notepad.

- Sections that seemed confusing
- Difficulties encountered in maintaining a daily log of foods consumed
- Questions that arose as you analyzed the food diary

REFERENCES

1. Touger-Decker R, Mobley C; Academy of Nutrition and Dietetics. Position of the academy of nutrition and dietetics: oral health and nutrition. *J Acad Nutr Diet* 2013;113:693–701.
2. Harper-Mallonee L. The scope of nutritional counselling in the dental practice setting. *CDE World* 2014.
3. Prochaska JO, DiClemente CC. Transtheoretical therapy: toward a more integrative model of change. *Psychother Theory Res Pract Train* 1982;19:276–288.

17

Nutritional Considerations for Special Population Groups

> You cannot achieve environmental security and human development without addressing the basic issues of health and nutrition.
>
> *Gro Harlem Brundtland—*
> *Former Director General*
> *of the WHO*

Learning Objectives

- Identify special patient groups that may present for dental nutritional counseling
- Discuss the influence of medical, dental, and lifestyle circumstances on nutritional counseling
- Identify challenges in eating when xerostomia is present
- List foods to avoid for patients with orthodontic appliances
- Describe a diet that assists with healthy immunity
- Understand diet limitations of the homeless
- Identify oral concerns for HIV+ patients that impact eating
- Discuss interventions to make eating more palatable for patients receiving cancer therapy

Key Terms

Dental Surgeries
Developmental Disabilities
HIV/AIDS
Meth-mouth
Mucositis

Necrotizing Ulcerative
  Periodontal (NUP)
Substance Abuse
Temporomandibular Joint
  (TMJ)

INTRODUCTION

Life is rarely perfect, which means *many* dental patients will present with circumstances outside the accepted norm. Just as we do not give the same exact oral hygiene instructions to every patient in our care, we do not give the same nutritional counseling advice to each patient in need. Nutritional counseling presentations should be tailored to address specific oral concerns, assessment findings, physical and mental abilities, likes/dislikes, and lifestyle/living arrangements. Patients may require special consideration while recovering from dental surgery, dealing with a chronic disease, uncertain living situations, or recovering from a life-threatening addiction. Being aware of these nutritional challenges will help you design individualized counseling sessions that will meet your patient's needs.

As a dental health care professional, you owe it to each patient to understand them as a *whole* person. If they have a chronic disease or diagnosed disability, research the condition with a depth and breadth you would appreciate if you were the patient. Visit reliable Web sites, research respected *professional* journals, or add current books of special population groups to your personal research library. Keep a three-ring binder with indexed information on the various diseases/disorders and their oral concerns in your operatory to provide accurate nutritional advice.

WOUND HEALING CONCEPTS

In the practice of dentistry, oral wounds present themselves on a daily basis. They can be the result of a disease process, surgery, neglect, or treatment. For example, dental abscess, bone graphs, extractions, traumatic injuries avulsed teeth; gingival curettage, heavy scaling, and root smoothing can inadvertently peel the inside lining of periodontal pockets, requiring the body to generate new epithelial tissue; elective oral or periodontal surgery can leave open tooth sockets, raw denuded tissue, incisions, and other situations that require tissue and bone to heal. Whatever the reason for oral wounds, better *post*-op healing occurs when the patient is well-nourished *pre*-op and has a healthy immune system to mitigate infection and is able to repair tissue in a timely manner. Below are some facts about wound healing:

- Wound repair increases metabolic function during the healing process. Increased metabolic function requires increase of nutrient dense calories.
- Increase in body temperature (fever) also increases metabolism, which equals more calories burned; there is a 12% increase in caloric nutrient requirement for every degree of temperature elevation.
- Adequate dietary protein is needed for repairing and making new tissue. With protein deficiency, the body will draw from its own structures (muscle).
- Vitamins A and C and zinc assist with oral wound healing (www.cleveland-clinic.org).

- Vitamins D and B complex keep the immune system healthy.[1]
- Aging negatively impacts the efficiency of wound healing. Older adults heal slower and with more complications.[2]

Oral/Maxillofacial and Periodontal Surgery Patient

Dental surgeries may include tooth extraction, site biopsy, orthognathic surgery, repair of facial trauma, bone grafting, crown lengthening, dental implants, gingivoplasty, gingival tissue graft, and pocket reduction. If not for pain medication, all postoperative surgery patients would feel significant pain in the area of operation. A wound has been created and will take time to heal. One way to assure greatest success for post-op wound healing is to have the patient complete a diet inventory *prior* to his or her surgery so similar foods can be recommended during the healing process. Increased caloric intake should include nutrient dense selections. Many specialty practices will recommend some type of liquid supplementation such as Ensure or Sustacal.

Patients with healthy immune function will heal faster than those who are undernourished. Multi vitamin/mineral supplementation may be recommended to assure adequate intake of vitamins D and B complex.[3–5] Solid foods can also be eaten as long as the patient feels comfortable, but if hard to tolerate, soft foods should be eaten for 3 to 4 days until *significant* healing has occurred. The following is a list of foods to *avoid* for the first 3 to 5 days after surgery:

- Spicy foods
- Salty foods
- Crunchy or hard foods
- Excessively hot foods and beverages
- Alcoholic beverages

If oral surgery involves tooth extraction, the following additional diet recommendations should be suggested:

- Avoid smoking and sucking through a straw as this action can dislodge the blood clot, creating a painful dry socket
- Drink plenty of fluids
- Eat only soft foods during the first 12 to 24 hours
- Chew on the opposite side of the wound

Necrotizing Ulcerative Periodontal Disease

Necrotizing ulcerative periodontal (NUP) disease is a destructive infection that causes necrosis of gingival tissues accompanied by bone loss. Tissues are fiery red, bleed spontaneously, and are extremely painful. Patients will present with elevated temperatures and lymphadenopathy and report a sense of lethargy. Dental treatment consists of aggressive debridement, patient education, and nutritional counseling. The following are diet suggestions that can help the patient through the first few critical days of healing:

- Increase caloric intake for increased metabolic function to modulate body temperature and tissue repair
- Choose a liquid or soft diet for the first few days
- Avoid all spicy or irritating foods
- Choose bland foods that feel soothing, such as gelatin, ice cream, applesauce, and pudding
- Eat frequent small meals
- Drink plenty of fluids
- Take vitamin/mineral supplements as recommended by the dentist

CHEWING CONSIDERATIONS

Not everyone can say that chewing is comfortable. Tooth loss and mobility, jaw pain, and oral appliances will limit the ability to tear and grind food and can have an effect on whether one chooses nutritious foods.

New Dentures

Despite best efforts through education and improvements in dental technology, patients continue to present with missing or mobile teeth due to oral neglect. With the rising cost of dental services, some patients will opt for less expensive extraction than a more expensive root canal and crown or implant. If a healthy diet is directly related to ability to chew, then the more teeth present, the better ability to chew and better nutrition.

Chewing (grinding food) with natural teeth can deliver a force of approximately 200 lb per square inch. Dentures are only 25% as effective. The **new denture** patient has to learn to talk and chew in a new way. Teaching the patient to accept limitations of new dentures requires an adjustment to *rules of eating*. The following is a list of suggestions that may be helpful during this time of change:

- Know that food will not taste the same—flavors are masked by the denture
- Cut solid food into small pieces
- Chew food evenly on right and left sides to prevent tipping of the denture
- Take small bites and chew slowly
- Initially, choose soft foods such as eggs, fish, cooked vegetables, and pudding

- Avoid sticky or very hard foods
- Be careful with hot food and drink as the covered palate will protect against high temperatures and the heat will not be felt until the food or drink hits the esophagus after swallowing

Temporomandibular Joint Disorder

Experiencing pain in the **temporomandibular joint (TMJ)**, one of the most frequently used and most complex joints in the body, can decrease quality of life. According to the American Dental Association, 15% of American adults experience TMJ disorder at one point in their lives with greater incidence reported in women than in men. Causes of this disorder can be from injury or trauma, tension and stress, poor tooth alignment, arthritis, and tumors. Problems with this joint can involve the muscles, ligaments, bone, and disc. Pain from this joint can be referred to the ear, face, and neck causing migraine-like headaches, earaches, and pain behind the eyes. Patients report annoying popping and clicking when opening, yawning, or chewing, and sometimes the jaw will get stuck in a certain position.

Degeneration of the joint will cause pain upon chewing. Learning to manage pain while eating is important as the patient collaborates with the dental professional for permanent relief. The following are helpful suggestions that can be made to alleviate pain while chewing:

- Avoid foods that require opening wide. Chewing ability is limited to how wide the mouth can open. Some patients will try to compress foods that are stacked higher than they can open.
- If the smallest movements during chewing are painful, liquid supplements offer all needed nutrients and calories.
- A soft diet is best with eating events divided into several small meals a day to limit amount of chewing time.

Orthodontic Appliances

The main concern about diet and **orthodontics** is that some foods will displace the brackets, loosen cement under bands, and bend the ligature wire. Plaque accumulates around appliances and takes conscious manipulation of cleaning aids to remove. If the patient has frequent eating episodes of carbohydrates, there is a greater opportunity for bacterial plaque to produce acid resulting in enamel demineralization. The patient should be instructed to avoid eating simple carbohydrates and hard or sticky foods. Most foods can be eaten, if cut into bite-sized pieces. Teeth are usually sore after adjustments, and soft foods are recommended. Plan ahead for adjustment days by preparing snacks and meals of soft consistency. Examples of foods to *avoid* are as follows:

- Popcorn (especially kernels), nuts, wasabi peas, and peanut brittle
- Ice
- Corn on the cob
- Sticky candy such a gummy bears, caramels, taffy, and jelly beans
- *All* soda
- Corn chips and crispy tacos
- Chewing gum
- Hard bagels, bread, rolls, or pizza crust
- Lemons
- Hard pretzels
- Whole pieces of fruit (cut into small pieces)

MEDICAL DISORDERS

Providing nutritional counseling to dental patients for improving oral health when a medical condition exists is more challenging than counseling someone with good general health. Tracking changes in a patient's medical condition by annually updating health forms can set the stage for wise nutritional counseling to prevent dental caries, maintain good periodontal health, and prevent or delay future complications. Understanding the medical disorder and related digestive or nutritional irregularities will support counseling efforts when addressing patients' diets. As a professional, staying current with the latest research regarding medical disorders is imperative and can improve counseling efforts that will lead to better compliance with nutritional suggestions.

Diabetes

There are approximately 29.1 million people in the United States diagnosed with diabetes; it is estimated that another 8.1 million have the disease but are undiagnosed.[6] Diabetes is a disease of ineffective production and/or utilization of insulin. Metabolism of glucose is altered; lipids in the body are mobilized and redistributed often in major blood vessels. An elevation in blood sugar causes inflammation in the body, taxing the immune system and eventually the cardiovascular, renal, and gastrointestinal systems. Chronic inflammation, over time, causes irreversible tissue damage and blocked blood vessels, which can lead to heart disease, stroke, kidney disease, blindness, and amputations and also lead to problems with the oral cavity. Individuals with diabetes are twice as likely to get gum disease as those without diabetes.[7-9]

There are three main types of diabetes:

- Type 1: autoimmune destruction of the cells that produce insulin in the pancreas
- Type 2: decreased cell sensitivity to insulin and/or declining production of insulin
- Gestational: glucose intolerance during pregnancy (usually temporary situation)

It is estimated that 25.9% of all adults older than 65 years are diabetic.[10] Ninety-five percent of diabetics have type 2 diabetes. With figures like these, it is probable that dental professionals will treat many diabetic patients in their practice. The following factors increase the risk of developing diabetes:

- Prolonged hyperglycemia
- Advancing age
- Obesity
- Long-term lack of physical exercise
- Hypertension
- Genetic predisposition—African American, Hispanic, or Native Americans are more prone to the disease

Microbes feed on glucose. The elevated glucose level in people with diabetes provides an ideal environment for growing bacteria and fungi. The diabetic patient is more likely to have halitosis, dental caries at the gingival third, oral candidiasis, angular cheilitis, and periodontal disease. Oral health management of diabetic clients should include the following:

- Obtaining a thorough and accurate medical history
- Inquiring about self-management of the disease:
  - Oral medications, including dosage and times
  - Eating patterns
  - Insulin injections
  - Frequency of blood glucose readings
  - Blood sugar goal range
- Education about oral manifestations of diabetes:
  - Oral burning sensation
  - Increased incidence of periodontal disease/dental caries
  - Xerostomia
- Education regarding warning signs that indicate a need to seek dental care:
  - Bleeding gums when brushing
  - Tender, red, and swollen gingiva
  - Purulent drainage between the teeth and gums
  - Loose teeth
  - Halitosis

When providing nutritional counseling in the health care setting to diabetic patients focus on the reduction of dental caries and periodontal disease. Within the scope of a dental health care worker, counseling for a diabetic should include the following:

- Sip on water or chew sugarless gum to help alleviate dry mouth and stimulate saliva flow.
- Follow a balanced diet as prescribed by the primary care practitioner (PCP), endocrinologist, or registered dietitian to ensure adequate nutrient intake.
- Include cariostatic foods as allowed in the daily diet.
- Add a multivitamin daily; if using a chewable tablet, brush afterward.
- Practice thorough, daily, plaque removal with sulcular brushing and some type of interproximal aid *twice* a day.
- Use a nonalcohol, antibacterial mouthwash daily, diluted ½ mouthwash and ½ water.

In addition, reinforce the following:

- Maintain control of goal hemoglobin A1C and daily blood glucose as set by the primary care provider.
- The importance of seeing PCP and dentist on a regular basis.
- Seek out diabetic education from a registered dietitian and/or certified diabetic educator.

Cancer

Cancer is a disease that can affect any tissue in the body causing cells to rapidly divide. The rapid generation of cells leads to the development of a tumor or mass, which creates pressure on blood vessels, nerves, crowding, and eventually destroying healthy cells surrounding the ensuing tumor or mass. It is estimated by the American Cancer Society that 1.6 million people will be diagnosed with cancer in 2016.[11]

Visit the American Cancer Society for further details on specific cancers, statistics per state, gender, and age group.[11]

Often, side effects of cancer treatment make eating difficult with loss of appetite, difficulty swallowing, mouth ulcers, nausea, constipation, and diarrhea. In addition, there may be altered taste and smell or a metallic taste in the mouth. Simply rinsing the mouth with a mixture of baking soda and water before eating may help. Also, using plastic utensils and avoiding canned foods may eliminate metallic taste.

The two most common complaints Precipitating cancer patients' dental visits are xerostomia and mouth ulcerations. Xerostomia may be a side effect of some medications used in cancer treatment or from an alteration in volume of salivary secretions, which occurs often if radiation is administered to the head and neck area. Nutritional counseling should include the following:

- Eat moist foods with extra sauce, gravy, or butter
- Chew sugar-free gum or suck on hard candies that contain xylitol
- Eat frozen fruits like berries, melon, and grapes or fruit popsicles
- Sip water throughout the day and rinse mouth often
- Avoid dry foods such as crackers, toast, and granola bars
- Cut food into small pieces

Chemotherapeutic and radiation therapies can cause painful ulcerations in the oral cavity lasting for the duration of treatment. See Food for Thought box for recommendation of mixing a soothing mouth rinse at home. Following are some helpful suggestions to offer patients in an effort to decrease pain and make eating more pleasant:

- Eat soft foods, such as pudding, applesauce, cottage cheese, mashed potatoes, scrambled eggs, cream of wheat, and gelatin.
- Puree meats and coarse vegetables such as corn or peas.
- Avoid spicy, salty, or acidic foods such as black pepper, cayenne, or salad dressing and pickles made with vinegar.
- Avoid citrus fruits and juices; choose fruit nectar as it is less acidic.
- Avoid high-fiber or crunchy foods that can scratch delicate tissues.
- Use a straw for beverages to decrease contact with inflamed mucosa.
- Consider nutritional supplements to add needed nutrients when eating food is difficult.

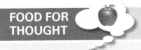 **FOOD FOR THOUGHT**   **HOME-MADE MOUTH RINSE FOR CLIENTS WITH INFLAMED MUCOSA**

Prepare the mixture prior to each use for freshness. Water should be filtered, bottled or boiled, and cooled. For the liquid antacid, use Mylanta, Maalox, or equivalent to coat the oral mucosa to protect and promote healing. When choosing a mouth wash, read the labels carefully to make sure there is no alcohol in it as alcohol will further injure the already inflamed tissues.
Combine the following ingredients using equal proportions of each item:

Size	Water	Liquid Antacid	N A Mouthwash
Small	1 teaspoon	1 teaspoon	1 teaspoon
Medium	2 teaspoons	2 teaspoons	2 teaspoons
Large	1 tablespoon	1 tablespoon	1 tablespoon

Good nutrition is imperative before, during, and after the course of treatment, and education should be provided to all involved in the care of the patient with cancer. Their diet needs to be rich in calories and high in lean protein for optimal healing and rejuvenation of healthy cells. With cancer treatments, a person's immune system becomes compromised as the white blood cells that normally fight off invading bacteria are destroyed. This becomes a concern when the diet includes fresh fruits and vegetables; they contain microbes that a healthy immune system can normally handle but a compromised system cannot. Fresh fruits and vegetables contain necessary nutrients for healing and should not be avoided. Clients with a compromised immune system may ask about foods they *should be eating*. Table 17-1 shows a list of foods that are considered safe for persons who are immune compromised due to disease, medications, or other medical treatments. This table, with a complete list of safe and unsafe foods, can be shared with patients whose immune systems are compromised. In addition, foods can be prewashed with commercial or homemade food wash sprays to decrease patient microbes on the food. See Food for Thought for a tip on preparing produce wash at home.

For more information on food preparation, storage, cooking, and shopping for cancer patients, visit: http://www.cancer.org/treatment/survivorshipduringand aftertreatment/nutritionforpeoplewithcancer/nutritionforthepersonwithcancer/ nutrition-during-treatment-weak-immune-system

FOOD FOR THOUGHT HOME-MADE FOOD WASH

This solution will remove the majority of the toxic chemicals from fruits and vegetables prior to eating or using in a recipe:

1 cup water
1 cup white vinegar
1 tablespoon baking soda
Juice of ½ lemon

Put all ingredients into a spray bottle large enough to accommodate the liquid. Spray produce and let stand 5 minutes. You can also make the mixture in a bowl and submerge the produce into the solution. No need to rinse the produce. Allow to set and air dry.

Do not soak delicate fruits such as strawberries or raspberries; these can be soaked in plain water for 2 minutes, drain, and allow to air dry.

Table 17-1	Food List for Immune Compromised	
Food Group	**Foods—Allowed**	**Foods—Not Allowed**
Dairy	All milk products that are pasteurized Commercially packaged cheese and cheese products made with pasteurized milk Pasteurized yogurt (including those with fruit and live cultures) Dry, refrigerated, and frozen pasteurized whipped topping Ice cream, frozen yogurt, sherbet, and ice cream bars Commercial nutritional supplements (liquid and powdered) Commercial eggnog, sour cream	Raw or unpasteurized milk products cheese, yogurt, or other milk products Cheese from delicatessens Cheeses containing chili peppers or other uncooked vegetables Cheeses with molds (e.g., blue, Roquefort, and gorgonzola) Sharp cheddar, brie, camembert, feta cheese, and farmer's cheese
Meat	Fully cooked or canned meats Thoroughly cooked eggs Commercially packaged salami, bologna, and other luncheon meats Canned and commercially packaged smoked fish—refrigerated after opening Commercially packaged peanut butter	Raw, undercooked, or aged meats Raw or undercooked eggs and egg substitutes Meats and cold cuts from delicatessens Hard cured salami in natural wrap Cold smoked salmon (fish); lox Pickled fish
Breads/grains/cereals	All breads, bagels, rolls muffins, pancakes, sweet rolls, or waffles Potato chips, corn chips, tortilla chips, pretzels, and popcorn Cooked pasta, rice, and other grains All cereals, cooked and ready-to-eat	Raw grain products
Vegetables	All cooked, frozen, or canned Fresh vegetables and potatoes that have been properly washed	Unwashed raw vegetables All raw vegetable sprouts (alfalfa, mung bean, etc.) Salads from delicatessens Commercial salsas stored in refrigerated case
Fruits	Canned or frozen fruits Raw fruits only if washed properly Dried fruits	Unwashed fruits Unpasteurized fruit juices
Nuts	Canned or bottled roasted nuts Nuts in baked products Commercially packaged peanut butter	Unroasted raw nuts Roasted nuts in the shell

(continued)

Table 17-1	Food List for Immune Compromised (*continued*)	
Food Group	**Foods—Allowed**	**Foods—Not Allowed**
Desserts	Refrigerated commercial and homemade cakes, pies, pastries, and pudding Homemade and commercial cookies Shelf-stable cream-filled cupcakes, fruit pies (e.g., Pop tarts, fruit pies), and canned pudding Ices, popsicle-like products	Unrefrigerated, cream-filled pastry products (not shelf-stable)
Beverages	Commercially bottled distilled, spring, and natural waters All canned, bottled, and powdered beverages Instant and brewed coffee, tea; cold-brewed tea made with boiling water Brewed herbal teas using commercially packaged tea bags Commercial nutritional supplements, liquid, and powdered	Tap water and ice made from tap water—unless tested and treated Well water (unless tested yearly and found to be free of bacteria) Cold-brewed tea made with warm or cold water Unpasteurized fruit and vegetable juices
Fats	Oil, shortening Refrigerated lard, margarine, and butter Commercial, shelf-stable mayonnaise and salad dressings (including cheese-based salad dressings; refrigerated after opening) Cooked gravy and sauces	Fresh salad dressings containing aged cheese (e.g., blue, Roquefort) or raw eggs, stored in refrigerated case
Miscellaneous	Salt, sugar, and brown sugar Jam, jelly, and syrups—refrigerated after opening Commercial (pasteurized) honey Catsup, mustard, BBQ sauce, and soy sauce—refrigerated after opening Pickles, pickle relish, and olives—refrigerated after opening Candy, gum	Raw or non–heat-treated honey; honey in the comb Herbal and nutrient supplement preparations Brewer's yeast, if uncooked

HIV/AIDS (Human Immunodeficiency Virus/Acquired Immune Deficiency Syndrome)

Human immunodeficiency virus (HIV) or acquired immune deficiency syndrome (AIDS) is a disease of the immune system. HIV is a virus that eventually becomes AIDS as the immune system is further destroyed, making it impossible for an infected individual to fight off bacteria and viruses. According to the United Nations Declarations and Goals, more than 36.9 million people are living with HIV in the world.[12] According to the Centers for Disease Control, 1.2 million are living with HIV just in the United States.[13]

Oral manifestations of HIV/AIDS are numerous, and the health care professional needs to be able to recognize, report, and assist in educating patients on the treatment plan. Oral manifestations may include but are not limited to the following: necrotizing periodontitis, candida, Kaposi sarcoma, oral hairy leukoplakia, and aphthous ulcers, all of which can make chewing and swallowing painful. Side effects of treatment medications include anorexia, nausea, and xerostomia.

Many AIDS patients will eat a diet high in simple carbohydrates for taste and palatability when their desire for food is minimal. Comfort foods like milkshakes, pudding, and ice cream help keep energy levels high when there is no appetite for other foods. The danger of a high-sucrose diet is that it puts patients at a higher risk for dental caries and candidiasis, as yeast fungi feed on sugar. In addition, many will seek dental treatments to help alleviate oral symptoms of bleeding, mucositis (painful inflammation and ulceration of mucosa), periodontal infection, and restoration of carious teeth. Treatment for prevention of caries and periodontal disease should be aggressive. Frequent oral hygiene therapy visits and fluoride treatments are recommended. HIV/AIDS patients can also benefit from information in Table 17-1.

General nutritional counseling for dental patients with HIV/AIDS should include staying well hydrated, increasing total caloric intake fortified with adequate servings of lean protein. Liquid dietary supplements may be used, when necessary, to fortify insufficient diets. Patients should be educated about the carious process and recommended a caries reduction diet. For specific help with mucositis, patients can be counseled to do the following:

- Suck on ice to numb tissues
- Eat a soft, bland diet
- Puree solid foods
- Avoid alcohol

For xerostomia, associated with HIV/AIDS, nutritional counseling should include the following:

- Eat moist foods with extra sauce, gravy, or butter
- Chew gum or suck on hard candies that contain xylitol

- Eat frozen fruits like berries, melon, and grapes or fruit popsicles
- Sip water throughout the day and rinse mouth often
- Avoid dry foods such as crackers, toast, and granola bars
- Cut food into small pieces

DEVELOPMENTAL DISORDERS

The Center for Disease Control and Prevention defines developmental disabilities as a group of severe chronic conditions caused by mental and/or physical impairments that impedes life activities such as language, mobility, learning, self-help, and independent living. Not all are discovered at time of birth as they can develop up to 22 years of age. Autism, cerebral palsy, vision and hearing impairment, Down syndrome, and Fragile X are examples of developmental disorders. There is no cure, but educational programs can teach individuals and their caregivers how to maximize potential. Oral concerns of children with developmental disabilities are different than for children without disabilities. Both children and adults with development disabilities are at higher risk for dental caries than the general population for various reasons unique to their group: inadequate oral hygiene due to poor eye–hand motor control, infrequent dental visits, trouble accessing care due to special transportation needs, higher percentage of malocclusion, and financial considerations.[14]

Parents who care for children with developmental disabilities may feed them a specific diet, which may or may not have a scientific foundation. Some proponents favor special diets for autistic children—avoid gluten and casein (wheat and dairy) to improve foggy thinking and eliminate food cravings. Also gastrointestinal complaints are not uncommon.[15] Suggest foods easy to digest, rich in good bacteria, naturally fermented bacteria (yogurt), and pureed vegetables. It is best not to interfere with what a parent feels is best for their child and is a conversation better left to the registered dietician or physician. However, educating about the process of dental caries and explaining the role nutrients have in maintaining healthy periodontium can only improve the diet they currently follow.

Many adults with developmental disabilities live in group homes with others who may have a different disability. Social services have organized educational programs that teach disabled individuals about good nutrition and will even provide lessons on how to prepare healthy meals. Patients with developmental disabilities often choose easy foods—finger food, ready-made, and store bought food, which do not take a lot of time, steps, or ingredients to prepare. Discovering favorite or preferred foods is an important first step in determining a diet that sustains oral health. If their favorite food is cariogenic, offer a healthier substitution. For example, if they eat donuts every day, encourage them to eat cold cereal with milk. If they drink soda, suggest tea sweetened with sugar substitute. Talk about colors on a plate—the more colors the healthier; for example, green and orange vegetables, piece of meat, and sliced toma-toes instead of one large bowl of macaroni and cheese. Keep the sessions simple and aim for small changes.

LIFESTYLE CONCERNS

Imagine not knowing where you will sleep tonight, where your next meal will come from, or not being able to go through a day without alcohol or drugs. Thankfully, the majority of individuals do not have to deal with these concerns. As a health care pro-fessional, it is imperative to have an understanding that some patients are not always where they want to be in their lives. Though we may not always agree or under-stand lifestyle choices a person makes, as a professional, we need to show empathy. Nutritional advice has to be practical and meet the needs of the patient. Instructing a patient to eat fresh fruits and vegetables who rely on a dumpster for his or her daily meals or telling a young mother that her child needs to have milk daily when there is no means to keep it cold, does not meet the needs of the individual.

Poverty/Homeless

According to the 2014 Current Population Reports, it is estimated that 47 million people live in poverty.[16] Poverty is determined based on a household income of less than $23,834 for a family of four and is further adjusted according to size of family.[17] Of the estimated number, the largest groups of persons in poverty are between the ages of 18 and 64 years, followed by children under 18 years of age.[17] See Table 17-2 for Incidence of Poverty. Poverty in the younger age is of concern to dental profes-sionals, as this is a critical time of permanent tooth development. Key nutrients, such as calcium, may be missing from the diet, and abundance of simple sugar consump-tion may be related to the low cost of processed foods.[18]

Table 17-2	Incidence of Poverty	
Age Range in Years	**Per Million**	
18–64	26.5	
65 and older	4.6	
<18	15.9	

U.S. Census Bureau.[17]

Exact statistics on homeless persons are more difficult to determine than incidence of poverty, as the numbers fluctuate daily. The National Coalition for the Homeless estimates that 3.5 million Americans are homeless at one point in their lives.[19] There are many circumstances that lead to homelessness: extended unemployment, domestic abuse, increased cost of living, lack of affordable housing, as well as natural disasters may force individuals and families to live in their cars, on the street, or in shelters. Runaway teens that fear being sent home and families who double up with relatives or friends are not present in calculations of homelessness rate. Homelessness can be long term (small proportion) or short term, which represents the majority. Either way, good nutrition remains a concern.

In January 2013, the United States Department of Housing and Urban Development conducted a count of homeless on a single night in the United States which resulted in 610,042 homeless individuals. Of this number, 65% were in shelters and 35% were unsheltered. Eighty-five percent were individuals, and 15% were families. Twenty-three percent were youths under the age of 18 years. In their research, they identified five states that account for more than 50% of the homeless population—California 22%, New York 13%, Florida 8%, Texas 5%, and Massachusetts 3%.[20] Further statistics can be found at https://www.hudexchange.info/resources/documents/ahar-2013-part1.pdf

When counseling individuals living in poverty or who are homeless, it is important to understand the challenges they face. Unlike middle-class patients who are concerned about the future and are ready to hear about prevention, the poor are most concerned with the present and how they can survive today. Food security is a primary issue; inability to store or cook food eliminates that reliable feeling of knowing where the next meal is coming from. Many strategies may be used to secure food, such as soup kitchens, federal food assistance programs, food banks at local churches, stealing food, eating inside grocery stores, or scavenging in dumpsters. Parents may skip meals so their children can eat. Many living in poverty understand and desire to eat healthfully; however, they have difficulty accessing affordable nutritious food.[21] Even though those without resources will not seek preventive dental care, they will seek palliative treatment for pain. Many communities have financial assistance programs or clinics available to those who need medical care that are supported through donations and/or have dentists, as well as other health professionals, who volunteer their time and skills. Begin the nutrition counseling dialogue by inquiring about the foods eaten within the last 24 to 72 hours. This is a good starting point to understand sources of food, oral effects of food choices, and determine possible changes for improvement. Nutritional counseling can include the benefits of foods that bring saliva into the mouth, difference between cariogenic and cariostatic foods, and nutrient dense foods to assist with healing and healthy immunity. In addition, offer suggestions and provide contact information for community resources that can help the individual and/or their family to secure nutritious food.

Substance Abuse

Mind altering drugs, alcohol, and tobacco are the three most abused substances. In 2009, over 23 million people (12 or older) needed treatment for an illicit drug or alcohol abuse problem. Visit www.drugabuse.gov (NIDA) for most current results of the National Survey of Drug Use and Health (NSDUH). Abuse is simply overindulgence in a substance that if used long enough will cause harm to the mind and body. **Substance abuse** may or may not lead to addiction. Addiction, also referred to as *dependence*, occurs when a physiological need for the substance develops; there is a gradual tolerance requiring increased amounts to get desired effect and withdrawal symptoms when use is stopped. When *addicted*, an individual will experience mental and physical cravings that occur from substance residues that stay in the body long after the last episode of use. According to NIDA, addiction is a disease for which there is no *absolute* cure; addicted individuals simply go into remission and learn to manage the cravings and urges to start using again.

Oral health needs of individuals with an addiction stem from poor oral hygiene and neglect, bruxism, and poor diets that consist mainly of simple carbohydrates.[22-24] During recovery, patients may use food as a substitute for their craving for drugs or alcohol. They give in to binge eating, gain weight, and then struggle with establishing normal eating patterns. Extensive nutritional counseling is recommended for patients in recovery and should include suggestions for overall good health:

- Take a daily multivitamin/mineral supplement
- Set routine schedules for meals
- Establish parameters for between meal snacking
- Counsel about the caries process and eliminate barriers to reduce potential acid production to less than 60 minutes a day
- Suggest foods that stimulate saliva production
- Chew gum with xylitol

According to the 2015 National Survey on Drug Use and Health, daily marijuana use now exceeds daily cigarette smoking among twelfth graders, and alcohol abuse is in a downward trend. Unfortunately, the abuse of methamphetamines is still of serious concern worldwide.[25,26] Effects of the drug elicit a sense of euphoria, exceptional energy, increased attention, decreased fatigue, and a sense of invulnerability. Anorexia is one of the side effects of methamphetamine abuse, and because of nonstop movement, users will look emaciated and undernourished. **Meth-mouth** is an accepted term to describe a cluster of oral finding on someone who abuses the drug[27-31]:

- Fast developing rampant caries (within a year)
- Teeth most affected are maxillary central incisors and posterior molars
- Stained and crumbling teeth

- Tooth fracture and muscle trismus from bruxing
- Tooth loss
- Periodontal disease
- Enamel erosion
- Xerostomia

In a 2015 study by National Institute on Drug Abuse that examined mouths of 571 methamphetamine abusers, 96% had cavities, 31% had missing teeth, and 58% had untreated dental caries. The more meth they used, the worse their dental decay. Rampant caries in methamphetamine users results mainly from xerostomia caused by the acidic nature of the drug, increase in soda consumption due to carbohydrate craving, and lack of oral hygiene. Methamphetamine users are more likely to snack instead of having set meal-times.[32] Visit http://www.ada.org/public/topics/meth-mouth.asp to read the American Dental Association's information on meth-mouth. Figure 17-1A–C is example of meth-mouth caries.

Seeking relief from oral pain precippitates dental visits for methamphetamine abusers. Many are not amenable to recommendations for cessation of drug abuse, but

A   **B**

C

Figure 17-1   A–C: Meth-mouth caries. (Courtesy of Dr. Rick Foster, Jamestown, NC.)

it is an opportune time to talk with them about the process of dental caries and make suggestions for small changes in their diet. As long as the patient continues to abuse methamphetamines, it is difficult to plan for future appointments. It is recommended that patients who abuse methamphetamines be given oral hygiene instructions and *extensive* nutritional counseling.[33] A 24-hour diet recall can identify the most destructive diet habits and can open a conversation on how to mitigate the damages. The following are some diet changes that may be easy to implement and acceptable to patients:

- Limit sugar intake
- Drink tea with artificial sweeteners instead of soda
- Drink one can of flavored diet supplement per day (Ensure or Sustical) instead of soda
- Sip on water and rinse the mouth often
- Apply fluoride varnish/prescribe chlorhexidine rinse
- Chew gum with xylitol

When the patient is in recovery, suggestions for general nutritional health should be made.

CHAPTER REVIEW

  PRACTICE FOR PATIENTS

A 42-year-old female with uncontrolled type 2 diabetes made an appointment for a recare visit. She is questioning why her teeth feel so sensitive to hot and cold. Upon exam, there is evidence of gingival inflammation and mild tenderness with palpation. Her mucous membranes appear dry, and her tongue is furrowed. She is not sure of her blood glucose level but she is sure they are elevated because she "feels thirsty all the time."

1. What other information do you need to know?

2. What counseling will you give this patient?

3. What recommendations do you have for her?

RELATE TO YOU

Assignment #1

Choose two of the special patient groups and make information sheets for your dental practice to give the client as take home instructions. Include the following:

a. Description of the service just provided at the office
b. What to expect in the next 24 hours
c. Suggestions of foods to avoid
d. Suggestions of foods to include in the diet
e. Any special oral care instructions

Assignment #2

Make a list of referral agencies to use as a resource for patients.

a. Include organizations that serve free meals
b. Alcoholics Anonymous and Al-Anon
c. Homeless shelters
d. Shelters for battered women
e. Shelters that accept families
f. Contacts at public schools to sign-up children for free breakfast and lunch

REFERENCES

1. Stein SH, Livada R, Tipton DA. Re-evaluating the role of vitamin D in the periodontium. *J Periodontol Res* 2014;49(5):545–553.
2. Smith PC, Cáceres M, Martínez C, et al. Gingival wound healing: an essential response disturbed by aging? *J Dent Res* 2015;94(3):395–402.
3. Lau BY, Johnston BD, Fritz PC, et al. Dietary strategies to optimize wound healing after periodontal and dental implant surgery: an evidence-based review. *Open Dent J* 2013;7:36–46.
4. Bauer JD, Isenring E, Waterhouse M. The effectiveness of a specialised oral nutrition supplement on outcomes in patients with chronic wounds: a pragmatic randomised study. *J Hum Nutr Diet* 2013;26(5):452–458.
5. Lee J, Park J-C, Jung U-W, et al. Improvement in periodontal healing after periodontal surgery supported by nutritional supplement drinks. *J Periodontal Implant Sci* 2014;44(3):109–117.
6. Centers for Disease Control. *National Diabetes Statistics Report, 2014.* 2015. Retrieved from http://www.cdc.gov/diabetes/pubs/statsreport14/national-diabetes.

7. Foltz-Gray D. Diabetes and your mouth. *Diabetes Self Manag* 2015;4:16–18.
8. Jindal A, Parihar AS, Sood M, et al. Relationship between severity of periodontal disease and control of diabetes in patients with Type I DM. *J Int Oral Health* 2015;7(S-2): 17–20.
9. Garcia D, Tarima S, Okunseri C. Periodontitis and glycemic control in diabetes: NAHANES 2009–2012. *J Periodontol* 2015;86(4):499–506.
10. American Diabetes Association. Position statement on evidence based nutrition principles and recommendations for the treatment and prevention of diabetes and related complications. *Diabetes Care* 2002;25(1):202–212.
11. American Cancer Society. *Cancer Facts.* 2016. Retrieved from http://www.cancer.org/research/cancerfactsstatistics/cancerfactsfigures2016/
12. UNAIDS. *United Nations Declarations and Goals.* 2014. Retrieved from http://www.unaids.org/enresourcescampaigns/HowAIDSchangedeverything/factsheet
13. Centers for Disease Control. *Living with HIV.* 2016. Retrieved from http://www.cdc.gov/hiv/basics/livingwithhiv/index.html
14. Estrella MR, Boynton JR. General dentistry's role in the care for children with special needs: a review. *Gen Dent* 2010;58(3):222–229.
15. Chaidez V, Hansen R, Hertz-Picciotto I. Gastrointestinal problems in children with autism, developmental delays or typical development. *J Autism Dev Disord* 2014;44(5):1117–1127.
16. Short K. *Current Population Reports. The Supplemental Poverty Measure: 2014.* 2015. Retrieved from http://census.gov/
17. U.S. Census Bureau. *U.S. Census Bureau American Community Survey, 2014.* 2015. Retrieved from http://www.census.gov/content/dam/census/library/publication/2015/demo
18. Kaur J, Lamb MM, Ogden CL. The association between food insecurity and obesity in children—The National Health and nutrition Examination Survey (NHNES). *J Acad Nutr Diet* 2015;115(5):751–758.
19. National Coalition for the Homeless. *Building a Movement to End Homelessness.* 2014. Retrieved from http://nationalhomeless.org/about-homelessness
20. HUD. *United States Department of Housing and Urban Development.* 2014. Retrieved from https://www.hudexchange.info/resources/documentahar-2013-part1.pdf
21. Wicks R, Trevena LJ, Quine S. Experiences of food insecurity among urban soup kitchen consumers: insights for improving nutrition and well-being. *J Am Diet Assoc* 2006;106(6):921–924.
22. Shekarchizadeh H, Khami MR, Mohebbi SZ, et al. Oral health of drug abusers: a review of health effects and care. *Iran J Public Health* 2013;42(9):929–940.
23. O'Sullivan EM. Dental health of Irish alcohol/drug abuse treatment centre residents. *Community Dent Health* 2012;29(4):263–267.
24. Fan J, Hser YI, Herbeck D. Tooth retention, tooth loss and use of dental care among long-term narcotics abusers. *Subst Abus* 2006;27(1–2):25–32.
25. Smit DA, Naidoo S. Oral health effects, brushing habits and management of methamphetamine users for the general dental practitioner. *Br Dent J* 2015;218: 531–536.
26. Shetty K. Meth-mouth. *Med J Aust* 2006;185(5):292.
27. Rommel N, Rohleder NH, Wagenpfeil S, et al. The impact of the new scene drug "crystal meth" on oral health: a case–control study. *Clin Oral Investig* 2016;20(3): 469–475.

28. Rommel N, Rohleder NH, Wagenpfeil S, et al. Evaluation of methamphetamine-associated socioeconomic status and addictive behaviors and their impact on oral health. *Addict Behav* 2015;50: 182–187.

29. De-Carolis C, Boyd GA, Mancinelli L, et al. Methamphetamine abuse and "meth-mouth" in Europe. *Med Oral Patol Oral Cir Bucal* 2015;20(2):e205–e210.

30. Ravenel MC, Salinas CF, Marlow NM, et al. Methamphetamine abuse and oral health: a pilot study of "meth-mouth". *Quintessence Int* 2012;43(3):229–237.

31. Shetty V, Harrell L, Clague J, et al. Methamphetamine users have increased dental disease: a propensity score analysis. *J Dent Res* 2016;95(7):814–821.

32. Morio KA, Marshall TA, Qian F, et al. Comparing diet, oral hygiene and caries status of adult amphetamine users and nonusers: a pilot study. *J Am Dent Assoc* 2008;139(2): 171–176.

33. Wakeen B. Nutritional concerns related to chemical dependency and drug addiction—specifically methamphetamines. *ACFSA*, Summer 2008.

Nutrients at a Glance

CARBOHYDRATES AT A GLANCE

Molecular Structure	Primary Role in Body	Source in Diet	Recommended Dietary Intake	Digestion/ Absorption	kcal/g
$C_6H_{12}O_6$	Energy Maintain steady blood glucose levels Spare protein Provide bulk	Grains, fruits, vegetables, and dairy products	55%–65% total daily calories	Begins in the mouth when mixed with amylase, passes through the wall of the small intestines, and absorbed by the body	4

PROTEINS AT A GLANCE

Molecular Structure	Primary Role in Body	Source in Diet	Recommended Dietary Intake	Digestion/ Absorption	Kcal/gm
COOH (carboxyl group) NH_2 (amino radical) Carbon and hydrogen side groups	GMR Growth Maintenance (enzymes, antibodies) Repair	Meat Dairy	40–65 g/d Depends on weight	Begins in the stomach when mixed with pepsin, passes to the small intestines where it mixes with trypsin and chymotrypsin, then passes through the wall and is absorbed by the body; liver controls ratio of amino acids in the blood stream	4

LIPIDS AT A GLANCE

Molecular Structure	Primary Role in Body	Source in Diet	Recommended Dietary Intake	Digestion/ Absorption
Carbon atom with a carboxyl end (COOH) and methyl end (CH$_3$)	Insulates against cold Cushion organs Energy Cell structure Provides fat-soluble vitamins	Butter, oil Marbleized meat Dairy products Sauces and salad dressing	<30% of total daily calories consumed	Begins in the mouth when mixed with lipase and continues in stomach when mixed with gastric lipase. Emulsified by bile and pancreatic lipase in small intestines. Passes through wall of small intestines where absorbed by body

WATER AT A GLANCE

Molecular Structure	Primary Role in Body	Source in Diet	Recommended Dietary Intake	Digestion/ Absorption
H$_2$O	Solvent for metabolic processes Removes toxins Transports nutrients Builds tissue Regulates temperature Cushions organs Lubricates mucous membranes	Drinking water Liquid Beverages Food	64 oz	Freely passes through small intestine membranes and is absorbed; can be reabsorbed by the colon

VITAMINS AT A GLANCE

Water-Soluble Vitamins		Function	RDI	Food Sources	Deficiency	Excess	Oral Deficiency Symptoms
Thiamin	B$_1$	Energy metabolism	1.1 mg	Pork, fortified cereal, grains, meat, poultry, peanut butter, and eggs	Beriberi	—	—
Riboflavin	B$_2$	Production of ATP	1.1 mg	Milk, meat, poultry, fish, enriched whole grains, and cereals	Ariboflavinosis	—	Red swollen lips; vertical fissures; cheilosis; burning, smooth red tongue; atrophied lingual papillae; red, burning gingival tissues
Niacin	B$_3$	Cell function Coenzyme to B$_2$ RBC formation	12 mg	Meat, poultry, fish, dark green leafy vegetables, enriched grains, peanut butter, and peas	Pellagra	Causes facial flushing Decreased blood lipids	—
Pyridoxine	B$_6$	Coenzyme in reactions for amino acid, fatty acid, and CHO metabolism	1.4 mg	Meat, poultry, fish, liver, eggs, brown rice, lentils, and peanuts	Microcytic anemia Depression Convulsions	Permanent neurologic damage Numbness in extremities Uncoordinated muscle movement	Deficiency causes angular cheilitis and glossitis
Folate	B$_9$	Synthesize amino acids RBC maturation Synthesis of DNA and RNA	400 µg	Fortified grains, yeast, kidney, and dark green leafy vegetables	Fetal neural tube defects Macrocytic anemia	—	—
Cobalamin	B$_{12}$	RBC production DNA synthesis	2.4 µg	Meat, poultry, fish, eggs, and dairy	Pernicious anemia Permanent nerve and brain damage	—	—
Ascorbic acid	C	Collagen formation Strengthens immune system Iron and calcium absorption	60 mg	Kiwi, citrus, strawberries, cantaloupe, leafy greens, and cruciferous vegetables	Scurvy	GI upset Diarrhea Orange urine Interferes with anticoagulants Iron toxicity	Red purplish, swollen, bleeding gingival tissues Loose teeth Slow healing

(continued)

VITAMINS AT A GLANCE *(continued)*

Fat-Soluble Vitamins	Function	RDI	Food Sources	Deficiency	Excess	Oral Deficiency Symptoms
A	Formation of epithelium, skin, and mucous membranes; Healthy eyes; Bone remodeling	800 µg	Carrots, yellow and orange fruits and vegetables, spinach, broccoli, liver, eggs, butter, and fortified foods	Hypovitaminosis A; Xerophthalmia; Night blindness	Headache; Vomiting; Double vision; Hair loss; Bone abnormalities; Liver damage	Xerostomia; Oral leukoplakia; Hyperkeratosis; Hyperplastic gingival tissue
D	Absorption of calcium and phosphorus; Bone formation	5–10 µg	Liver, egg yolks, and fish oil	Rickets; Osteomalacia	Kidney stones; Calcified blood vessels	Failure of bone wounds to heal; Enamel hypocalcification; Loss of alveolar bone; Thinning trabeculation
E	Antioxidant; Protects RBCs	15 mg	Margarine, vegetable shortening, salad dressing, whole grains, nuts, and legumes	Hemolytic anemia	Nausea; Diarrhea; Cramps; Interferes with anticoagulants	No known deficiency symptoms; May delay clotting
K	Synthesis for prothrombin	100 µg	Dark green leafy vegetables	Prolonged bleeding; Hemorrhage	Increased clotting time	Failure of wounds to stop bleeding

RDI, recommended daily intake; ATP, adenosine triphosphate; RBC, red blood cell; GI, gastrointestinal.

MINERALS AT A GLANCE[a]

Major Minerals	Major Functions	RDI/Day (Adult)	Food Source	Deficiency State	Excess States
Calcium	Mineralization of calcified structures Contracting muscles Nerve conduction Cofactor in blood-clotting protein	1,200 mg	Dairy Animal bones Stone-ground meal Tofu Broccoli Legumes Fortified orange juice	Rickets Osteomalacia Osteoporosis	
Chloride	Anion that partners with sodium to maintain extracellular water balance	750 mg	Table salt Processed foods Meat Eggs	Rare	
Magnesium	Mineralization of calcified structures Protein synthesis Neuromuscular activity	400 mg	Nuts Meat Green leafy vegetables Legumes Grains	Occurs from dieting, gastric bypass, drinking soft water, or loss during body functions; causes muscle spasms, hallucinations, mental derangement	Occurs with long-term antacid use
Phosphorous	Mineralization of calcified structures Energy metabolism Protein synthesis Muscle contractions	700 mg	Meat Eggs Fish Poultry Legumes Dairy	Occurs with use of antacids	
Potassium	Cation that works to balance fluid inside cells Muscle contractions Neurologic transmissions	2,000 mg	Processed food Meat Grains Fruits and vegetables	Occurs during dehydration Muscle cramps Cardiac arrest Respiratory failure	Numbness of extremities, face, and tongue Dilation of heart
Sodium	Cation in extracellular fluid for regulation of fluid balance	500 mg	Table salt Processed foods Meat Eggs Dairy	Rare	Hypertension
Sulfur	Part of biotin and thiamin Part of enzymes that detoxify Liver function Acid–base balance of body fluid	None	Meat Poultry Fish Legumes	Rare	Rare

[a]Based on National Institutes of Health Medline Plus.
NIH, National Institutes of Health; RDI, recommended daily intake.

Glossary

A

acid production—a period during the caries process when bacteria secrete acid

alveolar bone—bone of the human skull that contains the tooth sockets

amino acid—a molecule containing both an amine and carboxyl group

ana—modern abbreviation for anorexia nervosa, eating disorder

anion—negatively charged ion

antidiuretic hormone (ADH)—hormone released by the pituitary gland that has an antidiuretic action that prevents the production of dilute urine

antioxidant—substance that reduces damage to cells caused by free radicals attaching oxygen to molecules

B

B-complex—group of several B vitamins

binge—unrestrained excessive indulgence

bioavailability—rate at which a substance is absorbed into a living system or is made available at the site of physiological activity

biologic value—measure of proportion of absorbed protein from food that gets incorporated into the body

C

calcium—major mineral predominant in dairy products used by the body for formation of strong teeth and bones

caries equation—plaque bacteria + fermentable carbohydrate = acid production, which demineralizes teeth

caries risk—high or low potential for developing dental caries

cariogenic—ability to contribute to formation of dental caries

cariostatic—does not contribute to the initiation or development of dental caries

cations—positively charged ion

CHO—abbreviation for carbohydrate

421

chylomicron—a lipoprotein rich in triglyceride and common in the blood during fat digestion and assimilation

collagen—fibrous proteins in connective tissue

complementary protein—a protein that is incomplete by itself, but together with another protein will provide all the amino acids for a complete protein

complete protein—contains all the amino acids necessary for protein metabolism

complex carbohydrate—a polysaccharide consisting of hundreds or thousands of monosaccharides

consumption norm—the perceived amount of food portion to consume; a form of portion control on food intake

critical period—time during fetal development where the environment has the greatest impact

critical pH—acidic pH of 5.5 where enamel demineralization begins

cruciferous—a family of plants whose leaf structure resemble a cross

crunchy foods—hard dry food that emits sound when chewed

D

defecation—elimination of solid waste

dehydration—abnormal depletion of body fluids

density of bone—thickness of bone mass

detergent foods—foods thought to remove plaque during the action of chewing them

diet—food and drink regularly provided and consumed

dietary guidelines—list of suggestions for healthy eating

dietary supplement—substance that enhances a regular diet

dipeptide—a peptide containing two amino acids

disaccharide—a carbohydrate consisting of two monosaccharide molecules

DRI—abbreviation for dietary reference intake

DRV—British dietary reference value

DV—abbreviation for daily value reported on nutrition labels

dysphagia—difficulty swallowing

E

early childhood caries—syndrome characterized by severe dental caries in teeth of infants and young children

ectomorph—large bone structure

edema—excess accumulation of fluid in body tissues

endomorph—small bone structure

energy balance—an equal amount of energy in (food) and energy out (exercise)

enriched—add nutrients that were lost during food processing

enzymes—proteins that catalyze chemical reactions; assist with breaking apart food molecules during the digestive process

essential amino acids (EAA)—amino acids that must be obtained in the diet

essential fatty acid (EFA)—fatty acid that must be obtained in the diet

essential nutrient—a nutrient the body must get by consuming food

excretion—elimination of toxic waste through body fluids

extracellular—occurring outside a body cell

F

fat soluble—capable of being dissolved in or absorbed by fat

fatty acids—saturated or unsaturated monocarboxylic acids that occur naturally in the form of glycerides in fats and oils

fluoride—compound of fluorine that strengthens tooth enamel and makes it less susceptible to dental caries

food-borne illnesses—sickness that happens due to food laden with bacteria

fortification—adding vitamins and minerals to food products

fruitan—an individual who consumes only raw fruits

functional food—foods or dietary components that may provide a health benefit beyond basic nutrition and impart health benefits or desirable physiological effects

G

gingivitis—inflammation of gingival tissues

glycemic index—rate at which ingested food causes the level of glucose in the blood to rise

goiter—enlargement of the thyroid gland visible from the front of the neck

H

health claims—statements made by food manufacturers that indicate their product will prevent or reduce the risk of certain diseases

heme iron—the type of iron that is readily absorbed by the body; found in animal food products

hemochromatosis—inherited disease where iron builds up in excess in the body

herbal supplement—natural substance thought to heal or improve the human condition

high-density lipoprotein (HDL)—lipoproteins that carry fatty acids and cholesterol from body tissues to the liver

homeostasis—stable state of equilibrium

host factors—issues precipitated by the person's own body

hydro—prefix meaning water

hydrogenation—infusing hydrogen at an unsaturated bond between two carbons in a fatty acid to prolong shelf life

I

immune response—how the body recognizes and defends itself against harmful invading bacteria, viruses, and other detrimental substances

immune system—all the mechanisms within a body that protect against disease by identifying and killing pathogens and tumor cells

incomplete protein—a protein that is missing amino acids to make it complete

inorganic—molecule does not contain carbon

insoluble—does not dissolve in liquid

intracellular—occurring inside a body cell

ionic compound—two or more ions are held next to each other by electrical attraction

K

ketosis—state of metabolism when the liver converts fats to fatty acids and ketones, which are then used for energy

kilocalorie—scientific term for calorie

kitchen dangers—anything that might occur in the kitchen that can cause harm to people; fire, illness, injury, and so on

Kwashiorkor—severe malnutrition in infants and children caused by diets that are low in protein

L

lactic acid—most predominant acid formed from bacteria metabolism of carbohydrate

lacto—prefix meaning milk

Lactobacillus—type of oral bacteria responsible for dental caries

lacto-ovo vegetarian—an individual who consumes a vegetarian diet that includes dairy products and eggs

lactovegetarian—an individual who consumes a vegetarian diet that includes dairy products

lanugo—soft, downy growth of hair seen on faces of individuals who starve themselves

lipid—fats and oils

lipoprotein—spherical particles that contain cholesterol, fat, and protein that circulate in the blood

low carb—proportion of carbohydrate in a food product is low compared to protein and fat

low-density lipoprotein (LDL)—lipoprotein that transports cholesterol and triglycerides from the liver to peripheral tissues

lysis—suffix meaning split apart

M

magnesium—fourth most abundant mineral in the human body

major mineral—minerals that are required in the amounts of 100 mg or more

marasmus—chronic malnourishment due to a calorie-deficient diet mastication—chewing food

maternal nutrition—the diet a mother follows when she is pregnant

mesomorph—medium bone structure

methylmercury—methyl group bonded to mercury atom and is highly toxic to the human body

mia—modern abbreviation for bulimia nervosa eating disorder

monosaccharide—one molecule of carbohydrate; is the smallest unit and does not break into a lesser unit

monounsaturated fat—fatty acid that has a single double bond in the fatty acid chain

mucositis—painful inflammation and ulceration of mucous membranes

MyPyramid—the US government's pictorial graphic that can be individually customized to teach healthy eating habits

N

negative nitrogen balance—nitrogen output exceeds nitrogen intake

neutral pH—7.0 on the pH scale; level at which acid production ceases

NLEA—abbreviation for Nutrition Labeling Education Act of 1990

nonessential amino acids—amino acids made by the body

nonessential nutrient—a nutrient the body produces

nonheme iron—iron that is not well absorbed by the body; found in flour and grains

noxious substance—a substance physically harmful to a human body

nutrition—the sum of the processes by which an animal or plant takes in and utilizes food substances

nutrient—a nutritive substance or ingredient

nutrition facts—name for design of food labels that contain information about a food product

O

oligosaccharide—a carbohydrate containing 3 to 10 monosaccharides

organic—molecule has a carbon-to-carbon bond or carbon-to-hydrogen bond

osmosis—diffusion of fluid through a cell wall

ovo—prefix meaning eggs

P

partially hydrogenated—adding hydrogen to fatty acid to make them more saturated; also called a "trans fat"

peptide—amide derived from two or more amino acids

peptide bond—chemical bond between two molecules formed when a carboxyl group bonds with an amino group

periodontal disease—infection of supporting tissues around teeth

peristalsis—successive waves of involuntary contraction passing along the walls of a hollow muscular structure (as the esophagus or intestine) and forcing the contents onward

phosphate—mineral that helps remineralize enamel

phospholipid—major class of lipid that looks like a triglyceride with a phosphate group

phosphoric acid—ingredient in diet and regular soda that drops the oral pH to acidic levels and contributes to formation of dental caries

plaque biofilm—the layer of microorganisms that accumulates at the gingival 1/3 in the oral cavity

plaque fluid—solution in and around oral bacterial colonies

polypeptide—chains of amino acids linked by peptide bonds

polysaccharide—a carbohydrate containing many monosaccharide molecules

polyunsaturated fat—a fatty acid that has two or more double bonds

portion distortion—replacement of proper food consumption norms with larger portions

positive nitrogen balance—nitrogen intake exceeds nitrogen output

posteruptive—period of human development that occurs after teeth are present in the oral cavity

potable—water fit for human consumption

precursor—a biochemical substance from which another more stable substance is formed

pre-eruptive—period of human development before teeth appear in the oral cavity

premature—birth of a child before complete gestation

prenatal—period of development when the child is still a fetus

PRO—abbreviation for protein

purging—to evacuate something unwanted

R

RDA—abbreviation for recommended daily allowance

RDI—abbreviation for recommended daily intake

remineralize—state of repairing demineralized areas of enamel

retentive factor—that which causes food to stick to teeth and not clear the oral cavity readily

roughage—food that contains a lot of fiber

S

safe food handling—practice of keeping, handling, and preparing food so it remains safe for human consumption

saliva—secretion of water, mucin, protein, salts secreted into the mouth by salivary glands

salivary gland hypofunction (SGH)—inadequate saliva production causing dry mouth

satiety—state of feeling full or gratified by food

saturated—having no double or triple bonds between carbons simple sugar—monosaccharide

SLPI—abbreviation for secretory leukocyte peptidase inhibitor; protective factor in saliva

sodium bicarbonate—baking soda; substance found in saliva that keeps the pH at neutral 7.0

soft foods—food that does not require chewing before swallowing

soluble—able to be dissolved in liquid

solute—a dissolvable substance

starch—category of carbohydrate; plant storage of glucose

sterols—lipids formed with carbon rings instead of chains and fatty acids

Strep mutans—abbreviation for *Streptococcus mutans*, which is a gram-positive, anaerobic bacteria commonly found in the human oral cavity and is a significant contributor to dental caries

sugar—common name for simple carbohydrate and significant contributor to dental caries

sugar alcohol—hydrogenated form of carbohydrate commonly used for replacing sucrose in food recipes and does not contribute to tooth decay

supplementary protein—a high-quality protein that is added to a meal that is otherwise marginal in protein value

synthesis—combining separate elements to form a whole

synthetic sweetener—noncaloric chemical sweetener that provides sweet taste in a diluted form

T

trace mineral—minerals required in very small amounts

trans fat—fatty acid that has been partially hydrogenated

triglycerides—chemical form in which most fat exists in food as well as in the body

tripeptide—a peptide consisting of three amino acids connected by a peptide bond

V

vegan—an individual who excludes food from their diet that has any animal product in it

very-low-density lipoprotein (VLDL)—subclass of lipoprotein that is assembled in the liver from cholesterol and converted in the bloodstream to LDL

W

water soluble—capable of being dissolved in water

X

xylitol—sugar alcohol that is obtained from birch bark, used as a sweetener, and does not contribute to dental caries

Prefixes

mono = one
di= two
tri = three
poly = many
hyper = over
hypo = under
endo = inside
meso = middle
ecto = outside

Suffixes

-ase = enzyme
-ose = carbohydrate
-ine = amino acid

Index

Page numbers in *italics* denote figures; numbers with "t" denote tables.